Esophageal Cancer

Francisco Schlottmann · Lorenzo Ferri ·
Daniela Molena · Marco G. Patti
Editors

Esophageal Cancer

Diagnosis and Treatment

Second Edition

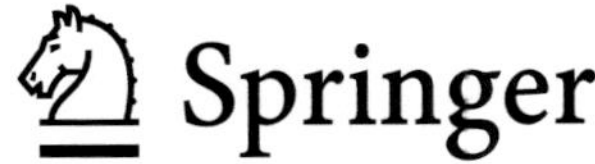 Springer

Editors
Francisco Schlottmann
Hospital Alemán of Buenos Aires
University of Buenos Aires
Buenos Aires, Argentina

Daniela Molena
Thoracic Surgery Service
Department of Surgery
Memorial Sloan Kettering
Cancer Center
New York, NY, USA

Lorenzo Ferri
Department of Surgery and Oncology
McGill University
Montreal, QC, Canada

Marco G. Patti
Department of Surgery
University of Virginia
Charlottesville, Virginia, USA

ISBN 978-3-031-39088-3   ISBN 978-3-031-39086-9   (eBook)
https://doi.org/10.1007/978-3-031-39086-9

This Springer imprint is published by the registered company Springer Nature Switzerland AG
The registered company address is: Gewerbestrasse 11, 6330 Cham, Switzerland

Paper in this product is recyclable.

Contents

About the Editors

Francisco Schlottmann received his medical degree with honors at the University of Buenos Aires in Argentina. He then completed his general surgery residency at the Hospital Alemán of Buenos Aires. After his surgical training, Dr. Schlottmann completed the Soudavar fellowship at Memorial Sloan Kettering Cancer Center, focusing his research on esophageal cancer. He then did a 2-year gastrointestinal surgery fellowship at the University of North Carolina, focusing his clinical and research activities on foregut disorders. Dr. Schlottmann obtained his Master of Public Health at the University of North Carolina Gillings School of Global Public Health. He also completed a 1-year Minimally Invasive and Robotic Surgery Fellowship at the University of Illinois at Chicago. He currently serves as Clinical Instructor at the University of Illinois at Chicago and as Affiliate Professor of Surgery at the Hospital Alemán of Buenos Aires with an active clinical and research interest in esophageal disorders, gastroesophageal reflux disease, obesity, esophageal cancer, and gastric cancer. Dr. Schlottmann is editor of 7 books, has published over 250 journal articles, and has written more than 60 book chapters.

Lorenzo Ferri is the David S. Mulder Chair in Surgery and a Professor in the Departments of Surgery and Oncology at McGill University in Montreal Canada. He is director of the Division of Thoracic and Upper Gastrointestinal Surgery Surgery and heads the Upper Gastrointestinal Cancer Program at McGill University, one of North America's largest and most comprehensive. Dr Ferri couples this clinical activity with an active translational and fundamental research program investigating the mechanisms of therapy resistance in gastroesophageal adenocarcinoma and the inflammatory basis of cancer progression. He is the recipient of numerous peer review grants, including from the Canadian Institutes of Health Research, Canadian Cancer Society, United States Department of Defense, and a Grand Challenge from Cancer Research UK. Through this work he has identified the important role of bacterial antigens - pattern recognition proteins (TLRs and NODs) and host neutrophils/Neutrophil Extracellular Traps in propagating cancer dissemination, thus representing a new paradigm in the metastatic process.

Daniela Molena received her medical degree from the University of Padova in Italy. She completed her general surgery residency at the University of Padova and at the University of Rochester Medical Center. She then completed the following fellowships: Gastrointestinal Surgery (University of California San Francisco); Minimally Invasive Surgery (University of Padova); Cardiothoracic Surgery (New York Presbyterian/Weill Cornell Medical Center); and Cardiothoracic Surgery (Memorial Sloan Kettering Cancer Center). After completing her training, Dr. Molena was appointed as Assistant Professor at John Hopkins Medical Center. Currently, she serves as Director of Memorial Sloan Kettering's Esophageal Program, where she strives to provide excellent and individualized care to patients and to integrate new technology and novel approaches to the Thoracic Oncology Service.

Marco G. Patti was born and raised in Catania, Italy. He graduated from the University of Catania, School of Medicine in 1981. Between 1983 and 1986 he did research at the University of California San Francisco, studying gastrointestinal physiology (Dr. Carlos Pellegrini and Dr. Lawrence Way). Between 1986 and 1993, he completed a Residency in General Surgery at UCSF. After completion of his residency, he did a fellowship in esophageal cancer at the Queen Mary Hospital in Hong Kong (Professor John Wong). Subsequently he practiced at the University of California San Francisco, the University of Chicago, and the University of North Carolina. Presently he is involved with mentoring in the Department of Surgery at the University of Virginia. Dr. Patti's clinical activity focuses on foregut disorders. Over the years, he has given major contribution to the diagnosis and treatment of GERD and achalasia. Dr. Patti has published more than 300 manuscripts in peer review journals and 10 books. He has been an invited speaker more than 220 times in the US. He is Past President of the International Society for Digestive Surgery and Past President of the International Society of Surgery. He was President for the World Congress of Surgery in August 2017 in Basel, Switzerland. He has been an invited speaker in North and South America, Europe, and Asia, giving more than 160 lectures.

Esophageal Anatomy

Mariano A. Menezes, Francisco Schlottmann and Fernando A. M. Herbella

Abstract

The esophagus has a peculiar anatomy: (a) it is surrounded by important organs and structures, (b) it crosses three cavities: neck, thorax and abdomen, (c) its lymphatic distribution is abundant and erratic, (d) the organs and structures of the mediastinum frequently present anatomic variations, and (e) the classic anatomic description is different from clinical presentation. In addition, minimally invasive surgery also brought a restricted but magnified view of the esophagus, and available imaging technology forces the understanding of sectional and regional anatomy. For all these reasons, the knowledge of the surgical anatomy of the esophagus is essential for surgeons before performing an esophagectomy. This chapter reviews the surgical anatomy of the esophagus and neighbor structures of interest to perform an esophagectomy.

Keywords

Esophagus · Anatomy · Esophagectomy · Lymph nodes · Radiology

Introduction

The esophagus has a peculiar anatomy. It is the only digestive organ that does not digest or absorb nutrients and lacks a serosa layer. From a surgical anatomy point of view, the esophagus has an exuberant lymphatic drainage able to spread metastasis quickly and far but is short of vascularization without a single artery bearing its name. The esophagus crosses three cavities (neck, thorax and abdomen) and it is surrounded by vital organs in a small container called mediastinum [1]. All these characteristics make the resection of the esophagus and the subsequent alimentary tract reconstruction a challenging procedure.

Anatomists frequently portrait the esophagus in didactic books in a stylized fashion commonly not useful for surgeons. In addition, minimally invasive surgery also brought a restricted but magnified view of the esophagus, and available imaging technology forces

M. A. Menezes
Department of Surgery, Pontifical Catholic University of Paraná, Londrina, Brazil
e-mail: mariano.menezes@pucpr.br

F. Schlottmann
Department of Surgery, Hospital Alemán of Buenos Aires, University of Buenos Aires, Buenos Aires, Argentina

F. A. M. Herbella (✉)
Department of Surgery, Escola Paulista de Medicina, Federal University of Sao Paulo, Rua Diogo de Faria 1087 cj 301, Sao Paulo 04037-003, Brazil
e-mail: herbella.dcir@epm.br

the understanding of sectional and regional anatomy. Thus, a strong knowledge of the anatomy of the esophagus is essential to all esophageal surgeons interested in performing an esophagectomy.

Esophageal Anatomy

The esophagus is a hollow organ with a four-layer structure: mucosa, submucosa, muscularis propria, and adventitia [2]. The mucosa is made of squamous epithelium overlying a lamina propria and a muscularis mucosa. The submucosa is made of elastic and fibrous tissue and is the strongest layer of the esophageal wall. The esophageal muscle is composed of an inner circular and outer longitudinal layer. The upper third of the esophageal musculature consists of skeletal muscle and the lower two thirds consist of smooth muscle. The adventitia consists in connective tissue that merges with connective tissue of surrounding structures. Unlike the remainder of the gastrointestinal tract, the esophagus does not have a serosal layer.

The upper esophageal sphincter is formed by the cricopharyngeus muscle along with the inferior constrictors of the pharynx and fibers of the esophageal wall. The lower esophageal sphincter is not a distinct anatomic structure.

Microscopic anatomy of the esophageal wall is further divided for diagnostic and therapeutic purposes to allow a more refined staging and guide endoscopic resection in early esophageal cancer [3, 4]. Thus, mucosa layer is subdivided in: (a) M1—epithelium (defining a carcinoma in situ); (b) M2—lamina propria mucosae; and (c) M3—muscularis mucosae. Submucosal layer is also subdivided in three layers: (a) SM1—upper third of the submucosa; (b) SM2—middle third of the submucosa; and (c) SM3—lower third of the submucosa. Endoscopic resection is suitable for early cancers invading up to the SM1 [5].

Macroscopically, the esophagus is divided in three portions: cervical, thoracic/mediastinal, and abdominal, according to the boundaries of the cavities that it crosses (i.e. the thoracic outlet at the level of the manubrium and the diaphragm). The cervical esophagus lies left of the midline and posterior to the larynx and trachea. The thoracic portion may also be subdivided in: (a) Upper thoracic esophagus—from the sternal notch to the tracheal bifurcation; (b) Middle thoracic esophagus—the proximal half of the two equal portions between the tracheal bifurcation and the esophagogastric junction; and (c) Lower thoracic esophagus—the thoracic part of the distal half of the two equal portions between the tracheal bifurcation and the esophagogastric junction (Fig. 1). The upper thoracic esophagus passes behind the trachea and tracheal bifurcation, while the middle and lower thoracic esophagus passes behind the left atrium and then enters the abdomen through the esophageal hiatus of the diaphragm. The abdominal portion may be absent in the case of a hiatal hernia.

Vascularization and Lymphatic Drainage

Esophageal vascularization is shared by small branches from adjacent organs. Arterial blood supply comes from branches of the inferior thyroid arteries, unnamed vessels originating directly from the thoracic aorta, bronchial arteries, inferior phrenic arteries, and left gastric artery. Blood is drained into the inferior thyroid, hemiazygos, azygos and left gastric vein [6].

Anatomy textbooks rarely describe a specific lymphatic drainage of the esophagus. Abundant lymphatics form a dense submucosal plexus. Thoracic lymph nodes are shown in a regular disposition seldom seen in an operation. Gray's anatomy textbook simply describes esophageal lymphatic drainage as "a plexus around that tube, and the collecting vessels from the plexus drain into the posterior mediastinal glands" [7]. Lymph from the cervical and upper-mid thoracic esophagus drains mostly into the cervical, paratracheal and subcarinal lymph nodes, whereas the lower thoracic and abdominal esophagus drains preferentially into the diaphragmatic, paracardial, left gastric, and celiac nodes [8].

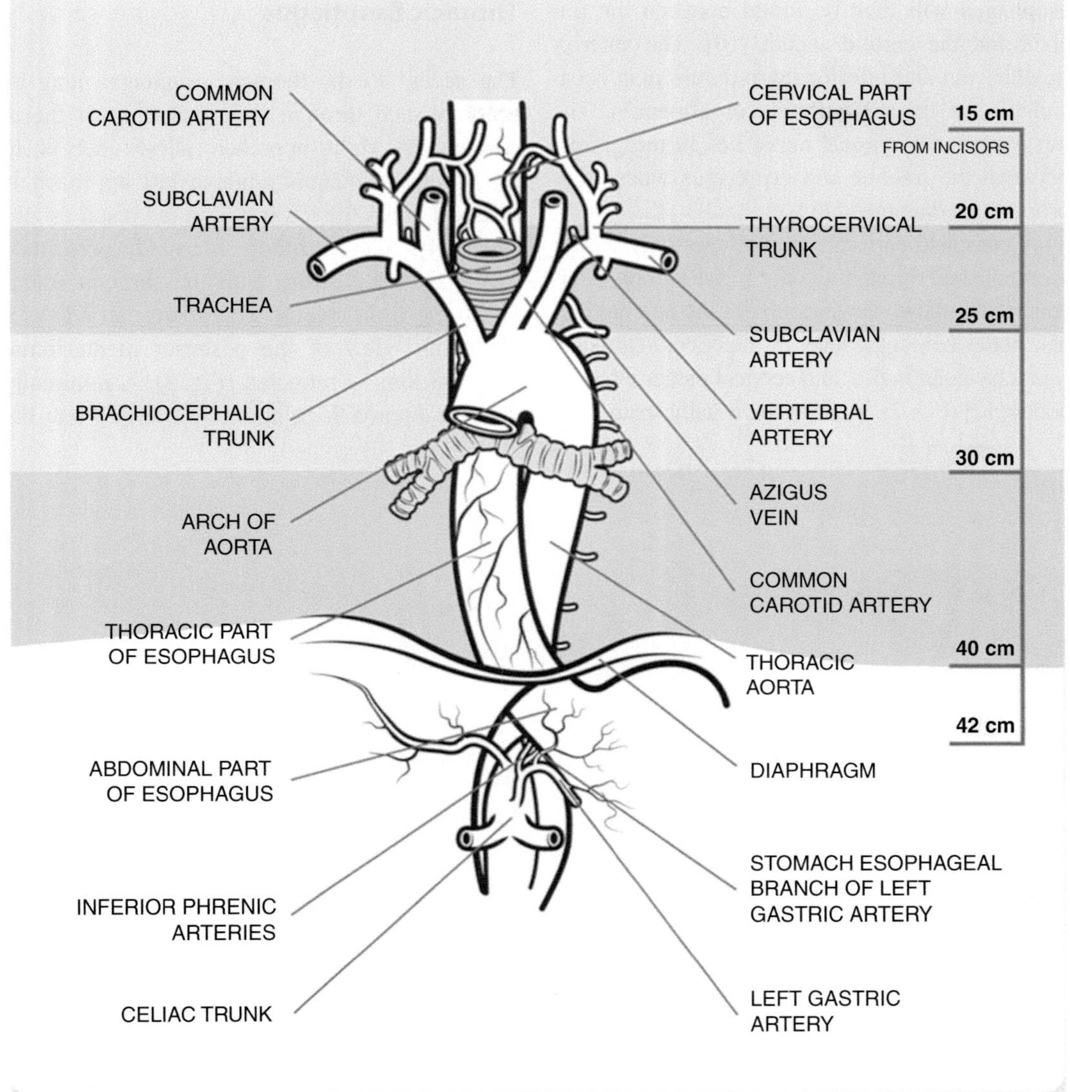

Fig. 1 Esophageal anatomy: the three portions of the esophagus and surrounding structures in the posterior mediastinum

Esophageal Surgical Anatomy

Cervical Esophagus

The access to the cervical esophagus may be obtained through an oblique incision parallel to the medial border of the left sternocleidomastoid muscle or a necklace incision. The former is simpler and the latter allows bilateral access if a complete lymphadenectomy is anticipated. The oblique incision allows access to the esophagus after dividing the platysma muscle (in the subcutaneous) and the deep cervical fascia which will expose the infrahyoide muscles (sternothyroid muscle mainly) that are retracted or divided. These muscles are responsible for larynx depression and its division may impair swallowing and fonation thus preservation is preferred [9]. The esophagus will then be found between the trachea and the carotid sheath [10]. The anterior jugular vein and inferior thyroid vein may occasionally be ligated without consequences. The left recurrent laryngeal nerve lies in the groove between the trachea and esophagus where it is prone to be damaged [11].

A complete cervical lymphadenectomy is best accomplished through a collar incision. This bilateral access allows the resection of the internal jugular nodes below the level of the cricoid cartilage, supraclavicular nodes, and cervical paraesophageal nodes [12] (Fig. 2). Muscles are usually spared.

Thoracic Esophagus

The access to the thoracic esophagus may be accomplished through a thoracotomy or thoracoscopy. A right approach allows access to the whole esophagus while a left approach is reserved when the interest is in the distal esophagus only. A thoracotomy is usually performed in the lateral position with the surgeon standing in the right side of the patient that allows a panoramic view of the posterior mediastinum after the lung is retracted (Fig. 3). A minimally invasive approach brings a restricted view but

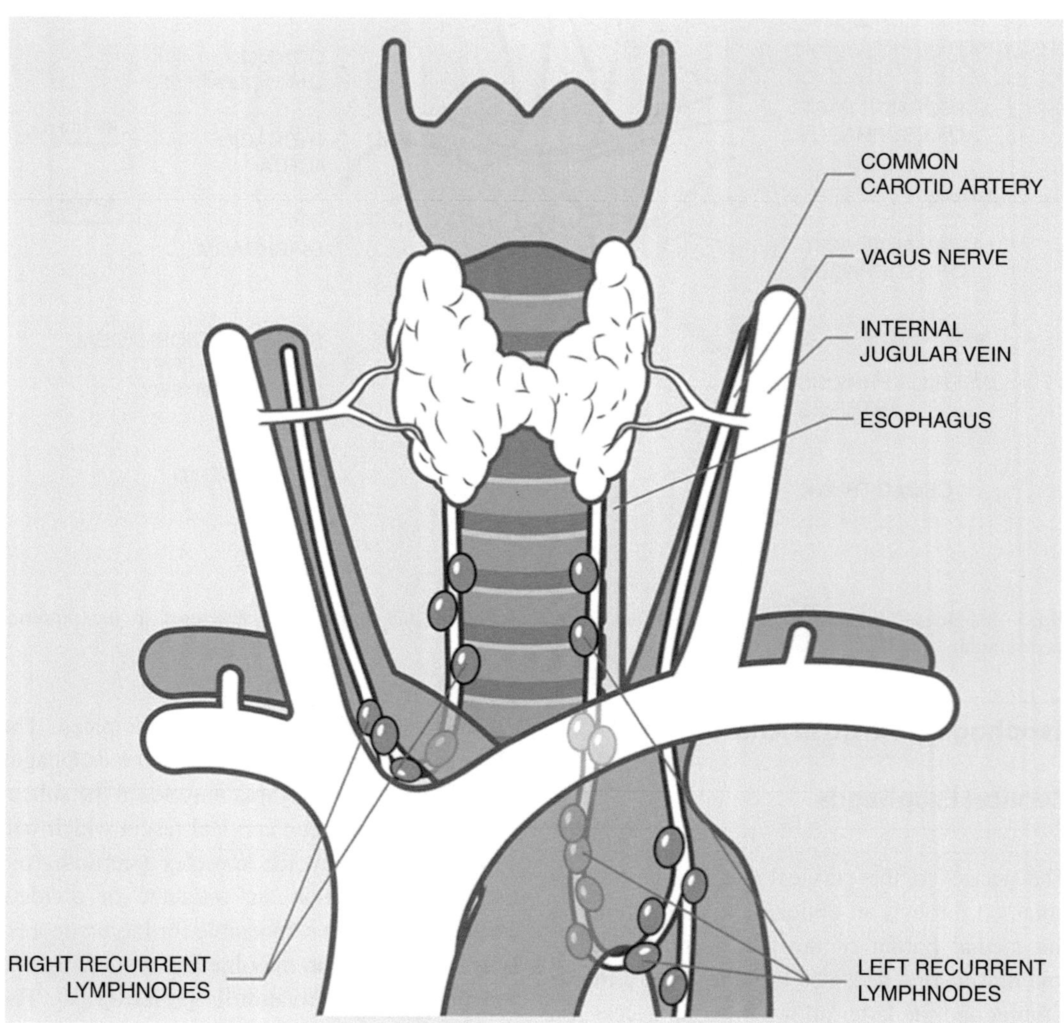

Fig. 2 Cervical lymph nodes of interest for esophagectomy and lymphadenectomy

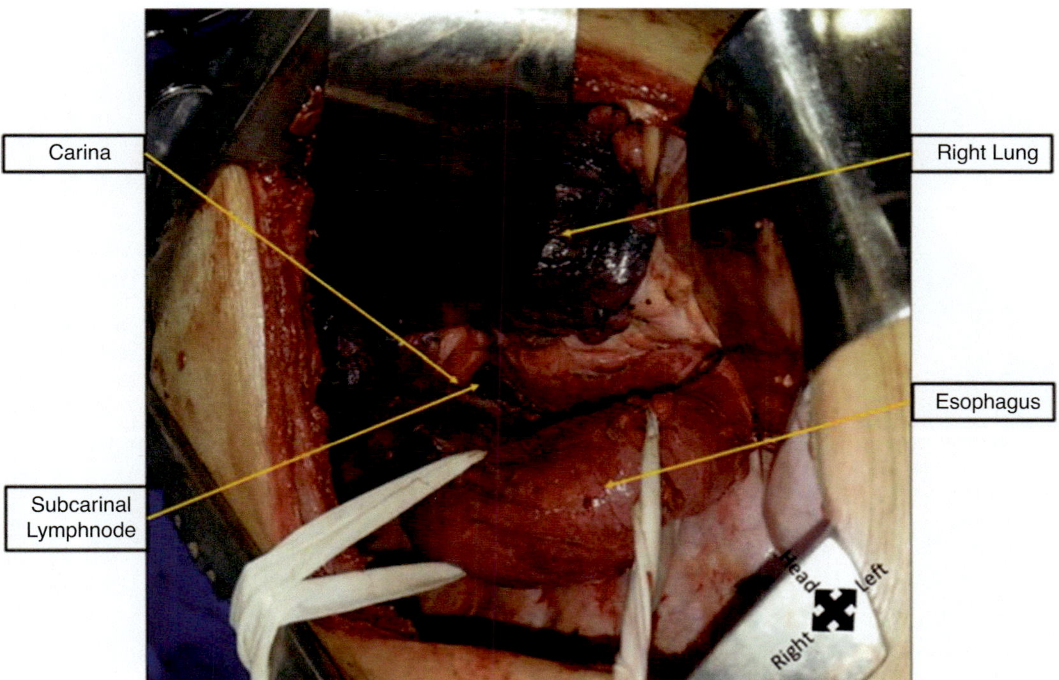

Fig. 3 Right thoracotomy. The access through the intercostal space limits the view and access to the esophagus in the posterior mediastinum. An adequate retraction of the lungs medially is mandatory

with a magnified image (Fig. 4). Some surgeons advocate the operation to be performed in prone position with putative advantages of lower pulmonary complications and increased number of resected lymph nodes [13] (Fig. 5).

The important structures that are intimately related to the thoracic esophagus are the trachea and pericardium ventrally; the azygos vein and right pleura on the right laterally, the spine and thoracic duct dorsally, and the aorta and left pleura left laterally [14].

The anatomy of the vagus had some relevance at the time when vagal-sparing esophagectomy was attempted in order to prevent morbidity related to vagotomy [15]. Currently, this procedure is seldom performed but a selective preservation of pulmonary vagal branches is proposed [16].

Pleural preservation is desired during a transhiatal esophagectomy to minimize the consequences of thoracic drainage. Pleural lesion may occur during dissection of the mid-thoracic esophagus if a recess of the pleura intervenes between the esophagus and the azygos vein

on the right side below the pulmonary veins. However, the pleura is more commonly injured during the dissection of the distal left esophagus where they are in close contact [11].

The azygos system anatomy is of interest during an esophagectomy since the arch of the azygos vein is divided to allow a better exposure of the upper thoracic esophagus, and these veins are resected during an en-bloc esophagectomy [17]. Some authors, on the other side, believe the resection of the azygos system is not considered essential since it does not affect the number of retrieved lymph nodes [18]. Variations of the azygos system are uncountable and related to the origin of the veins or the communication between the left and right-side systems. However, the clinical importance of these variations is negligible since they can be promptly recognized during an esophagectomy and comprise small caliber vessels that can be easily ligated without any consequences [11].

The recurrent laryngeal nerve has a thoracic course and can be injured during the dissection

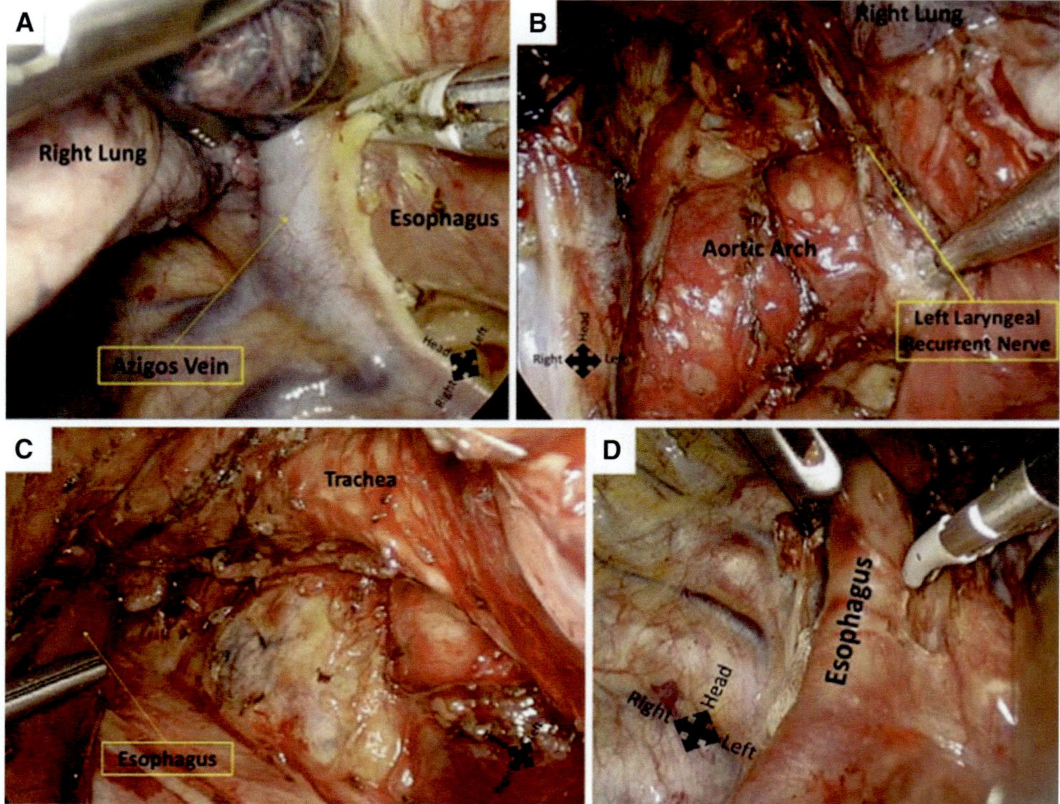

Fig. 4 Right thoracoscopy in lateral position. Minimally invasive surgery allows a magnified but restricted operative view but camera freedom of movement allows visualization of the complete thoracic cavity: upper part where the azigos vein crosses the esophagus (A) area of the aortic arch where left laryngeal nerve lymph nodes are located (B), trachea (C), the whole extension of the esophagus (D)

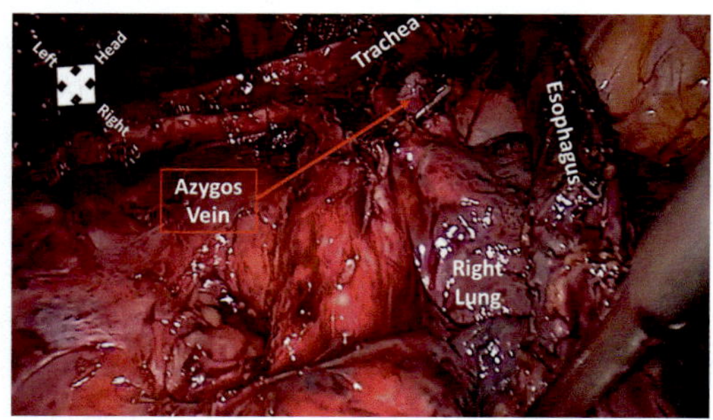

Fig. 5 Right thoracoscopy in prone position. Minimally invasive surgery allows a magnified but restricted operative view. The prone position has the advantage of removing the lungs from the operative view and allows good access to the respiratory tract to perform lymphadenectomy of peritracheal lymph nodes. The laryngeal recurrent nerves are; however, in an obstructed view

of the lymph nodes present along its course (node stations 2 and 4) [19]. The right recurrent nerve originates at the origin of the right subclavian artery behind the sternoclavicular joint, loops around the artery and ascends to the neck. The left recurrent nerve originates at the inferior border of the aortic arch, them it loops around the aorta and ascends to the neck [20]. Anatomic variations are uncommon. Non-recurrence may occur in 10% of the cases but since the nerve does not have a thoracic course in these cases, it is automatically protected from injury [11].

The thoracic duct origins in the cisterna chyli in the abdomen, ascends to the posterior mediastinum, to the right of the midline, between the descending thoracic aorta on the left and the azygos vein on the right. The duct inclines to the left, enters the superior mediastinum, and ascends toward the thoracic inlet along the left edge of the esophagus. The thoracic duct usually ends at the junction of the left subclavian and internal jugular veins [21]. There are commonly major anatomical variations that may lead to intraoperative injury during an esophagectomy [11]. The intraoperative identification of the injury and the duct itself may be difficult. Therefore, mass ligation of the duct including all tissue between the aorta, spine, esophagus, and pericardium is recommended in cases of suspect lesion of the duct [22]. Mass ligation is preferred over identification and individual ligation since duplication or plexiform ducts are common [11].

A proper lymphadenectomy is an essential part of an oncologic esophagectomy [23]. Thus, the knowledge of the anatomy of the lymph nodes that drain the esophagus is mandatory. Unfortunately, anatomy textbooks frequently show a regular disposition of nodes not useful for surgeons (Fig. 6). In addition, there is no standard classification and nomenclature of

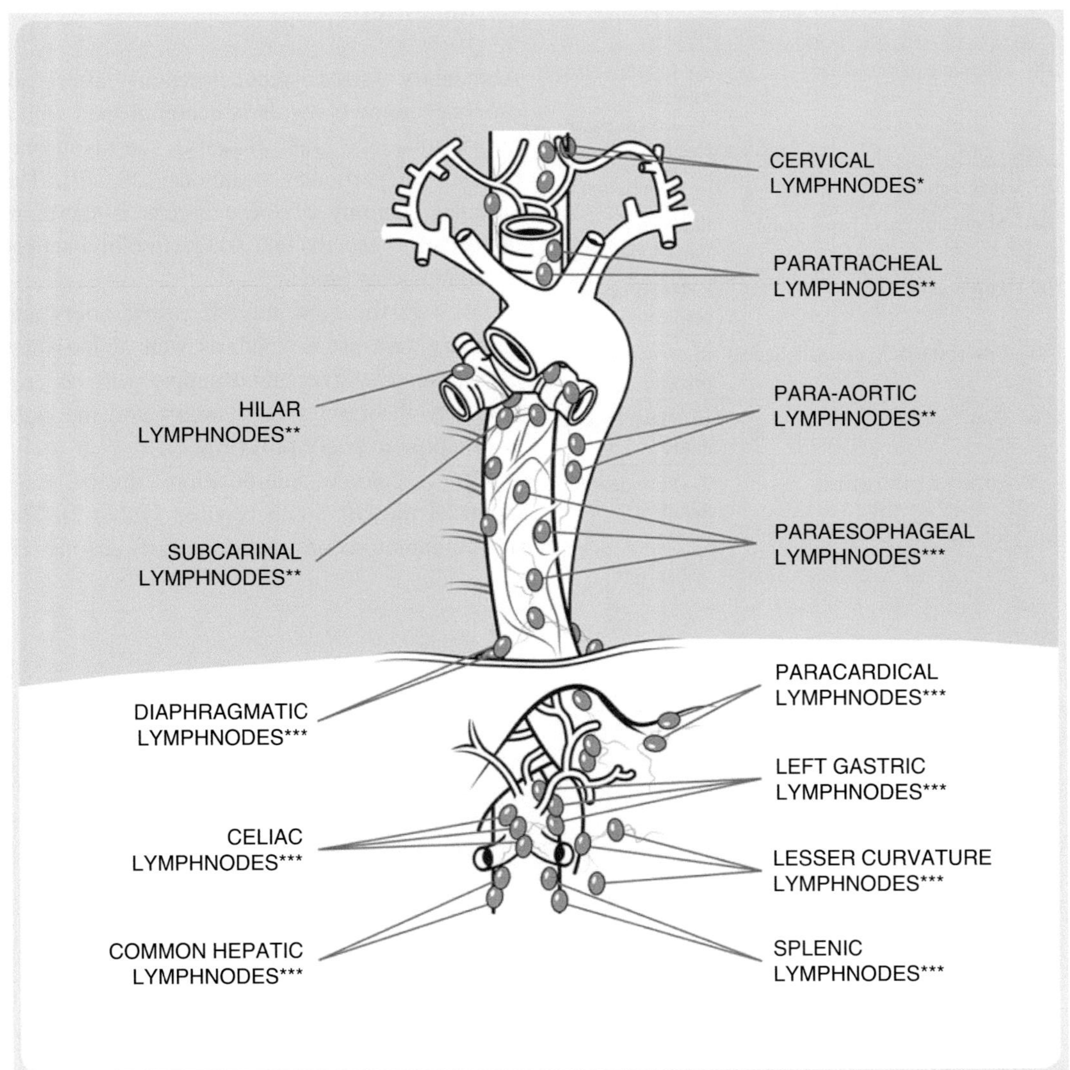

Fig. 6 Lymph nodes of interest to esophagectomy and lymphadenectomy. The exuberant lymphatic drainage of the esophagus may lead to metastasis in cervical (*), thoracic (**) and abdominal (***) periesophageal lymph nodes

mediastinal lymph nodes, and the number and location of lymph nodes is commonly erratic (Table 1) [24].

Table 1 Mediastinal Lymph Nodes Classification according to a Japanese society of esophageal disease and American joint committee for cancer and their correlations

Japanese society for esophageal disease	American joint committee for cancer
102—Deep cervical	1—Highest mediastinal
105—Upper thoracic esophaggeal	2—Upper paratracheal
106—Thoracic paratracheal	2—Upper paratracheal 4—Lower paratracheal
107—Bifurcation	7—Subcarinal
108—Middle thoracic paraesophageal	8M/8Lo—Paraesophageal
109—Pulmonary hilar	8M—Paraesophageal
110—Lower thoracic paraesophageal	8Lo—Paraesophageal
111—Diaphragmatic	15—Diaphragmatic
112—Posterior mediastinal	9—Pulmonary ligament

Abdominal Esophagus

The esophagus has a constant and short course in the abdomen that is familiar to surgeons used to laparoscopic surgery of benign esophageal disorders at the esophagogastric junction [25].

A 2 or 3-field lymphadenectomy will include the lymph nodes of the upper abdomen in a similar fashion to the D2 lymphadenectomy of the gastric cancer [26, 27] (Fig. 6).

Anatomy for Esophageal Replacement

Alimentary tract reconstruction after an esophagectomy is regularly accomplished with a gastric tube as a graft. However, the colon may be used in particular situations [28, 29]. The vascular anatomy of these organs is therefore important to establish an adequate blood supply to the replacing organ.

For a gastric tube, the left gastric artery and coronary vein are divided, as well as the short gastric vessels. The blood supply will be provided by the right gastric artery and the right gastroepiploic artery [30] (Fig. 7).

For a colonic interposition, diverse segments of the colon can be used (Table 2). The most common reconstruction options are the left

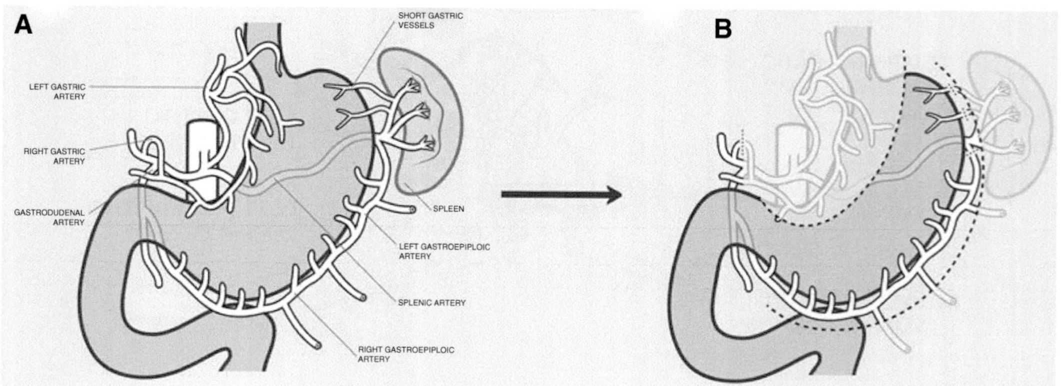

Fig. 7 Vascular anatomy of the stomach of interest to esophageal replacement (A). The greater curvature gastric tube is supplied by the right vessels (B)

Table 2 Relationship between blood supply, the segment of the colon used for esophageal replacement and type of peristalsis

Arterial supply	Colon conduit	Peristalsis
Ileocolic artery	Ascending + transverse	Antiperistalsis
Right colic artery	Cecum + ascending	Isoperistalsis
	Ascending + transverse	Antiperistalsis
Middle colic artery	Cecum + ascending + transverse	Isoperistalsis
	Ascending + transverse	Antiperistalsis
Left colic artery	Transverse + descending	Isoperistalsis

colon, with the ascending branch of the left colic vessels, and the right colon with the middle colic vessels or even with the left colic vessels [29–33] (Fig. 8). Since a segment of transverse colon is need irrespective if right or left colon is used, vascularization of the graft is dependent on anastomosis between the different colic pedicles. In a series of mesenteric arteriograms, the marginal artery in the right colon was present in only 30% of the cases, while in the left colon it was present in all cases [34]. Thus, the blood supply of the right colon is less reliable than that of the stomach and left colon [35]. Some surgeons prefer to have a preoperative angiography in order to identify the anatomy of the arteries and the continuity of the marginal artery [36] while others do not consider it necessary [37].

The replacing organ may reach the neck through different routes: posterior mediastinum, anterior mediastinum, transpleural (rare) and subcutaneous (rare). There are controversial results on the length of the anterior (retrosternal) as compared to the posterior route [39, 40]. The anterior path, however, is more constricted at the level of thoracic inlet [41].

Esophageal Radiologic Anatomy

The development of clinical imaging has allowed surgeons to better stage patients with esophageal cancer and plan the surgical approach. The old barium esophagram has been replaced by newer studies.

Endoscopic Ultrasound

Endoscopic ultrasound allows visualization of the esophageal wall and adjacent structures. The sonographic image distinguishes 5 distinct layers (Fig. 9): the innermost layer with increased echogenicity and a thin hypoechoic layer immediately deep to it correspond mainly to the mucosa and partly to the muscularis mucosae, and the next echogenic layer corresponds to the submucosa. The fourth hypoechoic layer is the muscularis propria layer and the outermost echogenic layer is the adventitia with fat appendage [42]. Lymph nodes can also be identified by endoscopic ultrasound [43].

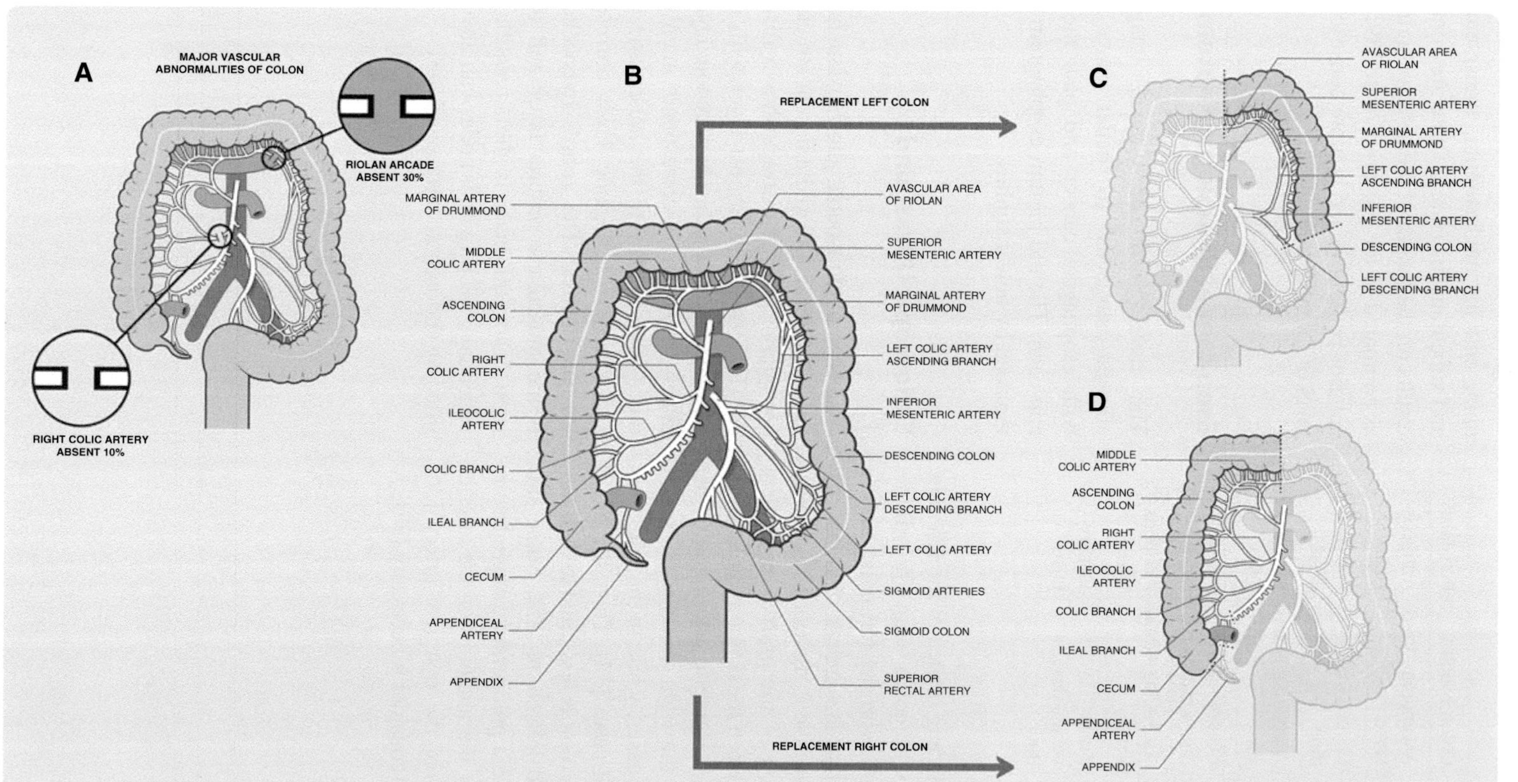

Fig. 8 Vascular anatomy of the colons of interest to esophageal replacement. A patent arcade communicating the superior and inferior mesenteric vessels is mandatory to supply the graft. This communication is absent in some cases but it can be tested during the operation (A). The vessels that supply the left or right colon used as a graft are represented in B, C, and D

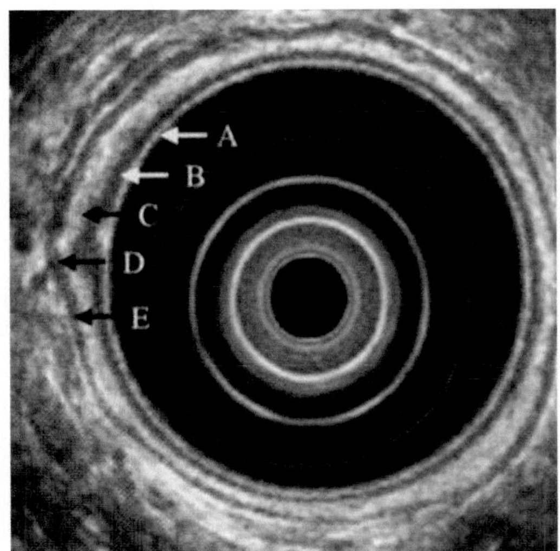

Fig. 9 Endoscopic ultrasound of the esophagus with five distinct layers: A) mucosa, B) muscularis mucosae, C) submucosa, D) muscularis propria, and E) adventitia

Computed Tomography

Computed tomography of the neck, chest and abdomen allows high quality imaging of the esophagus and 3D reconstruction [44] (Fig. 10).

The detection of lymph nodes by computed tomography correlates well to anatomic findings [24–45].

Magnetic Resonance

Dedicated techniques of magnetic resonance protocols increased esophageal anatomy visualization as compared to computed tomography. Magnetic resonance is able to detect individual layers of the esophageal wall, the thoracic duct, a connective tissue layer attaching the esophagus to the anterior wall of the aorta, and a fascial plane passing between layers of the right and left parietal pleura posterior to the esophagus [46]. Some surgeons believe the study of these planes and layers allow a more detailed dissection of the esophagus in order to preserve nerves and retrieve lymph nodes more efficiently [14].

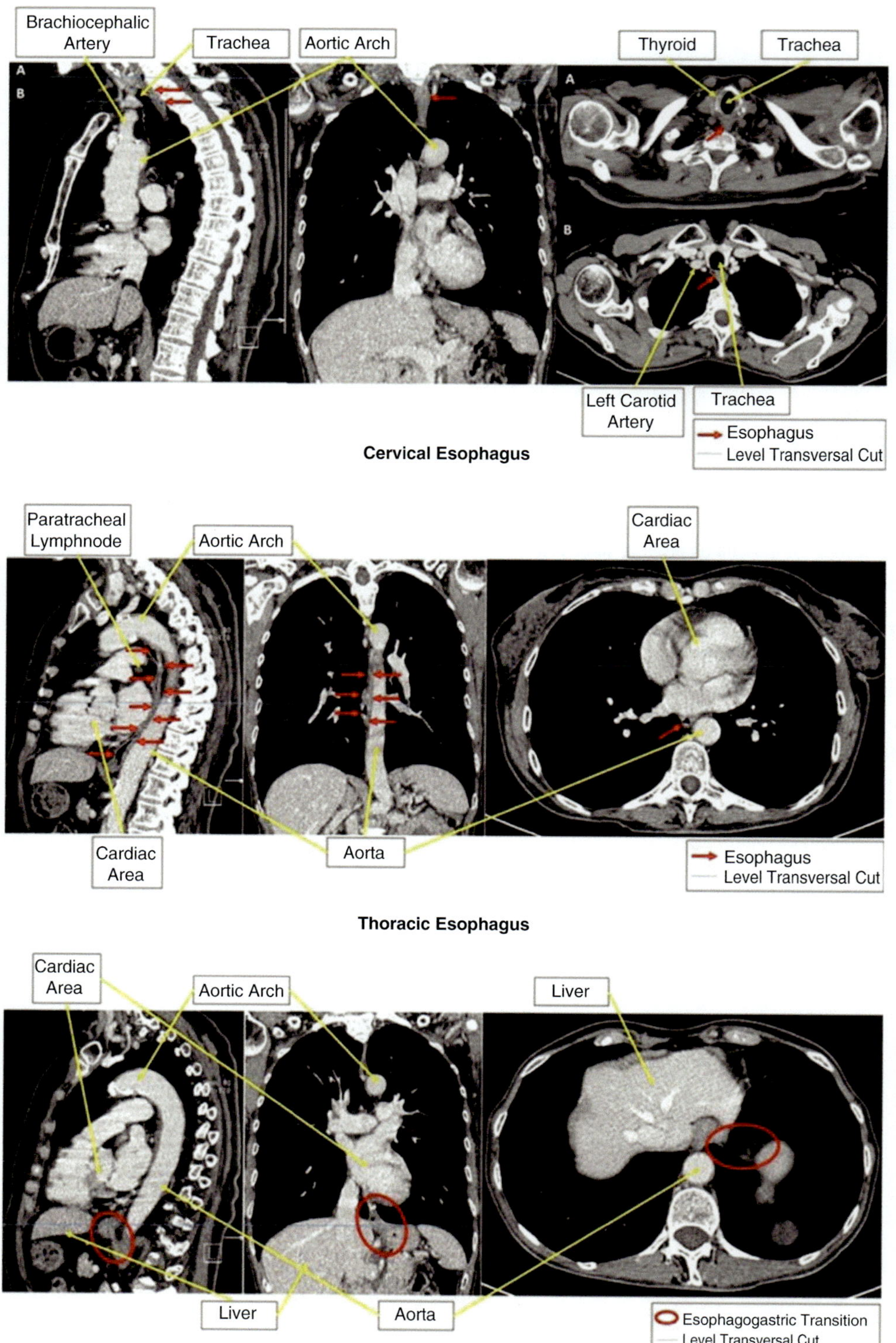

Fig. 10 Computerized tomography scans of the esophagus and surrounding structures. Tomography has a limited differentiation of tissues in the mediastinum as compared to magnetic resonance but the visualization of the esophagus and lymph nodes are adequate for clinical decisions

References

1. Oezcelik A, DeMeester SR. General anatomy of the esophagus. Thorac Surg Clin. 21(2):289–97, https://doi.org/10.1016/j.thorsurg.2011.01.003.
2. Rice TW, Bronner MP. The esophageal wall. Thorac Surg Clin. 2011;21(2):299–305. https://doi.org/10.1016/j.thorsurg.2011.01.005.
3. Japan Esophageal Society. Japanese classification of esophageal cancer, 11th edition: part I. Esophagus. 2017;14(1):1–36. DOI:https://doi.org/10.1007/s10388-016-0551-7.
4. Shimamura Y, Ikeya T, Marcon N, Mosko JD. Endoscopic diagnosis and treatment of early esophageal squamous neoplasia. World J Gastrointest Endosc. 2017;9(9):438–47. https://doi.org/10.4253/wjge.v9.i9.438.
5. Rizvi QU, Balachandran A, Koay D et al. Endoscopic management of early esophagogastric cancer. Surg Oncol Clin. 2017;26(2):179–191. https://doi.org/10.1016/j.soc.2016.10.007.
6. Patti MG, Gantert W, Way LW. Surgery of the esophagus. Anatomy and physiology. Surg Clin North Am. 1997;77(5):959–70. PMID: 9347826.
7. Gray H. Lymphatic drainage of thorax. In: Williams PL, editor. Gray's anatomy. 38th ed. New York, Edinburgh, London, Tokyo, Madrid and Melbourne: Churchill Livingstone; 1995. p. 1624–6.
8. Wang Y, Zhu L, Xia W, et al. Anatomy of lymphatic drainage of the esophagus and lymph node metastasis of thoracic esophageal cancer. Cancer Manag Res. 2018;26(10):6295–303. https://doi.org/10.2147/cmar.s182436.
9. Yasuda T, Yano M, Miyata H, et al. Evaluation of dysphagia and diminished airway protection after three-field esophagectomy and a remedy. World J Surg. 2013;37:416. https://doi.org/10.1007/s00268-012-1822-7.
10. Orringer MB. Transhiatal esophagectomy without thoracotomy. Operative Tech Thorac Cardiovasc Surg. 1984;10(1):63–83. https://doi.org/10.1053/j.optechstcvs.2005.03.001.
11. Takassi GF, Herbella FAM, Patti MG. Anatomic variations in the surgical anatomy of the thoracic esophagus and its surrounding structures. ABCD. Arquivos Brasileiros de Cirurgia Digestiva (São Paulo). 2013;26(2):101–6. https://doi.org/10.1590/S0102-67202013000200006.
12. Yajima S, Oshima Y, Shimada H. Neck dissection for thoracic esophageal squamous cell carcinoma. Int J Surg Oncol. 2012;2012:750456. https://doi.org/10.1155/2012/750456.
13. Markar SR, Wiggins T, Antonowicz S et al. Minimally invasive esophagectomy: Lateral decubitus vs. prone positioning; systematic review and pooled analysis. Surg Oncol. 2015;24(3):212–219. ISSN 0960-7404. https://doi.org/10.1016/j.suronc.2015.06.001.
14. Weijs TJ, Ruurda JP, Luyer MDP, et al. New insights into the surgical anatomy of the esophagus. J Thorac Dis. 2017;9(Suppl 8):S675–80. https://doi.org/10.21037/jtd.2017.03.172.
15. Herbella FA, Regatieri CV, Moreno DG et al. Vagal integrity in vagal-sparing esophagectomy: a cadaveric study. *Diseases of the Esophagus*, Volume 19, Issue 5, 1 October 2006, 406–9. https://doi.org/10.1111/j.1442-2050.2006.00595.x.
16. Weijs TJ, Ruurda JP, Luyer MD, et al. Preserving the pulmonary vagus nerve branches during thoracoscopic esophagectomy. Surg Endosc. 2016;30:3816–22. https://doi.org/10.1007/s00464-015-4683-y.
17. Altorki N, Skinner D. Should en bloc esophagectomy be the standard of care for esophageal carcinoma? Ann Surg. 2001;234(5):581–7.
18. Boone J, Schipper MEI, Bleys RLAW, et al. The effect of azygos vein preservation on mediastinal lymph node harvesting in thoracic esophagolymphadenectomy. Dis Esophagus. 2007. https://doi.org/10.1111/j.1442-2050.2007.00760.x.
19. Gelpke H, Grieder F, Decurtins M, Cadosch D. Recurrent laryngeal nerve monitoring during esophagectomy and mediastinal lymph node dissection. World J Surg. 2010;34:2379–82. https://doi.org/10.1007/s00268-010-0692-0.
20. Wang J, Li J, Liu G, Deslauriers J. Nerves of the mediastinum. Thorac Surg Clin. 2011;21:239–49. https://doi.org/10.1016/j.thorsurg.2011.01.006.
21. Hematti H, Mehran RJ. Anatomy of the thoracic duct. Thorac Surg Clin. 2011;21(2):229–238. (ix). https://doi.org/10.1016/j.thorsurg.2011.01.002.
22. Crucitti P, Mangiameli G, Petitti T, et al. Does prophylactic ligation of the thoracic duct reduce chylothorax rates in patients undergoing oesophagectomy? A systematic review and meta-analysis. Eur J Cardio-Thorac Surg. 2016;50(6):1019–1024. https://doi.org/10.1093/ejcts/ezw125.
23. Tong D, Law S. Extended lymphadenectomy in esophageal cancer is crucial. World J Surg. 2013;37:1751–6. https://doi.org/10.1007/s00268-013-2068-8.
24. Herbella FA, Del Grande JC, Colleoni R, Japanese society for diseases of the esophagus. Anatomical analysis of the mediastinal lymph nodes of normal Brazilian subjects according to the classification of the Japanese society for diseases of the Esophagus. Surg Today. 2003;33:249–53. https://doi.org/10.1007/s005950300056
25. Bello B, Herbella FA, Allaix ME, Patti MG. Impact of minimally invasive surgery on the treatment of benign esophageal disorders. World J Gastroenterol: WJG. 2012;18(46):6764–70. https://doi.org/10.3748/wjg.v18.i46.6764.
26. Ma G-W, Situ D-R, Ma Q-L, et al. Three-field vs two-field lymph node dissection for esophageal cancer: a meta-analysis. World J Gastroenterol: WJG.

2014;20(47):18022–30. https://doi.org/10.3748/wjg.v20.i47.18022.

27. Giacopuzzi S, Bencivenga M, Cipollari C, et al. Lymphadenectomy: how to do it? Transl Gastroenterol Hepatol. 2017;2:28. https://doi.org/10.21037/tgh.2017.03.09.

28. Irino T, Tsekrekos A, Coppola A, et al. Long-term functional outcomes after replacement of the esophagus with gastric, colonic, or jejunal conduits: a systematic literature review. Dis Esophagus. 2017;30(12):1–11. https://doi.org/10.1093/dote/dox083.

29. Marks JL, Hofstetter WL. Esophageal reconstruction with alternative conduits. Surg Clin North Am. 2012;92:1287–97. https://doi.org/10.1016/j.suc.2012.07.006.

30. Liebermann-Meffert DM, Meier R, Siewert JR. Vascular anatomy of the gastric tube used for esophageal reconstruction. Ann Thorac Surg. 1992;54:1110–5.

31. Peters JH, Kronson JW, Katz M, DeMeester TR. Arterial anatomic considerations in colon interposition for esophageal replacement. Arch Surg. 1995;130(8):858–62; discussion 862–3.

32. Hamai Y, Hihara J, Emi M, Aoki Y, Okada M. Esophageal reconstruction using the terminal ileum and right colon in esophageal cancer surgery. Surg Today. 2012;42:342–50. https://doi.org/10.1007/s00595-011-0103-7.

33. Fürst H, Hartl WH, Löhe F, Schildberg FW. Colon interposition for esophageal replacement: an alternative technique based on the use of the right colon. Ann Surg. 2000;231(2):173–8.

34. Ventemiglia R, Khalil KG, Frazier OH, Mountain CF. The role of preoperative mesenteric arteriography in colon interposition. J Thorac Cardiovasc Surg. 1977;74:98–104.

35. Rice TW, Right colon Interposition for esophageal replacement. Operative Tech Thorac Cardiovasc Surg. 1999;4(3):210–21. https://doi.org/10.1016/S1522-2942(07)70118-6.

36. Predescu D, Popa B, Gheorghe M, et al. The vascularization pattern of the colon and surgical decision in esophageal reconstruction with colon. A selective SMA and IMA arteriographic study. Chirurgia (Bucur). 2013;108:161–71.

37. Fisher RA, Griffiths EA, Evison F, et al. A national audit of colonic interposition for esophageal replacement. Dis Esophagus. 2017;30(5):1–10. https://doi.org/10.1093/dote/dow003.

38. Chen H, Lu JJ, Zhou J, Zhou X, Luo X, Liu Q, Tam J. Anterior versus posterior routes of reconstruction after esophagectomy: a comparative anatomic study. Ann Thorac Surg. 2009;87:400–4. https://doi.org/10.1016/j.athoracsur.2008.11.016.

39. Hu H, Ye T, Tan D, et al. Is anterior mediastinum route a shorter choice for esophageal reconstruction? A comparative anatomic study. Eur J Cardiothorac Surg. 2011;40:1466–9. https://doi.org/10.1016/j.ejcts.2011.03.038.

40. Coral RP, Constant-Neto M, Silva IS, et al. Comparative anatomical study of the anterior and posterior mediastinum as access routes after esophagectomy. Dis Esophagus. 2003;16(3):236–8.

41. Cooke DT, Calhoun RF. Distance alone does not define the value of the posterior mediastinal route for esophageal reconstruction. Ann Thorac Surg. 2009;88(4):1390. https://doi.org/10.1016/j.athoracsur.2009.03.036

42. Fukuda M, Hirata K, Natori H. Endoscopic ultrasonography of the esophagus. World J Surg. 2000;24:216–26.

43. Dietrich CF, Liesen M, Buhl R, et al. Detection of normal mediastinal lymph nodes by ultrasonography. Acta Radiol. 1997;38:965–9.

44. Ba-Ssalamah A, Zacherl J, Noebauer-Huhmann IM, et al. Dedicated multi-detector CT of the esophagus: spectrum of diseases. Abdom Imaging. 2009;34:3–18. https://doi.org/10.1007/s00261-007-9290-5.

45. Quint LE, Glazer GM, Orringer MB, et al. Mediastinal lymph node detection and sizing at CT and autopsy. AJR Am J Roentgenol. 1986;147:469–72. https://doi.org/10.2214/ajr.147.3.469.

46. Riddell AM, Davies DC, Allum WH, et al. High-resolution MRI in evaluation of the surgical anatomy of the esophagus and posterior mediastinum. AJR Am J Roentgenol. 2007;188:W37–43. https://doi.org/10.2214/AJR.05.1795.

Esophageal Squamous Cell Cancer: Pathogenesis and Epidemiology

Claudia Wong and Simon Law

Abstract

Esophageal cancer is a highly lethal disease. Despite an increasing incidence of adenocarcinoma in last decades, squamous cell carcinoma remains the predominant cell type worldwide. The majority of squamous cell cancers are from the East. Risk factors for the development of esophageal squamous cell carcinoma differ between high- and low-incidence regions. Tobacco and alcohol intake are the two major risks factors for esophageal squamous cell carcinoma. They also have a synergistic effect; the mechanism of which is now better understood. Other dietary factors include lack of certain micronutrients, consumption of food with carcinogenic ingredients, eating habits and food preservation methods. Genetic factors, viral infection and other premalignant conditions also play a role. Studying epidemiology and pathogenesis of the disease allows policymakers to enact public health policies to prevent the disease through health education and risk factors avoidance. Screening for early disease detection in high-risk populations could improve overall outcome.

Keywords

Squamous cell cancer · Esophageal cancer · Epidemiology · Pathogenesis · Tobacco · Alcohol

Introduction

Esophageal cancer is a disease of dismal prognosis. The two major histologic types of tumors, squamous cell carcinoma and adenocarcinoma, differ substantially in epidemiology, and pathogenesis. Squamous cell carcinoma remains the main cell type worldwide and most are found in Eastern populations. The cancer is characterized by late presentation and rapidly fatal course. This makes study on modifiable risk factors for esophageal cancer particularly important in the context of disease prevention. The present chapter addresses the epidemiology and pathogenesis with emphasis on esophageal squamous cell carcinoma (ESCC).

Epidemiology

Esophageal cancer is the 8th most common cancer globally and the 6th most common cause of cancer-related deaths [1]. Despite advances in diagnostic methods and multimodal therapy in high-income countries, survival rate at 5 years

C. Wong · S. Law (✉)
Department of Surgery, School of Clinical Medicine, The University of Hong Kong, Queen Mary Hospital, 102 Pokfulam Road, Pokfulam, Hong Kong
e-mail: slaw@hku.hk

from esophageal cancer remains low. The reported five-year survival rates for esophageal cancer are 21% in China [2], 20% in the United States [3], 9.8% in Europe [4], and < 5% in places where resources are limited [5, 6]. There were an estimated 512,500 new cases of ESCC in 2020, representing 85% of all esophageal cancers [7, 8]. Although there has been a decline in the incidence of ESCC in certain parts of the world, probably related to improvement in living standard and lifestyle habits, ESCC remains the predominant histologic type worldwide.

ESCC is a male-predominant disease and is the most common histological type for both men and women. There is significant variation of incidence among different geographic regions and various ethnic groups. The incidence rates of ESCC are highest in Eastern and South-Central Asia and South Africa. In Asian countries, it is commonly found in the *"Asian esophageal cancer belt"*, bounded by eastern Turkey and east of Caspian Sea through northern Iran, northern Afghanistan, and southern areas of the former Soviet Union, such as Turkmenistan, Uzbekistan, and Tajikistan, to northern China and India. In high-incidence areas worldwide, including Linxian province in China, Golestan province in Iran, Western Kenya south to Malawi, the Eastern Cape province of South Africa, Calvados in France, Southern Brazil and Uruguay, the occurrence of esophageal cancer is 50–100-fold higher than that in the rest of the world.

In China, ESCC is the 4th most frequently diagnosed cancer and the 4th leading cause of cancer deaths. The age-standardized incidence rate of ESCC in China is 12.5 per 100,000 person-years, compared to 5.6 in the rest of the Eastern Asia, 1.8 in Northern Europe, 2.3 in Western Europe, 0.9 in North America, and 1.2 in Australia/New Zealand. The crude age-adjusted mortality is up to 12.7 per 100,000 person-years [1]. Incidence is generally higher in rural areas, of which provinces like Henan, Hebei and Shanxi have the highest incidence rates in the world. Esophageal cancer most commonly presents in the sixth and seventh decades of life and is rare before the fourth decade. About 70% of the patients in Japan are in their 60 s and 70 s at the time of diagnosis according to the Population-Based Cancer Registry. Similarly, the incidence of ESCC peaks at 70–80 years of age according to National Central Cancer Registry of China [9, 10].

Pathogenesis

Several etiological factors are in association with ESCC, of which, consumption of tobacco, alcohol, hot beverages and nitrosamines, genetic factors, and personal history of squamous cell carcinoma in the head and neck region and the esophagus are most studied (Table 1).

Alcohol and Smoking

Tobacco and alcohol consumption are the two major risks factors for ESCC. Smoking is regarded by the International Agency for Research on Cancer (IARC) as a cause of esophageal cancer [11]. Compared to non-alcohol drinkers, the risk of ESCC increases by 38%, 260% and 550% among those who drink alcohol 1–1.5 L/day, 1.5–6 L/day and > 6L/day, respectively [12, 13]. Alcohol and smoking have synergistic effect on the risk of ESCC. The mechanism is well studied. Alcohol damages cellular DNA by decreasing metabolic activity within cells, thereby reduces detoxification function and promotes oxidation [14]. It acts as a solvent for fat-soluble carcinogens such as aromatic amines, nitrosamines, polycyclic aromatic hydrocarbons, phenols, and aldehyde. Therefore, these substances from tobacco can easily diffuse to the esophageal tissue. A meta-analysis showed that the combined effect of drinking and smoking doubled the sum of their effects individually [15]. In low- or medium-incidence populations like in Europe and the United States, ESCC is largely attributed to

Table 1 Etiology factors for esophageal squamous cell cancer

Factor	Contribution
Alcohol	+++
Smoking	+++
Diet related	
Deficiencies of fresh green vegetables, fruits and vitamins	+
N-nitroso containing food (e.g. pickled vegetables)	+
Chewing betel nut and mate drinking	+
Hot beverages	+
Fungal toxin	+
Infection	
Human papilloma virus	±
Pre-malignant conditions	
History of aerodigestive malignancy	+++
History of radiation to mediastinum	+
Achalasia	+
Lye corrosive stricture	+
Genetic factors	
Aldehyde dehydrogenase deficiency	++
Tylosis	+
Plummer-Vinson syndrome	+
Others	
Low socioeconomic class	+

smoking and alcohol [16, 17]. In the United States, United Kingdom, and France, population attributable risks of 57–73% have been reported for squamous cell carcinoma, based on reduction of smoking and alcohol use, and consumption of fruits and vegetables [17–20]. Similarly, studies in high incidence countries in Asia such as China estimated that 48.5% of esophageal cancers were attributable to the combined effect of alcohol, smoking and low fruit and vegetable intake [21].

Genetic Factors

Genetic predisposition may be related to the pathogenesis of ESCC. Genome-wide association studies have demonstrated a high heritability of ESCC when compared to other cancers [22], and there is an increased risk of ESCC in people who have a positive family history [23–25]. Mitochondrial studies have proved historical population migrations from central / northern to southern-eastern China; the two regions share the same high risk of ESCC and yet environmentally they are quite different [26].

Tylosis, characterized by hyperkeratosis of palms and soles, is a familial esophageal cancer syndrome inherited as an autosomal dominant trait. It has been reported to be associated with genetic mutations in RHBDF2 [27].

Genetic polymorphism is important in individuals with chronic alcohol consumption. Polymorphisms in alcohol dehydrogenase 1B (ADH1B), alcohol dehydrogenase (ADH7), and aldehyde dehydrogenase 2 (ALDH2) are known to alter ethanol metabolism. Approximately 36% of East Asians show a physiologic response to drinking that includes facial flushing, nausea, and tachycardia [28]. This facial flushing response is predominantly related to an inherited deficiency in the enzyme ALDH2. Alcohol is metabolized to acetaldehyde by alcohol dehydrogenase and the acetaldehyde is in turn metabolized by ALDH2 to acetate. Two main variants for ALDH2 exist, resulting from the replacement of glutamate with lysine at position 487. Only individuals homozygous with the glutamate allele have normal catalytic activity. Homozygotes with the lysine alleles have no detectable activity, while heterozygotes with Glu/Lys alleles have much reduced ALDH2 activity. The inability to fully metabolize acetaldehyde results in its accumulation in the body leading to the facial flushing and unpleasant side effects. Lys/Lys homozygotes cannot tolerate much alcohol because of the intensity of the side effects, and so paradoxically they do not have increased risk because they simply would not consume a significant amount of alcohol. Individuals who are Glu/Lys heterozygotes may become habitual drinkers because they could become tolerant to the side effects of alcohol and yet they had suboptimal catalytic activity and thus the acetaldehyde accumulates. These are the individuals most susceptible to the carcinogenic effects of alcohol consumption, which is related to acetaldehyde causing DNA damage and other cancer-promoting effects [29]. A simple questionnaire that elicits the history of a flushing response can be useful in identifying at-risk individuals, who could be advised against drinking or to undergo screening endoscopy. The risk of developing cancer may be reduced, or an earlier diagnosis could be possible [30].

Diet and Environment

In Asian countries, dietary and environmental factors certainly play a role in the development of ESCC. Studies have investigated the effects of dietary patterns, specific food and nutrients on the disease [31, 32]. Nitrosamines and their precursors such as nitrate, nitrite, and secondary amines, are found in pickled vegetables, which in turn have been shown to increase risk [33]. Nutritional depletion of certain micronutrients, particularly vitamins A, C, E, niacin, riboflavin, molybdenum, manganese, zinc, magnesium selenium, as well as fresh fruits and vegetables, together with an inadequate protein intake, predisposes the esophageal epithelium to neoplastic transformation [34]. While the lack of fresh fruit and vegetables is associated with increased risk of ESCC [35], meta-analyses showed that eating fruits and vegetables significantly reduced ESCC risk [36, 37]. The Nutrition Intervention Trial conducted in Linxian county in China showed that consumption of vitamin B2 and nicotinic acid decreased the incidence of esophageal cancer by 14%, while beta-carotene, vitamin E, and selenium intake could reduce esophageal cancer mortality by 17% in patients less than 55 years old [38].

Consumption of red meat, processed meat, and hot mate were shown to be associated with increased risk of ESCC [39, 40]. A meta-analysis showed that the cancer risk was 57% higher in people who consumed a large amount of red meat and 55% higher in people who took a large amount of processed meat [40]. Mate drinkers have a 60–260% increased ESCC risk compared to non-drinkers in South American countries [41, 42].

Change in specific dietary habits, such as replacing traditional methods of food preservation and storage with refrigeration, together with consumption of vitamin-rich food, may have produced a reduction in incidence rates in certain areas of China, especially in urban cities such as Shanghai [43, 44]. Consumption of hot food and beverages is associated with an increased risk of esophageal cancer, particularly squamous cell cancer [45, 46].

Infection

Infective pathogens including human papillomavirus (HPV), *Fusarium, Alternaria, Geotrichum, Aspergillus, Cladosporium, and Penicillium* species are found to be associated with esophageal cancer in some studies. The role of HPV, debated in more recent studies, is now controversial. Therefore, HPV vaccines may not be beneficial in ESCC prevention [47–51].

Premalignant/Neoplastic Condition

Patients with other aerodigestive malignancies have a particularly high risk of developing ESCC, presumably because of exposure to similar environmental carcinogens and "field cancerization". This concept was introduced by Slaughter and colleagues. It was postulated that clonal expansion develops in mucosa adjacent to an initial area of genetic and epigenetic alternations. This results in a proliferating field of early genetic changes that is at risk of future cancer development [52–54]. Using esophageal cancer as the index tumor, multiple primary cancers were found in 9.5% of patients, of whom 70% were in the aerodigestive tract [55]. The overall incidence of synchronous or metachronous esophageal cancer in patients with primary head and neck cancer is estimated to be 3–6% [56, 57].

Diseases that are known to predispose to esophageal cancer are few. The risk from achalasia is estimated to be 7- to 33-fold, but symptoms of achalasia are present for an average of 15–20 years before the emergence of cancer [58]. Other diseases include lye corrosive strictures, Plummer-Vinson syndrome, tylosis, and celiac disease.

Other Factors

Low socioeconomic status is associated with increased risk of ESCC. It is believed to be an interplay of many factors including poorer nutritional status, lacking of fresh food and produce, poor oral hygiene and tooth loss. Studies showed that tooth brushing exerts protective effects against ESCC and that tooth loss is associated with increased risk of ESCC [59–61]. These findings, however, should be interpreted carefully as poor oral hygiene may also be confounded by other lifestyle habits like smoking and drinking.

Prevention

ESCC is notorious for its poor prognosis. Being asymptomatic at an early stage, the majority of patients are diagnosed at an advanced stage. The disease tends to spread early compared to other gastrointestinal tract cancers at an equivalent depth of invasion. Identifying modifiable risk factors allows potential prevention and screening at high-incidence regions. This will facilitate early diagnosis and improve prognosis.

ESCC as aforementioned has been demonstrated to be linked with several environmental risk factors. To reduce the risk of ESCC, it is advisable to abstain from smoking and excessive alcohol drinking, consume more fresh vegetables and fruits, and minimize exposure to food carcinogens like nitrites or nitrosamine.

Early detection potentially improves survival outcome. Screening strategies and prediction models have been developed and reported [62]. Currently there is no international consensus on ESCC screening, probably because of the substantial geographic variations in

prevalence and concerns on cost-effectiveness. Chromoendoscopic examination using Lugol's iodine solution has been shown to be effective in Korea, Japan and China for screening of esophageal cancer. Magnifying endoscopy with narrow-band imaging (NBI) enables detection of superficial, early-stage cancers with high sensitivity but requires specialized training [63, 64]. These screening strategies and techniques are less applicable in low incidence regions.

Conclusion

ESCC is a fatal disease and a significant burden to the healthcare system especially in regions of high prevalence. Public health education, nutritional intervention and risk-stratified screening potentially reduce incidence rate and cancer-related deaths in high-incidence areas. Understanding of the epidemiology and pathogenesis of ESCC is essential for policymakers and stakeholders of healthcare systems to implement appropriate measures to improve the outlook of this lethal disease.

References

1. Sung H, Ferlay J, Siegel RL, et al. Global Cancer Statistics 2020: GLOBOCAN estimates of Incidence and mortality worldwide for 36 cancers in 185 countries. CA Cancer J Clin. 2021;71(3):209–49. https://doi.org/10.3322/caac.21660.
2. Cao W, Chen H-D, Yu Y-W, et al. Changing profiles of cancer burden worldwide and in China: a secondary analysis of the global cancer statistics 2020. Chin Med J. 2021;134(7).
3. Siegel RL, Miller KD, Jemal A. Cancer statistics, 2016. CA Cancer J Clin. 2016;66(1):7–30. https://doi.org/10.3322/caac.21332.
4. Gavin AT, Francisci S, Foschi R, et al. Oesophageal cancer survival in Europe: a EUROCARE-4 study. Cancer Epidemiol. 2012;36(6):505–12. https://doi.org/10.1016/j.canep.2012.07.009.
5. White RE, Parker RK, Fitzwater JW, et al. Stents as sole therapy for oesophageal cancer: a prospective analysis of outcomes after placement. Lancet Oncol. 2009;10(3):240–6. https://doi.org/10.1016/s1470-2045(09)70004-x.
6. Dawsey SP, Tonui S, Parker RK, et al. Esophageal cancer in young people: a case series of 109

cases and review of the literature. PLoS ONE. 2010;5(11):e14080. https://doi.org/10.1371/journal. pone.0014080.

7. Morgan E, Soerjomataram I, Rumgay H, et al. The global landscape of esophageal squamous cell carcinoma and esophageal adenocarcinoma incidence and mortality in 2020 and projections to 2040: new estimates from GLOBOCAN 2020. Gastroenterology. 2022;163(3):649-58.e2. https://doi.org/10.1053/j. gastro.2022.05.054.

8. Uhlenhopp DJ, Then EO, Sunkara T, et al. Epidemiology of esophageal cancer: update in global trends, etiology and risk factors. Clin J Gastroenterol. 2020;13(6):1010–21. https://doi. org/10.1007/s12328-020-01237-x.

9. Japan ES. Japanese classification of esophageal cancer, 11th edition: part I. Esophagus. 2017;14(1):1–36. https://doi.org/10.1007/s10388-016-0551-7.

10. Wang Y, Yan Q, Fan C, et al. Overview and countermeasures of cancer burden in China. Sci China Life Sci. 2023:1–12. https://doi.org/10.1007/s11427-022-2240-6.

11. Cogliano VJ, Baan R, Straif K, et al. Preventable exposures associated with human cancers. JNCI: J National Cancer Inst. 2011;103(24):1827–39. https://doi.org/10.1093/jnci/djr483.

12. Islami F, Fedirko V, Tramacere I, et al. Alcohol drinking and esophageal squamous cell carcinoma with focus on light-drinkers and never-smokers: a systematic review and meta-analysis. Int J Cancer. 2011;129(10):2473–84. https://doi.org/10.1002/ijc.25885.

13. Bagnardi V, Rota M, Botteri E, et al. Light alcohol drinking and cancer: a meta-analysis. Ann Oncol. 2013;24(2):301–8. https://doi.org/10.1093/annonc/mds337.

14. Muwonge R, Ramadas K, Sankila R, et al. Role of tobacco smoking, chewing and alcohol drinking in the risk of oral cancer in Trivandrum, India: a nested case-control design using incident cancer cases. Oral Oncol. 2008;44(5):446–54. https://doi.org/10.1016/j.oraloncology.2007.06.002.

15. Prabhu A, Obi KO, Rubenstein JH. The synergistic effects of alcohol and tobacco consumption on the risk of esophageal squamous cell carcinoma: a meta-analysis. Am J Gastroenterol. 2014;109(6):822–7. https://doi.org/10.1038/ajg.2014.71.

16. Tuyns AJ. Oesophageal cancer in non-smoking drinkers and in non-drinking smokers. Int J Cancer. 1983;32(4):443–4. https://doi.org/10.1002/ijc.2910320408.

17. Wang SM, Katki HA, Graubard BI, et al. Population attributable risks of subtypes of esophageal and gastric cancers in the United States. Am J Gastroenterol. 2021;116(9):1844–52. https://doi.org/10.14309/ajg.0000000000001355.

18. Engel LS, Chow WH, Vaughan TL, et al. Population attributable risks of esophageal and gastric cancers. J Natl Cancer Inst. 2003;95(18):1404–13. https://doi.org/10.1093/jnci/djg047.

19. Shield KD, Marant Micallef C, Hill C, et al. New cancer cases in France in 2015 attributable to different levels of alcohol consumption. Addiction. 2018;113(2):247–56. https://doi.org/10.1111/add.14009.

20. Brown KF, Rumgay H, Dunlop C, et al. The fraction of cancer attributable to modifiable risk factors in England, Wales, Scotland, Northern Ireland, and the United Kingdom in 2015. Br J Cancer. 2018;118(8):1130–41. https://doi.org/10.1038/s41416-018-0029-6.

21. Wu Y, Li Y, Giovannucci E. Potential impact of time trend of lifestyle risk factors on burden of major gastrointestinal cancers in China. Gastroenterology. 2021;161(6):1830-41.e8. https://doi.org/10.1053/j.gastro.2021.08.006.

22. Sampson JN, Wheeler WA, Yeager M, et al. Analysis of heritability and shared heritability based on genome-wide association studies for thirteen cancer types. J Natl Cancer Inst. 2015;107(12):djv279. https://doi.org/10.1093/jnci/djv279.

23. Tran GD, Sun XD, Abnet CC, et al. Prospective study of risk factors for esophageal and gastric cancers in the Linxian general population trial cohort in China. Int J Cancer. 2005;113(3):456–63. https://doi.org/10.1002/ijc.20616.

24. Gao Y, Hu N, Han X, et al. Family history of cancer and risk for esophageal and gastric cancer in Shanxi China. BMC Cancer. 2009;9:269. https://doi.org/10.1186/1471-2407-9-269.

25. Akbari MR, Malekzadeh R, Nasrollahzadeh D, et al. Familial risks of esophageal cancer among the Turkmen population of the Caspian littoral of Iran. Int J Cancer. 2006;119(5):1047–51. https://doi.org/10.1002/ijc.21906.

26. Li XY, Su M, Huang HH, et al. mtDNA evidence: genetic background associated with related populations at high risk for esophageal cancer between Chaoshan and Taihang Mountain areas in China. Genomics. 2007;90(4):474–81. https://doi.org/10.1016/j.ygeno.2007.06.006.

27. Blaydon DC, Etheridge SL, Risk JM, et al. RHBDF2 mutations are associated with tylosis, a familial esophageal cancer syndrome. Am J Hum Genet. 2012;90(2):340–6. https://doi.org/10.1016/j.ajhg.2011.12.008.

28. Brooks PJ, Enoch MA, Goldman D, et al. The alcohol flushing response: an unrecognized risk factor for esophageal cancer from alcohol consumption. PLoS Med. 2009;6(3):e50. https://doi.org/10.1371/journal.pmed.1000050.

29. Baan R, Straif K, Grosse Y, et al. Carcinogenicity of alcoholic beverages. Lancet Oncol. 2007;8(4):292–3. https://doi.org/10.1016/s1470-2045(07)70099-2.

30. Yokoyama A, Kumagai Y, Yokoyama T, et al. Health risk appraisal models for mass screening

for esophageal and pharyngeal cancer: an endoscopic follow-up study of cancer-free Japanese men. Cancer Epidemiol Biomarkers Prev. 2009;18(2):651–5. https://doi.org/10.1158/1055-9965.Epi-08-0758.

31. World Cancer Research Fund/American Institute for Cancer Research. Diet, Nutrition, Physical Activity and Cancer: a Global Perspective. Continuous Update Project Expert Report 2018.

32. Li WQ, Park Y, Wu JW, et al. Index-based dietary patterns and risk of esophageal and gastric cancer in a large cohort study. Clin Gastroenterol Hepatol. 2013;11(9):1130-36.e2. https://doi.org/10.1016/j.cgh.2013.03.023.

33. Cheng KK, Day NE, Duffy SW, et al. Pickled vegetables in the aetiology of oesophageal cancer in Hong Kong Chinese. Lancet. 1992;339(8805):1314–8. https://doi.org/10.1016/0140-6736(92)91960-g.

34. Yang CS. Research on esophageal cancer in China: a review. Cancer Res. 1980;40(8 Pt 1):2633–44.

35. Vingeliene S, Chan DSM, Vieira AR, et al. An update of the WCRF/AICR systematic literature review and meta-analysis on dietary and anthropometric factors and esophageal cancer risk. Ann Oncol. 2017;28(10):2409–19. https://doi.org/10.1093/annonc/mdx338.

36. Zhao W, Liu L, Xu S. Intakes of citrus fruit and risk of esophageal cancer: a meta-analysis. Medicine (Baltimore). 2018;97(13):e0018. https://doi.org/10.1097/md.0000000000010018.

37. Liu J, Wang J, Leng Y, et al. Intake of fruit and vegetables and risk of esophageal squamous cell carcinoma: a meta-analysis of observational studies. Int J Cancer. 2013;133(2):473–85. https://doi.org/10.1002/ijc.28024.

38. Qiao YL, Dawsey SM, Kamangar F, et al. Total and cancer mortality after supplementation with vitamins and minerals: follow-up of the Linxian general population nutrition intervention trial. J Natl Cancer Inst. 2009;101(7):507–18. https://doi.org/10.1093/jnci/djp037.

39. Zhao Z, Wang F, Chen D, et al. Red and processed meat consumption and esophageal cancer risk: a systematic review and meta-analysis. Clin Transl Oncol. 2020;22(4):532–45. https://doi.org/10.1007/s12094-019-02157-0.

40. Choi Y, Song S, Song Y, et al. Consumption of red and processed meat and esophageal cancer risk: meta-analysis. World J Gastroenterol. 2013;19(7):1020–9. https://doi.org/10.3748/wjg.v19.i7.1020.

41. Andrici J, Eslick GD. Maté consumption and the risk of esophageal squamous cell carcinoma: a meta-analysis. Dis Esophagus. 2013;26(8):807–16. https://doi.org/10.1111/j.1442-2050.2012.01393.x.

42. Lubin JH, De Stefani E, Abnet CC, et al. Maté drinking and esophageal squamous cell carcinoma in South America: pooled results from two large multicenter case-control studies. Cancer Epidemiol Biomarkers Prev. 2014;23(1):107–16. https://doi.org/10.1158/1055-9965.Epi-13-0796.

43. Ke L. Mortality and incidence trends from esophagus cancer in selected geographic areas of China circa 1970–90. Int J Cancer. 2002;102(3):271–4. https://doi.org/10.1002/ijc.10706.

44. He Y-T, Hou J, Chen Z-F, et al. Trends in incidence of esophageal and gastric cardia cancer in high-risk areas in China. Eur J Cancer Prev. 2008;17(2).

45. Andrici J, Eslick GD. Hot food and beverage consumption and the risk of esophageal cancer: a meta-analysis. Am J Prev Med. 2015;49(6):952–60. https://doi.org/10.1016/j.amepre.2015.07.023.

46. Wu M, Liu AM, Kampman E, et al. Green tea drinking, high tea temperature and esophageal cancer in high- and low-risk areas of Jiangsu Province, China: a population-based case-control study. Int J Cancer. 2009;124(8):1907–13. https://doi.org/10.1002/ijc.24142.

47. He D, Zhang DK, Lam KY, et al. Prevalence of HPV infection in esophageal squamous cell carcinoma in Chinese patients and its relationship to the p53 gene mutation. Int J Cancer. 1997;72(6):959–64. https://doi.org/10.1002/(sici)1097-0215(19970917)72:6<959::aid-ijc7>3.0.co;2-o.

48. Petrick JL, Wyss AB, Butler AM, et al. Prevalence of human papillomavirus among oesophageal squamous cell carcinoma cases: systematic review and meta-analysis. Br J Cancer. 2014;110(9):2369–77. https://doi.org/10.1038/bjc.2014.96.

49. Koshiol J, Wei WQ, Kreimer AR, et al. No role for human papillomavirus in esophageal squamous cell carcinoma in China. Int J Cancer. 2010;127(1):93–100. https://doi.org/10.1002/ijc.25023.

50. Sitas F, Egger S, Urban MI, et al. InterSCOPE study: Associations between esophageal squamous cell carcinoma and human papillomavirus serological markers. J Natl Cancer Inst. 2012;104(2):147–58. https://doi.org/10.1093/jnci/djr499.

51. Halec G, Schmitt M, Egger S, et al. Mucosal alpha-papillomaviruses are not associated with esophageal squamous cell carcinomas: Lack of mechanistic evidence from South Africa, China and Iran and from a world-wide meta-analysis. Int J Cancer. 2016;139(1):85–98. https://doi.org/10.1002/ijc.29911.

52. Braakhuis BJM, Tabor MP, Kummer JA, et al. A genetic explanation of slaughter's concept of field cancerization. Can Res. 2003;63(8):1727.

53. Mohan M, Jagannathan N. Oral field cancerization: an update on current concepts. Oncol Rev. 2014;8(1):244. https://doi.org/10.4081/oncol.2014.244.

54. Slaughter DP, Southwick HW, Smejkal W. Field cancerization in oral stratified squamous epithelium; clinical implications of multicentric origin. Cancer. 1953;6(5):963–8. https://doi.org/10.1002/1097-0142(195309)6:5<963::aid-cncr2820060515>3.0.co;2-q.

55. Poon RT, Law SY, Chu KM, et al. Multiple primary cancers in esophageal squamous cell carcinoma: incidence and implications. Ann Thorac Surg. 1998;65(6):1529–34. https://doi.org/10.1016/s0003-4975(98)00177-5.

56. Shaha AR, Hoover EL, Mitrani M, et al. Synchronicity, multicentricity, and metachronicity of head and neck cancer. Head Neck Surg. 1988;10(4):225–8. https://doi.org/10.1002/j.1930-2398.1988.tb00003.x.

57. Ho SY, Tsang RKY. Value of oesophagoscopy and bronchoscopy in diagnosis of synchronous malignancies in patients with head and neck squamous cell carcinomas. BMC Cancer. 2020;20(1):1172. https://doi.org/10.1186/s12885-020-07681-9.

58. Ribeiro U, Jr, Posner MC, Safatle-Ribeiro AV, et al. Risk factors for squamous cell carcinoma of the oesophagus. Br J Surg. 1996;83(9):1174–85.

59. Chen X, Yuan Z, Lu M, et al. Poor oral health is associated with an increased risk of esophageal squamous cell carcinoma—a population-based case-control study in China. Int J Cancer. 2017;140(3):626–35. https://doi.org/10.1002/ijc.30484.

60. Guha N, Boffetta P, Wünsch Filho V, et al. Oral health and risk of squamous cell carcinoma of the head and neck and esophagus: results of two multicentric case-control studies. Am J Epidemiol. 2007;166(10):1159–73. https://doi.org/10.1093/aje/kwm193.

61. Conway D. Oral health, mouthwashes and cancer–what is the story? Evid Based Dent. 2009;10(1):6–7. https://doi.org/10.1038/sj.ebd.6400624.

62. Li H, Sun D, Cao M, et al. Risk prediction models for esophageal cancer: A systematic review and critical appraisal. Cancer Med. 2021;10(20):7265–76. https://doi.org/10.1002/cam4.4226.

63. Ishihara R. Endoscopic Diagnosis and Treatment of Superficial Esophageal Squamous Cell Cancer: Present Status and Future Perspectives. Curr Oncol. 2022;29(2):534–43. https://doi.org/10.3390/curroncol29020048.

64. Morita FH, Bernardo WM, Ide E, et al. Narrow band imaging versus lugol chromoendoscopy to diagnose squamous cell carcinoma of the esophagus: a systematic review and meta-analysis. BMC Cancer. 2017;17(1):54. https://doi.org/10.1186/s12885-016-3011-9.

Esophageal Adenocarcinoma: Pathogenesis and Epidemiology

Manuela Monrabal Lezama, Francisco Schlottmann and Marco G. Patti

Abstract

Over the past 40 years, the incidence of esophageal adenocarcinoma (EAC) has increased more than six-fold in Western countries. The increase incidence of EAC has been attributed to the rising prevalence of obesity and gastroesophageal reflux disease (GERD). GERD affects an estimated 20% of the population in the US, and its prevalence is increasing worldwide. About 10% of patients with GERD will develop Barrett's esophagus (BE). This metaplastic lesion due to the chronic injury produced by repeated reflux episodes involves genetic mutations that can lead to a malignant transformation. The development of EAC is characterized by the progression from BE metaplasia to dysplasia, and ultimately invasive carcinoma.

M. Monrabal Lezama · F. Schlottmann (✉)
Department of Surgery, Hospital Alemán of Buenos Aires, 1640 Pueyrredon Ave,
Buenos Aires, Argentina
e-mail: fschlottmann@hotmail.com

F. Schlottmann
Department of Surgery, University of Illinois at Chicago, Chicago, IL, USA

M. G. Patti
Department of Surgery, University of Virginia, Charlottesville, VA, USA

Keywords

Esophageal adenocarcinoma · Epidemiology · Pathogenesis · Gastroesophageal reflux disease · Barrett's esophagus

Epidemiology

Esophageal cancer is the 8th most common cancer worldwide, with an estimated 604,000 new cases and 544,000 deaths in 2020 [1]. About 85% of all esophageal cancers globally are squamous cell carcinomas (SCC), with the highest incidence rates in populations within South-Eastern and Central Asia, Eastern Africa, and South America. Although only 14% of all esophageal cancers are esophageal adenocarcinomas (EAC), it is the dominant subtype particularly in male individuals in 21 mostly developed countries, with an elevated burden seen in Northern and Western Europe, Oceania, and Northern America (Fig. 1) [1, 2]. In these regions, the continuing declines in incidence rates of SCC are offset by rapid increases in the incidence of EAC since the late 1980s, surpassing the rate of SCC since the early 1990s [3]. Over the past 40 years, the incidence of EAC has increased more than six-fold in Western countries. EAC rates are substantially higher in men than in women, with a male to female ratio of 8.5 in Northern America [4].

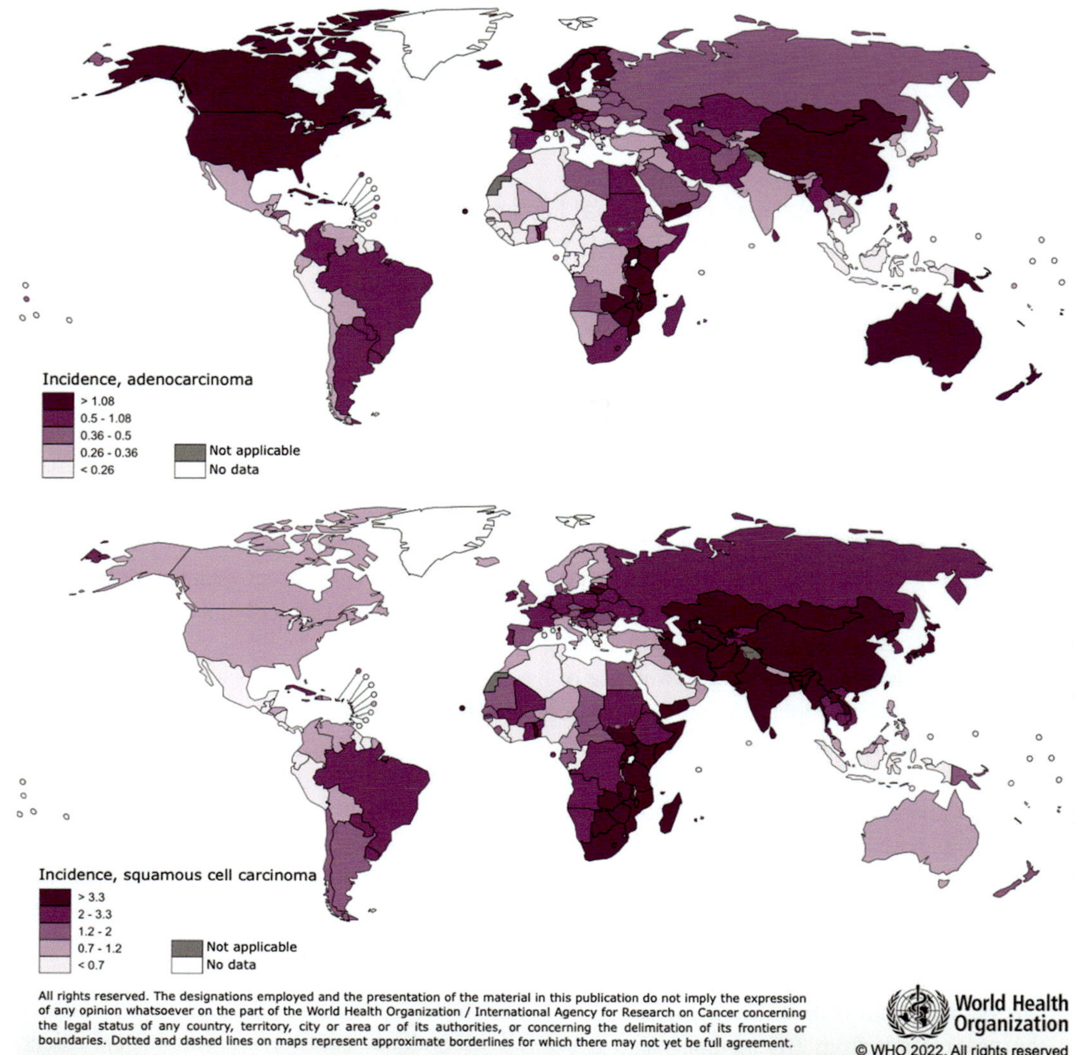

Fig. 1 Worldwide incidence of esophageal adenocarcinoma and squamous cell carcinoma in 2020 (age-adjusted according to the world standard population, per 100,000). Obtained with permission from the International Agency for Research on Cancer/World Health Organization (IARC/WHO)

The increase incidence of EAC has been attributed to the rising prevalence of obesity and gastroesophageal reflux disease (GERD). In fact, the strongest known risk factor for EAC is GERD, together with its more severe manifestation, Barrett's esophagus (BE). Although the real incidence of GERD is unknown due to its underdiagnosis, it is estimated that this disease affects around 20% of the adult population in the US, and its prevalence is increasing worldwide [5, 6]. It has been reported that high levels of urbanization may contribute to increased prevalence of GERD, such as in North America and Europe, compared to regions where rural areas predominate, such as in Asia, Latin America and the Caribbean [6]. While medical therapy has shown excellent results in controlling GERD symptoms, it has not averted the malignant complications of this disease. Increases in the prevalence of overweight and obesity have paralleled rises in the incidence of EAC in most countries. Although obesity also favors the development and severity of GERD, it has been shown to act as an independent risk factor for EAC, with a 52% increase in risk for every five units in body mass index [2, 4, 7, 8].

The total number of new EAC cases is expected to increase substantially. The United States and The United Kingdom are predicted to have the largest annual number of EAC diagnoses by 2030, with about 15,000 new cases in the US and about 8600 cases in The United Kingdom. By 2030, one in 100 men may be diagnosed with EAC in The United Kingdom and The Netherlands (Table 1). Globally, the estimated number of cases of esophageal cancer is expected to scale to 957,000 by 2040, with deaths uprising to 880,000 in the same year [1, 9].

Pathophysiology: From GERD to Barrett's Esophagus

About 10% of patients with GERD will develop BE. BE has been traditionally defined as the presence of at least 1 cm of metaplastic columnar epithelium that replaces the stratified squamous epithelium normally lining the distal esophagus. Currently, the presence of intestinal metaplasia (i.e. columnar epithelium with goblet cells) is also needed for the diagnosis of BE in the US [10]. The reason why intestinal metaplasia is mandated in the definition of BE is related to the higher risk of developing cancer in columnar epithelium containing goblet cells, as compared to columnar epithelium without intestinal metaplasia [11, 12].

The transformation of normal esophageal squamous mucosa into a simple columnar epithelium is thought to be due to the chronic injury produced by repeated reflux episodes. In fact, in patients with GERD, symptom duration has been shown to be a risk factor for the presence of BE. Lieberman [13] showed that compared with patients with GERD symptoms for less than one year, the odds ratio for BE in patients with GERD symptoms for 5 years was 3.0 and increased to 6.4 in patients with symptoms for more than 10 years. Interestingly, columnar mucosal metaplasia is also seen in the esophageal remnant in patients with a gastric pull-up following an esophagectomy, where the reflux of gastric contents into the residual esophagus is common because there is no lower esophageal sphincter. Oberg et al. [14] reported that 46.9% of patients had metaplastic columnar mucosa within their cervical esophagus following an esophagectomy, and the length of that metaplastic mucosa was significantly correlated with the degree of esophageal acid exposure. O'Riordan et al. [15] reported similar findings with 50% of patients developing columnar metaplasia in the remnant esophagus, with the duration of reflux being the most important factor influencing that transformation. Similarly, Dunn et al. [16] in a series of 134 patients, reported an

Table 1 Estimated number of new esophageal cancer cases in 2030, as compared to 2005 (Data extracted from "Predicting the Future Burden of Esophageal Cancer by Histological Subtype: International Trends in Incidence up to 2030. Am J Gastroenterol 2017")

Country	Population (million)		EAC		SCC		Total	
	2005	2030	2005	2030	2005	2030	2005	2030
Australia	19.9	28.5	537	1420	486	706	1023	2126
Canada	32.2	40.4	770	2043	462	379	1233	2423
France	61.1	68.0	1193	2863	3116	1930	4309	4793
Japan	126.8	120.1	670	1037	13,646	20,084	14,316	21,121
Netherlands	16.3	17.6	875	2652	514	714	1389	3366
UK	60.1	70.1	4278	8603	2708	3773	6986	12,376
US	277.5	316.8	8167	15,081	4736	4976	12,903	20,057

EAC Esophageal adenocarcinoma, *SCC* Squamous cell carcinoma, *UK* The United Kingdom, *US* The United States

incidence of 36% without any cases of progression to dysplasia.

The molecular pathway by which the normal squamous mucosa of the distal esophagus is transformed into a columnar mucosa remains uncertain. Tobey and colleagues [17] showed that acid damage of the esophageal epithelium produces dilated intercellular spaces, which in turn reduces the trans-epithelial resistance and increases trans-epithelial permeability. This change in permeability permits molecules as large as 20 kD to diffuse across the epithelium, exposing stem cells in the basal layer to refluxate. The intercellular acidification exposes the squamous basolateral membrane to acid, initiating a cascade of events leading to loss of cell osmoregulation, cell edema, and ultimately cell death [18]. Cell death is counterbalanced by tissue reparative processes, including restitution and replication. It is worth mentioning that during the normal growth process of the embryo, the esophageal cells undergo a columnar to squamous transition under the influence of a combination of active prosquamous and inactivated procolumnar homeobox genes. The cellular phenotype may reverse if the opposite set of cell patterning genes is reactivated. An acidic milieu, combined with other components of refluxate, may induce phenotypic transformation of squamous cells into columnar mucosal cells. The reason why pluripotent esophageal stem cells turn into columnar cells in this "acid environment" may be related to the better adaptability of this epithelium due to its acid resistance. Nevertheless, the origin of BE remains obscure. There are several hypotheses regarding the origin of stem cells that will give rise to BE [18–20]:

(1) Migration and differentiation of stem cells from the gastric cardia.
(2) Differentiation of stem cells residing in the crypts of the esophageal mucosal glands.
(3) Migration of stem cells from the bone marrow (circulating stem cells that can hone in to areas of injury to repair damaged tissue).

While the transition between squamous and columnar epithelium likely occurs within a few years, the development of intestinal metaplasia may take over 5–10 years [21]. Once the columnar epithelium is established, two possible pathways are observed. The first one, "*gastric differentiation*", implies the formation of parietal cells within glands and may represent a favorable change, as this mucosa is not thought to be premalignant. The second one, "*intestinal differentiation*", induces the expression of intestinalizing genes, causing the formation of goblet cells within the columnar epithelium. The development of intestinal metaplasia is considered a detrimental change because this mucosa is capable of further progression to epithelial dysplasia and adenocarcinoma.

The specific cellular event(s) that induce the "intestinalization" of the columnar epithelium is unknown. However, it is likely to occur in response to multiple noxious luminal contents rather than to acid reflux only. In fact, previous studies have demonstrated the association between BE and the exposure of a mixture of acid and bile salts on the esophagus [22–24]. The role of refluxed bile in the development of intestinal metaplasia was suggested by Oberg et al. [25] as patients with intestinal metaplasia had similar esophageal acid exposure to those with GERD and no BE, but significantly higher frequency of abnormal bilirubin exposure. It has been hypothesized that in a weakly acidic environment (pH 3–5), certain bile acids become non-ionized and are able to cross the cell membrane. Once inside the cell (pH 7) they become ionized and remain trapped causing mitochondrial injury, cellular toxicity, and mutagenesis [26]. The molecular mechanism by which bile acids promote the development of goblet cells may be related to the activation of the Caudal-related homeobox 2 (Cdx2) promoter via nuclear factor kappa B (NF-κB) with the consequent production of Cdx2 protein in esophageal immature keratinocytes, resulting in the production of MUC2 (intestinal-type protein found in Barrett's metaplasia) [27]. Further, bile acids have shown to enhance cytoplasmic expression of the signaling ligand Delta-like 1 (Dll1) which facilitates the intestinal metaplasia in conjunction with Cdx2 expression [28]. It was found that COX-2, an enzyme that plays a major role in inflammatory responses, has a substantially higher expression in human BE tissues than that in adjacent squamous cells and control tissues. Also, its presence was considerably higher in EAC tissues. Inhibition of NF-κB in esophageal squamous cells inhibits cell proliferation, followed by decreased COX-2 expression. Inhibition of NF-κB expression in EAC cells reduces the expression of COX-2 and CDX-2, and improves apoptosis of EAC cells. This suggests that COX-2 may be involved in the development of BE [29].

Pathophysiology: From Barrett's Esophagus to Esophageal Adenocarcinoma

BE is a premalignant mucosa with increased proliferation rates and decreased apoptosis rates compared to normal epithelium [30]. In fact, it is the only known precursor of EAC. However, only a small percentage of patients with BE will develop cancer, and more than 90% of patients with diagnosis of EAC have no prior history of BE [31, 32]. The question as to why some cases of BE progress to EAC and some do not remains unanswered. Currently, the presence and grading of dysplasia is the most important predictive factor for the development of adenocarcinoma. Known risk factors for development of dysplasia in BE include: increasing length of BE, advancing age, central obesity, tobacco usage, lack of nonsteroidal anti-inflammatory agent use, lack of proton-pump inhibitors (PPI) use, and lack of statin use [11]. Recently, caffeine intake and presence of colonic adenomas have been also described as risk factors for progression of BE to high grade dysplasia [33].

Gopal and colleagues [34] showed that the prevalence of dysplasia was strongly associated with age and length of BE. Patients with BE without dysplasia were younger than those with dysplasia (62 ± 0.8 years vs. 67 ± 1.7 years, p = 0.02), and the risk of dysplasia increased by 3.3%/year of age. Patients with BE length ≥ 3 cm also had a significantly greater prevalence of dysplasia compared to length < 3 cm (23% vs 9%, p = 0.0001), and the risk of dysplasia increased by 14% per cm of increased length. Hampel et al. [35] reported that obesity was associated with a significant increase of GERD complications and EAC. Interestingly, Singh et al. [36] found that, compared with patients with normal body habitus, patients with central adiposity had a higher risk of BE, even after adjusting for body mass index and presence of GERD, suggesting a reflux-independent association between truncal obesity and BE. Added to this, central adiposity was associated with higher risk of adenocarcinoma (OR 2.5, 95% CI 1.54–4.06) compared with normal body habitus. The relationship between BE and cigarette smoking was reported by Andrici and colleagues [37] who found that having ever smoked was associated with an increased risk of BE compared with non-GERD controls but not when compared with patients with chronic GERD, suggesting that the increased risk of BE associated with tobacco usage may be due to the increased incidence of GERD in cigarette smokers.

The presence of colonic adenomas and caffeine intake have been recently described as risk factors for high grade dysplasia in patients with BE. This could be explained by common genetic alterations between BE, EAC, colonic adenomas, and colonic adenocarcinomas such as a higher expression of COX-2 and other inflammation-mediators that can induce dysplasia. Additionally, the presence of a colonic adenoma may represent a genetic predisposition to the development of dysplasia. Caffeine intake stimulates gastric acid secretion and relaxes the LES, which ultimately aggravates GERD [33].

Some medications have shown to reduce the risk of progression to dysplasia or esophageal cancer in patients with BE. Singh and colleagues described that PPI use was associated with a substantial reduction in risk of high-grade dysplasia and/or esophageal adenocarcinoma in patients with BE (OR 0.29 95% CI 0.12–0.79) [38]. There was also a trend towards a dose–response relationship with PPI use for >2–3 years. On the contrary, a population-based study from Sweden showed an increased risk of esophageal carcinoma among PPI users, reporting that 5.4% of the esophageal cancer in the population could be attributed to PPI use. This could correlate with a disruption in the gastrointestinal microbiome, bacterial colonization and increase production of nitrosamines, which are all well-known gastric (and probably esophageal) cancer risk factors [39]. Albeit these findings, the relationship between esophageal cancer and PPIs intake remains controversial and needs further investigation.

Another meta-analysis reported that aspirin use also reduced the risk of high-grade dysplasia/adenocarcinoma, as well as non-aspirin cyclooxygenase inhibitors in patients with BE [40]. The chemopreventive effect seemed to be independent of duration of therapy. Finally, statin usage was also associated with a significant (41%) decrease in the risk of EAC within patients with BE [41]. Alexandre et al. also reported a meaningful reduction in esophageal cancer-specific mortality and all-cause mortality (39% and 37%, respectively) in patients with EAC taking statins [42]. In line with these findings, a multicenter retrospective study including 308,793 patients showed that the use of COX-2 inhibitors, statins, metformin, and PPIs may help preventing EAC [43].

There are four categories to stratify the dysplastic process: (1) no dysplasia; (2) indefinite for dysplasia; (3) low-grade dysplasia; (4) high-grade dysplasia. The development of EAC is characterized by the progression from BE metaplasia to dysplasia, and ultimately invasive adenocarcinoma (Fig. 2). Patients with non-dysplastic BE have very low risk for malignant progression and a meta-analysis of 24 studies and 2694 patients reported that the pooled annual incidence of adenocarcinoma was 0.2–0.5%. For patients with low-grade dysplasia, they described a pooled annual incidence of 0.5% for adenocarcinoma (95% CI 0.3–0.8). The annual incidence of either EAC or high-grade dysplasia was 1.73% (95% CI, 0.99–2.47%) [44]. Patients with high-grade dysplasia present an annual incidence of adenocarcinoma of 7% (95% CI 5–8) [10, 45, 46].

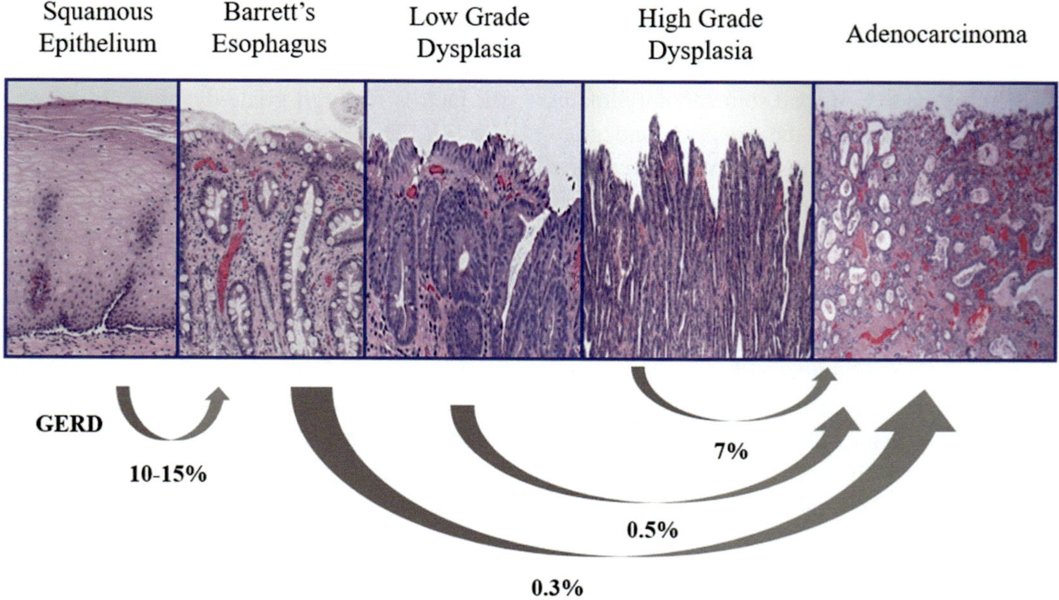

Fig. 2 Pathological progression from normal esophageal squamous epithelium to adenocarcinoma

Conclusions

The increase incidence of EAC has been attributed to the rising prevalence of obesity and GERD. The latter is considered the strongest risk factor for EAC, together with its more severe manifestation, Barrett's esophagus. This metaplastic lesion due to chronic injury produced by repeated reflux episodes involves genetic mutations that can lead to a malignant transformation. Therefore, the pathophysiology of EAC can be depicted by the progression from Barrett's esophagus metaplasia to dysplasia, and ultimately invasive adenocarcinoma.

References

1. Morgan E, Soerjomataram I, Rumgay H, et al. The global landscape of esophageal squamous cell carcinoma and esophageal adenocarcinoma incidence and mortality in 2020 and projections to 2040: new estimates from GLOBOCAN 2020. Gastroenterology. 2022;163(3):649-658.e2.
2. Huang J, Koulaouzidis A, Marlicz W, et al. Global burden, risk factors, and trends of esophageal cancer: an analysis of cancer registries from 48 countries. Cancers. 2021;13(1):141.
3. Devesa SS, Blot WJ, Fraumeni JF Jr. Changing patterns in the incidence of esophageal and gastric carcinoma in the United States. Cancer. 1998;83(10):2049–53.
4. Coleman HG, Xie SH, Lagergren J. The epidemiology of esophageal adenocarcinoma. Gastroenterology. 2018;154(2):390–405.
5. Nirwan JS, Hasan SS, Babar ZUD, et al. Global prevalence and risk factors of gastro-oesophageal reflux disease (GORD): systematic review with meta-analysis. Sci Rep. 2020;10:5814.
6. El-Serag HN, Sweet S, Winchester CC, et al. Update on the epidemiology of gastro-esophageal reflux disease: a systematic review. Gut. 2014;63:871–80.
7. Schlottmann F, Dreifuss NH, Patti MG. Obesity and esophageal cancer: GERD, Barrett´s esophagus, and molecular carcinogenic pathways. Expert Rev Gastroenterol Hepatol. 2020;14(6):425–33.
8. Bhaskaran K, Douglas I, Forbes H. Body-mass index and risk of 22 specific cancers: a population-based cohort study of 5·24 million UK adults. Lancet. 2014;384(9945):755–65.
9. Arnold M, Laversanne M, Brown LM, et al. Predicting the future burden of esophageal cancer by histological subtype: international trends in incidence up to 2030. Am J Gastroenterol. 2017;112(8):1247–55.
10. Shaheen NJ, Falk GW, Iyer PG, et al. Diagnosis and management of Barrett's esophagus: an updated ACG guideline. Am J Gastroenterol. 2022;117(4):559–87.
11. Bhat S, Coleman HG, Yousef F, et al. Risk of malignant progression in Barrett's esophagus patients: results from a large population-based study. J Natl Cancer Inst. 2011;103:1049–57.
12. Bandla S, Peters JH, Ruff D, et al. Comparison of cancer-associated genetic abnormalities in columnar-lined esophagus tissues with and without goblet cells. Ann Surg. 2014;260:72–80.
13. Lieberman DA. Risk factors for Barrett's esophagus in community-based practice. Am J Gastroenterol. 1997;92:1293–7.
14. Oberg S, Johansson J, Wenner J, et al. Metaplastic columnar mucosa in the cervical esophagus after esophagectomy. Ann Surg. 2002;235:338–45.
15. O'Riordan JM, Tucker ON, Byrne PJ, et al. Factors influencing the development of Barrett's epithelium in the esophageal remnant post-esophagectomy. Am J Gastroenterol. 2004;99:205–11.
16. Dunn LJ, Burt AD, Hayes N, et al. Columnar metaplasia in the esophageal remnant after esophagectomy: a common occurrence and a valuable insight into the development of barrett esophagus. Ann Surg. 2016;264(6):1016–21.
17. Tobey NA, Hosseini SS, Argote CM, et al. Dilated intercellular spaces and shunt permeability in nonerosive acid-damaged esophageal epithelium. Am J Gastroenterol. 2004;99:13–22.
18. Tobey NA, Orlando RC. Mechanisms of acid injury to rabbit esophageal epithelium. Role of basolateral cell membrane acidification. Gastroenterology. 1991;101:1220–8.
19. Souza RF, Krishnan K, Spechler SJ. Acid, bile, and CDX: the ABCs of making Barrett's metaplasia. Am J Gastrointest Liver Physiol. 2008;295:211–8.
20. Sarosi G, Brown G, Jaiswal K, et al. Bone marrow progenitor cells contribute to esophageal regeneration and metaplasia in a rat model of Barrett's esophagus. Dis Esophagus. 2008;21(1):43–50.
21. Nakagawa H, Whelan K, Lynch JP. Mechanisms of Barrett's oesophagus: intestinal differentiation, stem cells, and tissue models. Best Pract Res Clin Gastroenterol. 2015;29(1):3–16.
22. DeMeester SR, DeMeester TR. Columnar mucosa and intestinal metaplasia of the esophagus: fifty years of controversy. Ann Surg. 2000;231:303–21.
23. Oberg S, Ritter MP, Crookes PF, et al. Gastroesophageal reflux disease and mucosal injury with emphasis on short-segment Barrett's esophagus and duodenogastroesophageal reflux. J Gastrointest Surg. 1998;2:547–53.
24. Fein M, Ireland AP, Ritter MP, et al. Duodenogastric reflux potentiates the injurious effects of gastroesophageal reflux. J Gastrointest Surg. 1997;1:27–32.
25. Kauer WK, Peters JH, DeMeester TR, et al. Mixed reflux of gastric and duodenal juices is more

harmful to the esophagus than gastric juice alone. The need for surgical therapy re-emphasized. Ann Surg. 1995;222:525–531.
26. Oberg S, Peters JH, DeMeester TR, et al. Determinants of intestinal metaplasia within the columnar-lined esophagus. Arch Surg. 2000;135(6):651–5.
27. Theisen J, Peters JH, Fein M, et al. The mutagenic potential of duodenoesophageal reflux. Ann Surg. 2005;241:63–8.
28. Kazumori H, Ishihara S, Rumi MA, et al. Bile acids directly augment caudal related homeobox gene Cdx2 expression in oesophageal keratinocytes in Barrett's epithelium. Gut. 2006;55:16–25.
29. Tamagawa Y, Ishimura N, Uno G, et al. Bile acids induce Delta-like 1 expression via Cdx2-dependent pathway in the development of Barrett's esophagus. Lab Invest. 2016;96(3):325–37.
30. Jiangang S, Nayoung K, HongfangW, et al. COX-2 strengthens the effects of acid and bile salts on human esophageal cells and Barrett esophageal cells. BMC Mol Cell Biol. 2022;23(1):19.
31. Reid BJ, Sanchez CA, Blount PL, et al. Barrett's esophagus: cell cycle abnormalities in advancing stages of neoplastic progression. Gastroenterology. 1993;105:119–29.
32. Hvid-Jensen F, Pedersen L, Drewes AM, et al. Incidence of adenocarcinoma among patients with Barrett's esophagus. N Engl J Med. 2011;365:1375–83.
33. Dulai GS, Guha S, Kahn KL, et al. Preoperative prevalence of Barrett's esophagus in esophageal adenocarcinoma: a systematic review. Gastroenterology. 2002;122:26–33.
34. Kambhampati S, Tieu AH, Luber B, et al. Risk factors for progression of barrett's esophagus to high grade dysplasia and esophageal adenocarcinoma. Sci Rep. 2020;10:4899.
35. Gopal DV, Lieberman DA, Magaret N, et al. Risk factors for dysplasia in patients with Barrett's esophagus (BE): results from a multicenter consortium. Dig Dis Sci. 2003;48:1537–41.
36. Hampel H, Abraham NS, El-Serag HB. Meta-analysis: obesity and the risk for gastroesophageal reflux disease and its complications. Ann Intern Med. 2005;143:199–211.
37. Singh S, Sharma AN, Murad MH, et al. Central adiposity is associated with increased risk of esophageal inflammation, metaplasia, and adenocarcinoma: a systematic review and meta-analysis. Clin Gastroenterol Hepatol. 2013;11:1399–412.
38. Andrici J, Cox MR, Eslick GD. Cigarette smoking and the risk of Barrett's esophagus: a systematic review and meta-analysis. J Gastroenterol Hepatol. 2013;28:1258–73.
39. Singh S, Garg SK, Singh PP, et al. Acid-suppressive medications and risk of oesophageal adenocarcinoma in patients with Barrett's oesophagus: a systematic review and meta-analysis. Gut. 2014;63:1229–37.
40. Brusselaers N, Engstrand L, Lagergren J. Maintenance proton pump inhibition therapy and risk of oesophageal cancer. Cancer Epidemiol. 2018;53:172–177.
41. Zhang S, Zhang XQ, Ding XW, et al. Cyclooxygenase inhibitors use is associated with reduced risk of esophageal adenocarcinoma in patients with Barrett's esophagus: a meta-analysis. Br J Cancer. 2014;110:2378–88.
42. Singh S, Singh AG, Singh PP, et al. Statins are associated with reduced risk of esophageal cancer, particularly in patients with Barrett's esophagus: a systematic review and meta-analysis. Clin Gastroenterol Hepatol. 2013;11:620–9.
43. Alexandre L, Clark AB, Bhutta HY, et al. association between statin use after diagnosis of esophageal cancer and survival: a population-based cohort study. Gastroenterology. 2016;S0016508516000032.
44. Arai J, Niikura R, Hayakawa Y, et al. Chemoprevention of oesophageal squamous-cell carcinoma and adenocarcinoma: a multicentre retrospective cohort study. Digestion. 2022;103(3):192–204.
45. Singh S, Manickam P, Amin AV, et al. Incidence of esophageal adenocarcinoma in Barrett's esophagus with low-grade dysplasia: a systematic review and meta-analysis. Gastrointest Endosc. 2014;79:897–909.
46. Rastogi A, Puli S, El-Serag HB, et al. Incidence of esophageal adenocarcinoma in patients with Barrett's esophagus and high-grade dysplasia: a meta-analysis. Gastrointest Endosc. 2008;67:394–8.

Endoscopy and Endoscopic Ultrasound for Esophageal Cancer

Stephen Gowing

Abstract

Esophageal cancer is a serious malignancy and cause of cancer death worldwide with an ever-increasing incidence. The initial management and staging of esophageal cancer are crucial to determine optimal treatment and potential for cure. Optical endoscopy and endoscopic ultrasound (EUS) are key components of this, enabling tissue diagnosis, tumor localization, tumor characterization, and locoregional staging. Endoscopy is also employed in the treatment of dysplastic Barrett's esophagus and the resection of early-stage esophageal malignancies. Additionally, endoscopy can be utilized as a bridge for enteral nutrition as well as for palliation for unresectable disease.

Keywords

Esophageal cancer · Endoscopy · Endoscopic ultrasound · Barrett's esophagus · Endoscopic submucosal resection

S. Gowing (✉)
Thoracic Surgery, The University of Manitoba, Manitoba, Canada
e-mail: stephendonaldgowing@gmail.com

Introduction

Esophageal cancer remains one of the major causes of cancer death worldwide and its incidence is continuing to increase. While squamous cell carcinoma (SCC) remains a common diagnosis in Asia, in North America and Europe esophageal adenocarcinoma (EAC) remains the most common presentation [1]. Treatment of this aggressive cancer in its most common presentation requires multimodality treatments including chemotherapy, potential radiation therapy and esophagectomy. Tissue diagnosis, tumor location and clinical stage are paramount in determining potential therapies and often rely on an initial upper gastrointestinal endoscopy.

Initial Endoscopic Assessment for Esophageal Malignancy

The initial diagnosis and treatment of esophageal cancer most often begins with a traditional optical endoscopic assessment of the esophagus in response to patient clinical concerns such as dysphagia, odynophagia, esophageal stasis, regurgitation, weight loss, anemia, gastrointestinal bleeding, esophageal food bolus impaction or symptoms as benign as gastroesophageal reflux disease. Alternatively, upper gastrointestinal contrast swallow examination under fluoroscopy or computed tomography (CT) scanning may point towards this diagnosis and direct the clinician to perform endoscopy.

Initial assessment with an optical gastroscope begins with examining the entirety of the upper gastrointestinal tract from the upper esophageal sphincter/cricopharyngeal muscle passing into the esophagus, stomach and ending in the second or third stage of the duodenum. Retroflexion is performed in the stomach to assess the gastrointestinal junction for proximal gastric or distal esophageal tumors as well as hiatus hernia. Care must be taken on withdrawing the endoscope to examine for the presence of Zenker's diverticulum and the rare potential for esophageal cancer within.

Specific endoscopic findings alert the clinician to the potential for esophageal malignancy and will direct further sampling or investigations. These include but are not necessarily limited to: Barrett's esophagus, endoluminal nodules or masses, and mucosal or submucosal strictures that may prevent or hinder passage of the endoscope requiring esophageal dilation or stenting. Submucosal bulging or masses can alert to metastatic adenopathy or submucosal tumors to be further assessed with endoscopic ultrasound (EUS) or cross-sectional imaging.

When esophageal endoluminal masses suggestive of cancer are identified, the proximal and distal aspect of the lesion from the incisors are noted as well as the circumferential extent of the lesion. For lesions present close to the gastroesophageal junction (GEJ) the Siewert-Stein classification of GEJ adenocarcinomas (commonly denoted as Siewert) is additionally noted as follows:

- Siewert 1: epicentre 1–5 cm above the GEJ
- Siewert 2: epicenter up to 1 cm above and 2 cm below the GEJ
- Siewert 3: epicenter 2–5 cm below the GEJ

Siewert 3 lesions are most often referred to as gastric cancers and may treated with esophagectomy or total gastrectomy depending on patient and tumor characteristics [2].

High definition white light endoscopy (WLE) with targeted forceps biopsy remains the standard approach for diagnosis of mucosal based esophageal malignancies. Care must be taken to sample tissue from multiple areas of tumor to avoid non-diagnostic results in the event of necrotic tumor specimen. EUS linear fine needle aspiration (FNA) or core needle biopsy can be helpful as adjunct in assisting with tissue diagnosis sampling nodal metastases or through biopsying submucosal lesions. Tunneling deep endoscopic forceps biopsy in a bite-on-bite fashion with endoscopic clip mucosal closure remains an additional biopsy technique for submucosal lesions when linear EUS is not available or possible [3].

Barrett's Esophagus, Dysplasia and Early-Stage Esophageal Cancers

Barrett's esophagus (BE) (also known as intestinal metaplasia of the esophagus) is the conversion of the pale salmon pink squamous esophagus mucosa to a reddish columnar epithelium in response to chronic acid exposure to the esophagus. Unfortunately, these changes are known to predispose patients to the development of dysplastic Barrett's epithelium and eventually EAC. Thankfully, the incidence of progression of Barrett's epithelium to cancer remains low at a rate of 0.33% per year. However, the diagnosis of BE necessitates lifelong surveillance or the eradication of BE in event of the development of dysplasia or cancer [4]. Newer research has demonstrated that patients with higher aneuploidy (genomic copy number) in their Barrett's epithelium are at higher risk for progression to dysplasia and malignancy [5].

Barrett's esophagus is classified endoscopically according to the Prague Classification [6] denoting the circumferential extent (C) and the maximal extent (M) of BE. This measurement commences from the top of the gastric mucosal folds to denote the gastroesophageal junction. For example: Barrett's epithelium that is 4 cm in circumferential extent and 6 cm in maximal length (from non-circumferential tongues of Barrett's) would be classified as C4M6.

BE greater than or equal to 3 cm in length is referred to as long segment BE and has an increased risk of harboring dysplasia and malignancy. Short segment BE is consequently classified as less than 3 cm in maximal length [7].

High Definition WLE with 4 quadrant biopsies every one to two cm, according to the Seattle protocol [8], remains the standard method of assessment for dysplasia in Barrett's epithelium and for biopsy of endoluminal masses. Current recommendations for non-dysplastic BE surveillance are once every 3 years [9].

Optical Chromoendoscopy: Optical Chromoendoscopy works based on the principles of longer wavelengths of light such as red having deeper tissue penetration than shorter wavelengths of light such as green (540–560 nm) and blue (440–460 nm). Narrow-band imaging (NBI) utilizes green and blue wavelengths of light to improve visualization of mucosal patterns of capillaries and veins. NBI is easy to switch to and from WLE examination modes and does not require special staining for visualization. Mucosal bleeding, however, can quickly overwhelm NBI viewing models due to hemoglobin preferentially absorbing blue light [10]. Due to it's ease of use optical chromoendoscopy is strongly recommended to be combined with WLE and Seattle protocol biopsies for BE surveillance. Additionally, it is strongly beneficial for planning resection margins for endoscopic resection [9]. NBI classification schema exist for Barrett's esophagus indicating the presence of dysplasia and malignancy based on the presence or absence of mucosal pits and regularity/irregularity of vasculature. Similarly, classification schema exist for early esophageal squamous cell carcinoma regarding degree of vascular irregularity and presence/absence of vascular loop-like formations [11].

Chemical Chromoendoscopy: The addition of chemical washes to the esophagus and Barrett's epithelium can optically enhance malignant and dysplastic lesions to aid in their detection. Various washes and stains have been utilized in the detection of foregut malignancy including methylene blue (now replaced primarily by NBI techniques), crystal violet [12], Lugol's iodine and acetic acid [13].

The diagnosis of Barrett's esophagus as well as the detection of dysplasia and intramucosal adenocarcinoma in Barrett's epithelium are enhanced using a dilute acetic acid solution. A 2–3% acetic acid solution is sprayed onto the esophageal epithelium leading to acetowhitening of Barrett's epithelium. Combined with magnification endoscopy villous patterns of intestinal metaplasia characteristic of BE can be visualized versus the reticular mucosa characteristic of cardiac epithelium. With time the acetowhitening effect is lost and Barrett's epithelium returns to its characteristic reddish colour [14]. Importantly, dysplastic BE and intramucosal carcinoma demonstrates early loss of acetowhitening (LAW) compared to non-dysplastic BE resulting in the transient appearance of reddish lesions within whitened Barrett's epithelium allowing for the detection of dysplasia and malignancy [13].

For the detection of esophageal SCC, a dilute 2–3% Lugol's iodine solution can be used. Lugol's iodine stains normal mucosa brown or green–brown. Conditions that deplete cellular glycogen such as dysplasia and early squamous malignancy limit's Lugol's staining resulting in whitish appearing lesions. Lugol's staining is contraindicated in patients with iodine allergy [15].

Confocal Laser Endomicroscopy: Confocal laser endomicroscopy utilizes a catheter-based laser fluorescent probe allowing for microscopic real time imaging of live patient mucosal tissues. This technique allows for imaging for mucosal tissue only, unable to visualize the submucosa and deeper layers. Cellular architecture of squamous and Barrett's epithelium can be visualized allowing for the detection of mucosal dysplasia and malignancy. Currently, the widespread application of this emerging technology is limited by cost and expertise is only present in ultra-specialized centers [16].

Endoscopic Treatment of Dysplastic Barrett's Esophagus

In the event of the development of dysplastic BE, (either low-grade dysplasia (LGD) or high-grade dysplasia (HGD)) eradication of BE is recommended. An alternative to eradication of Barrett's remains intensive surveillance, elected for most commonly in cases of LGD where access to endoscopic eradication therapies such as radiofrequency ablation (RFA) are constrained by cost and reserved for HGD BE. For LGD BE, surveillance endoscopy once a year is commonly employed when endoscopic Barrett's eradication is not available [9].

Currently, BE with LGD or HGD is routinely treated with RFA. Any nodular Barrett's mucosa is excised by cap-based endoscopic mucosal resection (EMR) prior to RFA treatment to rule out invasive malignancy. Alternatively, short segment BE can also be treated with multiple EMRs, albeit with a higher rate of esophageal stricture post-resection [17]. Photodynamic therapy (PDT) and cryotherapy are alternative treatments for dysplastic BE. PDT has largely been abandoned due to high rates of esophageal stricture formation and the need for patients to take photosensitizing agents [18]. Cryotherapy appears to be less efficacious than RFA for eradicating dysplastic BE, however remains an alternative therapy when RFA fails or is contraindicated [19].

Extensive nodular HGD BE where suspicion of intramucosal carcinoma (IMC) is high is becoming more commonly treated with endoscopic submucosal dissection (ESD). With ESD the BE of concern is resected en bloc as a single specimen with dissection down to the level of the muscularis propria. This is accomplished through injection of a methylene blue saline solution into the submucosal space, thereby separating the mucosa from submucosa, allowing for resection via needle knife. Most commonly the high-risk areas of BE are excised with ESD followed by RFA treatment of the residual Barrett's epithelium [20, 21]. Circumferential ESD is performed in selected cases, often for salvage therapy, however significant stricture formation

is to be expected and managed afterwards [22, 23]. Although less commonly performed today, esophagectomy can still be performed for operable patients with dysplastic BE where endoscopic management has failed or is not available.

Endoscopic Resection of Early-Stage Esophageal Cancer

Early-stage esophageal cancers localized to the mucosa and upper submucosal space can be treated with endoscopic resection. Once esophageal cancers invade the submucosal space, they access the esophageal lymphatics, and are at significantly higher risk for lymph node metastases [24]. EMR remains an option for small mucosal only lesions less than 2 cm, however for larger lesions ESD is favored due its ability to obtain en bloc resection as well as deeper resection margins than EMR. ESD is also superior for resection of lesions that span across the GEJ (Fig. 1). Piecemeal EMR for lesions larger than 2 cm can be performed, however caution must be taken due to the inability to determine accurate lateral margins, as well as higher rates of R1 resection [20].

Determination of the suitability of solid esophageal lesions for endoscopic resection is dependent on tumor factors, clinical staging, as well as patient factors including operability. Various tumor characteristics including tumor size, differentiation, presence of lymphovascular invasion and depth of invasion are key for determination of the risks of lymph node metastasis [24]. Submucosal invasion is divided into three levels (SM1, SM2 and SM3) with increasing risk of lymph node metastases the deeper the tumor invades [25]. For comparable lesions based on size, depth of invasion, and degree of differentiation, SCC is noted to have much higher rates of lymph node metastasis compared to adenocarcinoma [24, 26]. Expert analysis of ESD specimens by specialized pathologists is critical as for patients with elevated risk of lymph node metastasis based on final pathology endoscopic resection alone is likely not sufficient for cure of disease.

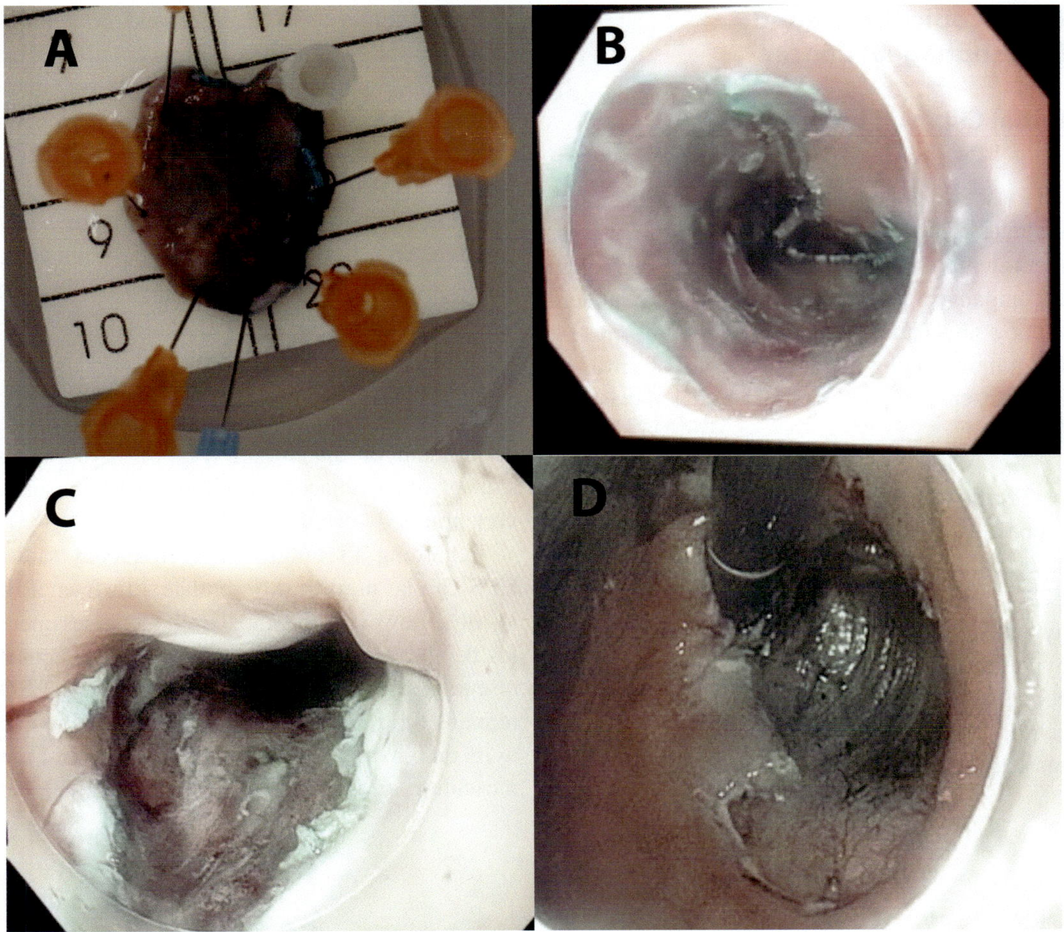

Fig. 1 Endoscopic Submucosal Dissection for Esophageal Cancer. (A, B) Pinned resection specimen (A) and resection bed (B) for T1a esophageal adenocarcinoma. (C, D) Resection bed for T1b Adenocarcinoma of the distal esophagus and gastroesophageal junction

Clinical staging investigations including CT scan, PET scan and EUS are preferred for solid luminal tumors prior to ESD whenever possible, however ultimately the determination of the risk of systemic metastasis is determined by the final pathology of the resection specimen. ESD functions as an excellent excisional biopsy and prognosticator in this regard. We often reserve staging investigations for patients with larger solid lesions whereas smaller superficial lesions are often selected for upfront ESD.

Operable patients who are found to be at elevated risk for lymph node metastasis following ESD routinely proceed with esophagectomy to excise the esophagus and surrounding lymphatic tissues. In our centre, despite elevated risks of lymph node metastases on final pathology, patients who are not otherwise operative candidates are often considered for adjuvant therapies including chemotherapy, radiation therapy and immunotherapy following ESD. Furthermore, patients with residual local mucosal disease only following induction chemotherapy or chemoradiation, and who are not found to be candidates for esophagectomy, may be considered for ESD to resect their residual mucosal disease.

Endoscopic Ultrasound for Esophageal Cancer

Initial Clinical Staging

The assessment of esophageal cancers often includes EUS for clinical staging. Initial assessment with radial endoscopic ultrasound often accompanies standard esophagogastroduodenoscopy and can provide important information for tumor staging including depth of invasion and presence of locoregional nodal metastases (Table 1).

Tumor (T) Stage: Using a 360° radial EUS scope depth of tumor invasion can be directly assessed. The layers of the esophagus on radial EUS are visualized as follows: mucosa (first hyperechoic layer), muscularis mucosa (first hypoechoic layer), submucosa (second hyperechoic layer), muscularis propria (second hypoechoic layer), adventitia (esophageal) or serosa (gastric) (third hyperechoic layer) (Fig. 2).

Solid tumors are visualized and their interface with the various mucosal layers allows for sonographic determination of depth of invasion [27]. Depth of esophageal tumor invasion is referred to as T-stage and is described as followsaccording to the TNM 8th edition: Tis—carcinoma in situ, T1a—mucosal lesion only invading lamina propria or muscularis mucosa, T1b—invading submucosa, T2—invading into but not through muscularis (Fig. 3), T3—invading through muscularis propria into adventitia (Fig. 4), T4—invasion of adjacent structures (T4a—invasion of azygous vein, pericardium, peritoneum or diaphragm (Fig. 5), T4b—invasion of other adjacent structures such as aorta, vertebral body or airway) [28].

Regarding T1 tumors, high frequency radial EUS can be used to differentiate T1a from T1b lesions, however, the most reliable assessment for depth of invasion remains complete mucosal resection with EMR or ESD. In this regard, ESD remains the superior determinant of T stage due to its en bloc dissection down to the level of the muscularis propria. EUS remains more reliable

Table 1 Esophageal TNM staging 8th edition [28]

Tumor invasion (T)	
T0	No evidence of primary tumor
Tis	Carcinoma in situ
T1a	Tumor invades the mucosa (lamina propria or muscularis mucosa)
T1b	Tumor invades the submucosa
T2	Tumor invades into but not through muscularis propria
T3	Tumor invades adventitia
T4a	Tumor invades pericardium, diaphragm, pleura, peritoneum, azygous vein
T4b	Tumor invades aorta, vertebral body, trachea
Lymph Nodes (N)	
N0	No lymph nodes metastases
N1	Metastases in ≤ 2 lymph nodes
N2	Metastases in 3–6 lymph nodes
N3	Metastases in ≥ 7 lymph nodes
Distant Metastases (M)	
M0	No evidence of distant metastases
M1	Distant metastases

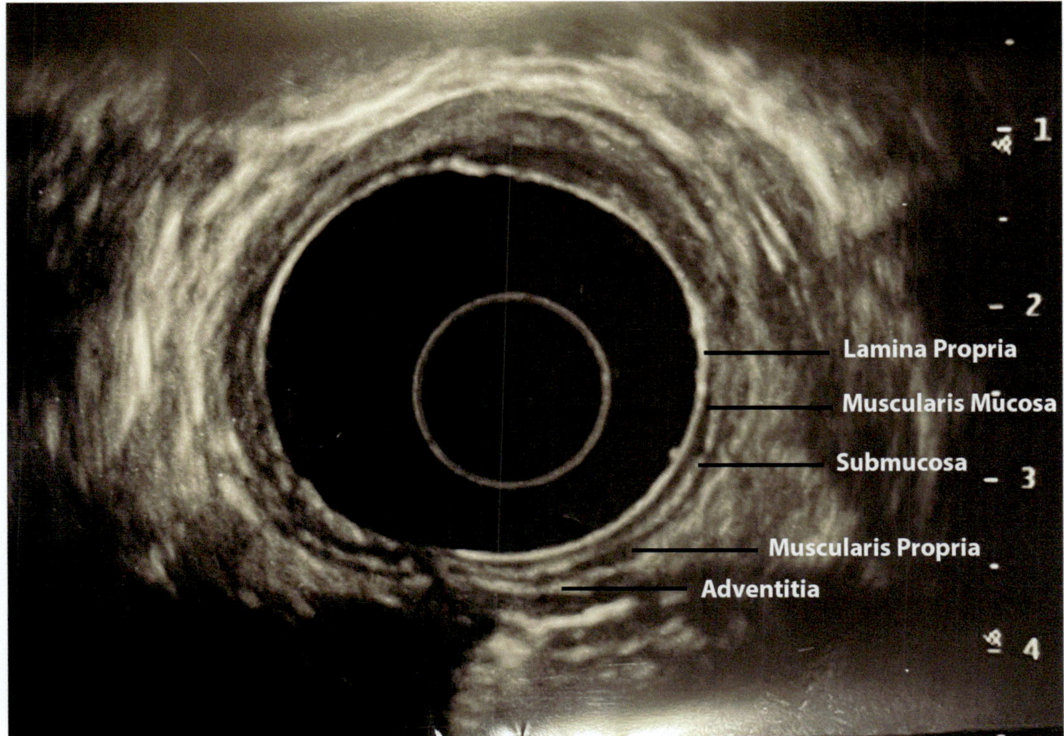

Fig. 2 Sonographic layers of the esophageal wall

for differentiation between numerical T stages (T1 from T2, T2 from T3, T3 from T4) [27].

Nodal (N) Staging: EUS allows for the assessment of locoregional lymph nodes for nodal staging. For esophageal cancer lymph nodal basins in the periesophageal, subcarinal, perigastric, celiac, splenic artery and hilum, left gastric artery and common hepatic artery are visualized and assessed for potential metastatic involvement. Sonographic features of nodal metastases include: size greater than 1 cm, round shape, hypoechoic, discrete borders, and absence of lymphatic hilar structures or intranodal vessels [27]. TNM 8th edition nodal staging is described as: NX—lymph node status cannot be assessed, N0—no nodal metastases, N1—metastases in ≤2 regional nodes, N2—metastases in 3–6 regional nodes, N3—metastases in ≥7 regional nodes [28] (Fig. 6).

Metastasis (M) Staging: EUS can occasionally be utilized to provide information regarding local metastatic disease to solid organs, predominantly the liver. However, this information is most commonly obtained from the complementary staging imaging investigations of CT and PET imaging [29].

Accuracy of EUS

The overall accuracy of radial EUS for T and N staging of esophageal cancer is approximately 90%, however there is significant variation according to stage [30]. EUS accuracy for T staging increases for more advanced compared to early disease, particularly for differentiating T1a from T1b tumors [31]. EUS restaging following chemoradiation is reported to be decreased potentially from radiation

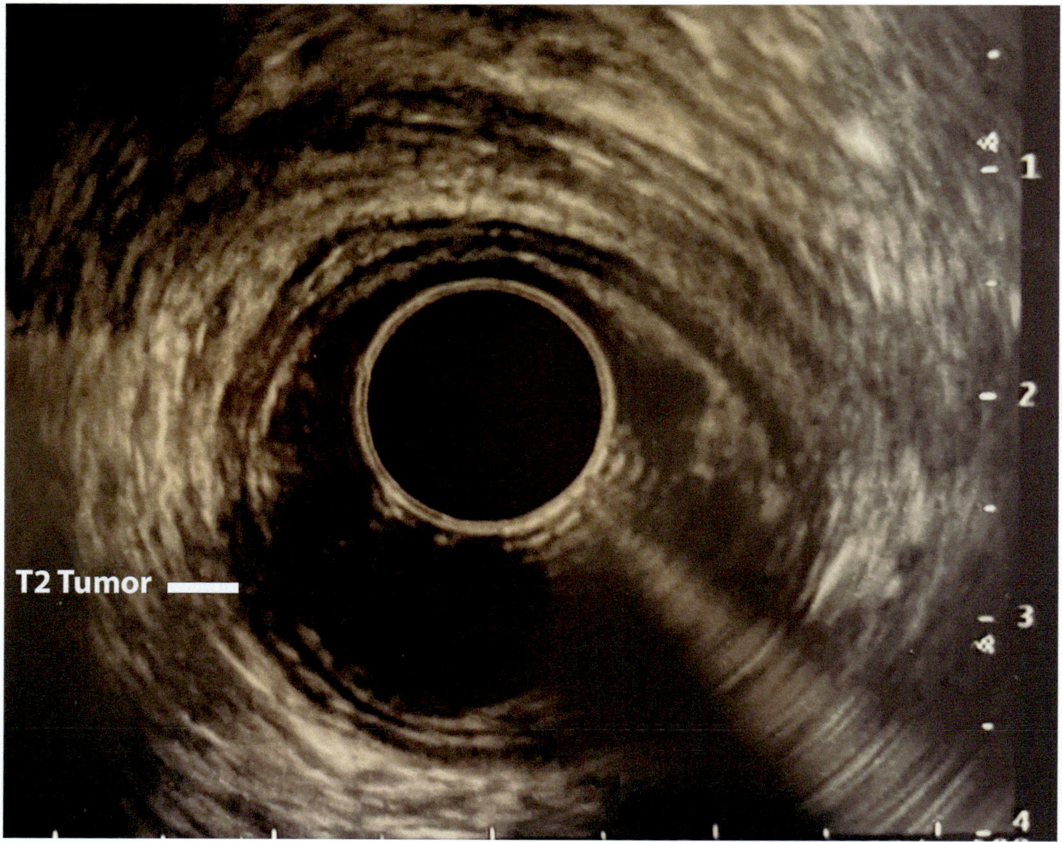

Fig. 3   Radial EUS example of T2 esophageal adenocarcinoma

induced changes in periesophageal tissues [32]. However, in our centre we perform routine EUS surveillance in the addition to cross-sectional CT imaging in higher risk patients following ESD resection or definitive chemoradiation therapy.

Limitations of EUS

EUS has limitations in staging for esophageal cancer in the presence of malignant strictures that prevent the passage of the echoendoscope beyond the lesion. This can necessitate endoscopic dilation to assist in endoscope passage or the use of EUS miniprobe as staging adjuncts. While EUS miniprobe can assist in the sonographic assessment of small mucosal lesions, their high frequencies diminish depth of tissue penetration. Unfortunately, this often prevents accurate EUS nodal assessment of the stomach and retroperitoneal lymph node basins beyond the malignant stricture [27]. It is often argued however, that given the high risk of nodal metastases from T3 lesions, and the supplemental staging information for nodal metastases given by CT/PET imaging, that once a T3 lesion is visualized, passage of the EUS scope beyond the cancer provides minimal treatment-plan impacting information. Other patient factors that can prevent EUS staging include benign esophageal strictures or patient factors that prevent the passage of the large EUS scope beyond the upper esophageal sphincter. Thankfully next-generation EUS scopes are slimmer in diameter reducing the incidence of these problems [33].

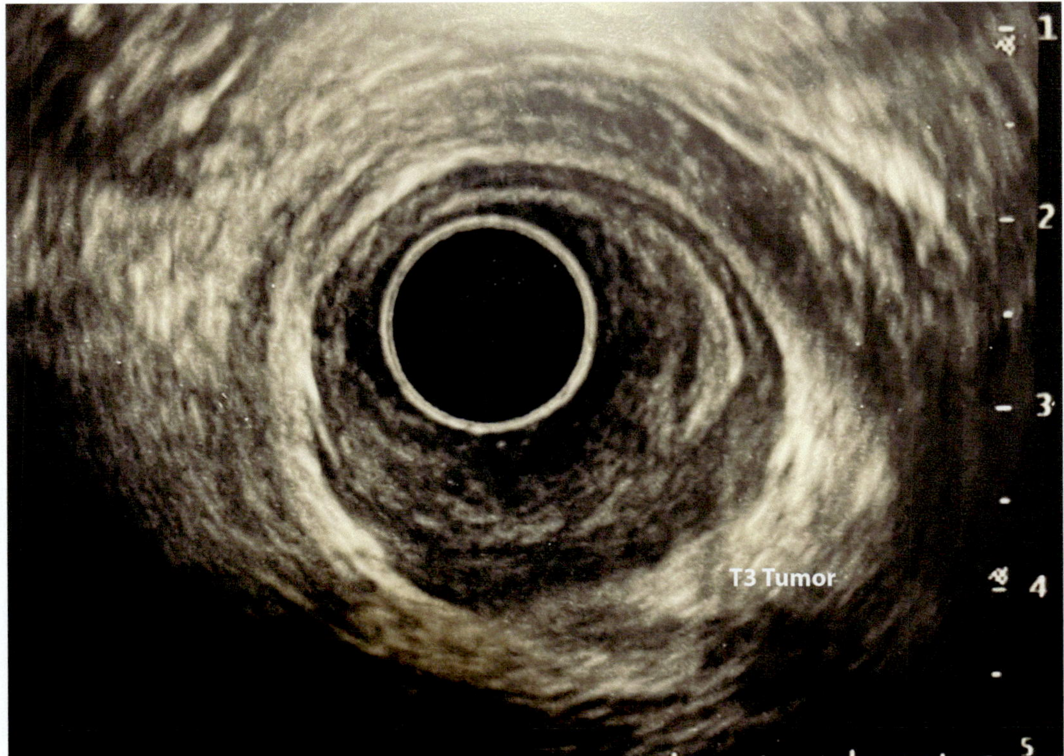

Fig. 4 Radial EUS example of T3 esophageal adenocarcinoma

EUS for Other Benign and Malignant Esophageal Tumors

Radial EUS is routinely utilized for the characterization and identification of benign and malignant lesions of the submucosal and muscularis propria. These most commonly include esophageal leiomyoma and gastrointestinal stromal tumors (GIST) but may also include other rarer benign and malignant tumor varieties. Additionally, congenital lesions such as esophageal duplication and bronchogenic cysts can be identified and characterized. EUS image characterization and esophageal layer localization are key components for lesion identification. Linear EUS FNA or Core Needle biopsy becomes a useful adjunct for tissue sampling when the diagnosis is not clear based on EUS and CT imaging characteristics alone and clinical management will be impacted [34] (Fig. 7).

Linear EUS and Linear Endobronchial Ultrasound (EBUS)

Mediastinal, periesophageal, hilar, pulmonary, perigastric and retroperitoneal adenopathy may be detected in patients during clinical staging for esophageal cancer. Occasionally lymph node enlargement may be secondary to infection and inflammation, autoimmune conditions such as sarcoidosis or low-grade malignancies unrelated to the patient's esophageal cancer. In this setting enlarged lymph nodes on CT or EUS or metabolically active lymph nodes on PET scan may require nodal sampling with linear EUS or linear EBUS guided FNA to determine the presence of esophageal cancer nodal metastases. While EBUS can biopsy pulmonary, hilar and mediastinal lymph nodes surrounding the airway, EUS can biopsy mediastinal, periesophageal, perigastric and retroperitoneal lymph nodes. Linear EUS and EBUS needles are offered in sizes

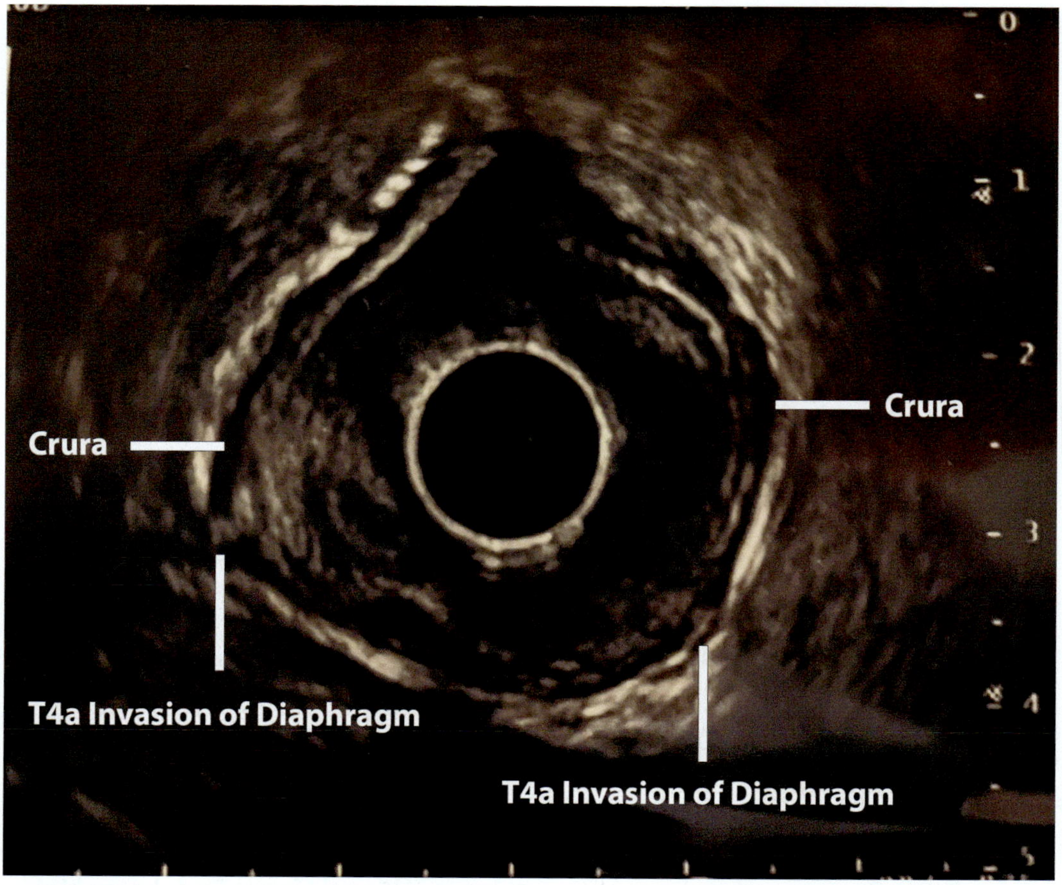

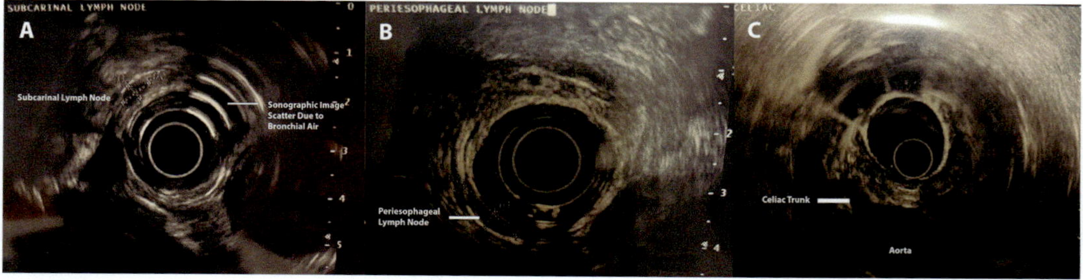

Fig. 5 Radial EUS example of T4a esophageal adenocarcinoma invading diaphragmatic crura

Fig. 6 Examples of Nodal Stations Evaluated for Radial EUS Nodal Staging. (A) Subcarinal lymph node (B) Periesophageal Lymph Node (C) Celiac Trunk location of Celiac lymph nodes

between 19 and 25 gauge depending on the clinical application suspected [35, 36].

EUS for Surveillance

Following endoscopic or surgical resection of esophageal cancer, surveillance EUS has been advocated to look for early signs of locoregional nodal metastases. Surveillance EUS performed at intervals of every six months following resection can result in earlier detection of disease recurrence. It remains unclear however if earlier detection of disease recurrence results in any improvement in long-term survival [37, 38]. Regarding the need for EUS surveillance

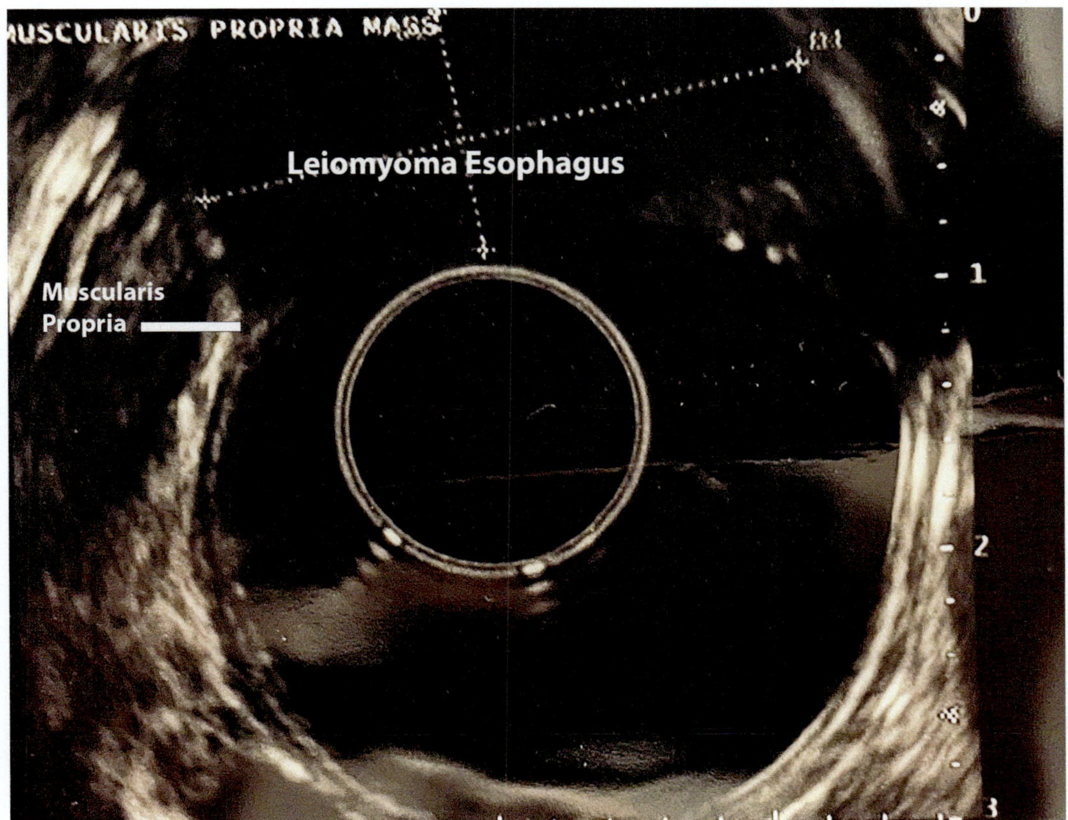

Fig. 7 Esophageal Leiomyoma arising from muscularis propria

following ESD tumor resection, when tumors resected are T1a or greater surveillance EUS in addition to cross-sectional imaging CT scan is suggested to monitor for locoregional nodal recurrence.[39] If suspicious enlarged lymph nodes are identified, linear EUS FNA biopsy can be performed for tissue diagnosis (Fig. 8).

Endoluminal Stenting

Esophageal Cancer and Endoluminal Stenting

A variety of partially and fully covered self-expanding metal (SEM) esophageal stents are available for the treatment of luminal stenosis induced by esophageal cancers. Stents are routinely inserted under direct endoscopic vision through proximal or distal release mechanisms. Fluoroscopy-guided stent insertion is also possible after endoscopic guide-wire placement and marking with radio-opaque materials on the patient's skin [40].

Fully covered stents have a silicone membrane covering and take longer for tissue ingrowth and are removable up to 4–6 weeks following insertion. Partially covered stents have coverage of most of the stent with proximal and distal ends uncovered and exposed to allow for tissue ingrowth. Once inserted for greater than 2 weeks times tissue ingrowth occurs and following this removal may not be possible or may cause significant mucosal injury with removal. Therefore, the use of partially covered esophageal stents are often reserved for patients with unresectable cancers [41].

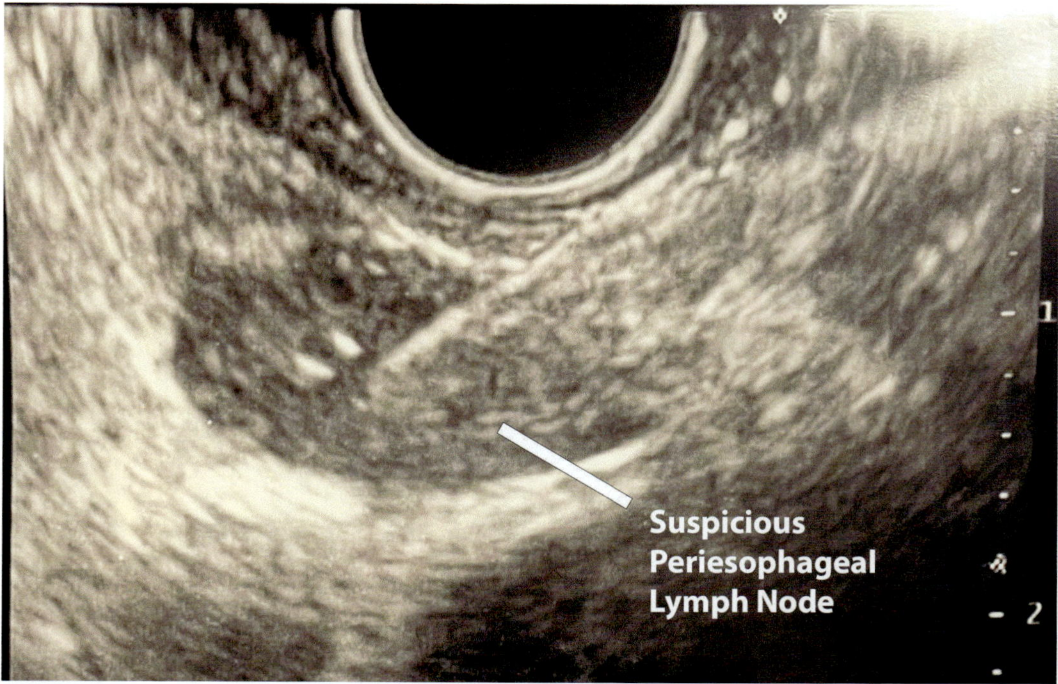

Fig. 8 An enlarging periesophageal lymph node detected by surveillance radial EUS. Sampled with 22-gauge linear EUS FNA. Note the size greater than 1 cm, sharp borders and lack of central hilar/vascular structures suggestive of malignant involvement

Treatment of Esophageal Perforations Related to Cancer

Perforated esophageal cancers induced by retching or iatrogenically through endoscopy by scope passage or dilation can be similarly treated with endoluminal esophageal stenting. Often, once perforation occurs related to a malignancy, esophageal stents may require permanent placement [42]. ESD of esophageal superficial mucosal cancers results in exposure of esophageal muscularis propria. Occasionally full thickness perforation occurs secondary todissection of submucosal fibrosis or injury. If these injuries are present in the esophagus and do not involve the gastroesophageal junction, fully covered esophageal stenting can be performed to allow for healing and stentremoval in approximately 4 weeks. In similar fashion, following fully circumferential ESD stricture formation can occur, leading to prophylactic fully covered esophageal stent placement following resection to reduce severity of stricturing [43].

Complications of endoluminal stenting for esophageal cancer include retrosternal chest pain, tissue ingrowth, tumor overgrowth, stent migration, stent food bolus obstruction and aspiration pneumonia (particularly when stents are placed across the GEJ). Rare complications include tracheoesophageal fistula formation, bleeding, and esophageal perforation. Incidence of complications from stenting is estimated to be between 40 and 50% [44].

Endoscopy and Enteral Nutrition

Endoscopy is important for the support of enteral nutrition in patients with resectable and non-resectable esophageal cancers. While esophageal stenting routinely allows for passage of orally ingested food into the stomach and small bowel, stenting is not always possible. This can commonly occur for proximal esophageal cancers involving the UES, esophageal collapse secondary to external compression from nodal metastases, or lengthy tumors that prevent esophageal stenting [41].

Upper gastrointestinal nutritional support can be re-established using endoscopy. Nasojejunal feeding tubes can be directed endoscopically with the potential addition of fluoroscopy to enter the proximal jejunum. Nasojejunal feeding tubes are problematic however as they can routinely be removed accidentally through traction. Percutaneous endoscopic gastrostomy (PEG) tubes can be placed with the aid for a gastro-scope or fluoroscopy as a palliative support for patients with unresectable cancers or for patients requiring neoadjuvant therapy with goal of curative intent esophagectomy. Care must be maintained to not injure the right gastroepiploic artery for any potential esophagectomy candidates. PEG tubes can also be modified to direct feeding tubes into thejejunum beyond the stomach. While PEG tubes have advantages, foreign body site infections can necessitate their removal. Insertion of PEG tubes can be complicated by gastric perforation necessitating endoscopic or surgical closure [45].

References

1. Huang J, Koulaouzidis A, Marlicz W, Lok V, Chu C, Ngai CH, Zhang L, Chen P, Wang S, Yuan J, Lao XQ, Tse SLA, Xu W, Zheng ZJ, Xie SH, Wong MCS. Global burden, risk factors, and trends of esophageal cancer: an analysis of cancer registries from 48 countries. Cancers (Basel). 2021;13(1). https://doi.org/10.3390/cancers13010141

2. Siewert JR, Hölscher AH, Becker K, Gössner W. Cardia cancer: attempt at a therapeutically relevant classification. Chirurg. 1987;58(1):25–32.

3. Koutsoumpas A, Perera R, Melton A, Kuker J, Ghosh T, Braden B. Tunneled biopsy is an underutilised, simple, safe and efficient method for tissue acquisition from subepithelial tumours. World J Clin Cases. 2021;9(21):5822–9. https://doi.org/10.12998/wjcc.v9.i21.5822.

4. Whitson MJ, Falk GW. Predictors of progression to high-grade dysplasia or adenocarcinoma in Barrett's esophagus. Gastroenterol Clin North Am. 2015;44(2):299–315. https://doi.org/10.1016/j.gtc.2015.02.005.

5. Killcoyne S, Gregson E, Wedge DC, Woodcock DJ, Eldridge MD, de la Rue R, Miremadi A, Abbas S, Blasko A, Kosmidou C, Januszewicz W, Jenkins AV, Gerstung M, Fitzgerald RC. Genomic copy number predicts esophageal cancer years before transformation. Nat Med. 2020;26(11):1726–32. https://doi.org/10.1038/s41591-020-1033-y.

6. Sharma P, Dent J, Armstrong D, Bergman JJ, Gossner L, Hoshihara Y, Jankowski JA, Junghard O, Lundell L, Tytgat GN, Vieth M. The development and validation of an endoscopic grading system for Barrett's esophagus: the Prague C & M criteria. Gastroenterology. 2006;131(5):1392–9. https://doi.org/10.1053/j.gastro.2006.08.032.

7. Sharma P, Morales TG, Sampliner RE. Short segment Barrett's esophagus–the need for standardization of the definition and of endoscopic criteria. Am J Gastroenterol. 1998;93(7):1033–6. https://doi.org/10.1111/j.1572-0241.1998.00324.x.

8. Spechler SJ, Sharma P, Souza RF, Inadomi JM, Shaheen NJ. American Gastroenterological Association technical review on the management of Barrett's esophagus. Gastroenterology. 2011;140(3):e18–52; quiz e13. https://doi.org/10.1053/j.gastro.2011.01.031

9. Qumseya B, Sultan S, Bain P, Jamil L, Jacobson B, Anandasabapathy S, Agrawal D, Buxbaum JL, Fishman DS, Gurudu SR, Jue TL, Kripalani S, Lee JK, Khashab MA, Naveed M, Thosani NC, Yang J, DeWitt J, Wani S. ASGE guideline on screening and surveillance of Barrett's esophagus. Gastrointest Endosc. 2019;90(3):335–59.e332. https://doi.org/10.1016/j.gie.2019.05.012.

10. Gono K, Obi T, Yamaguchi M, Ohyama N, Machida H, Sano Y, Yoshida S, Hamamoto Y, Endo T. Appearance of enhanced tissue features in narrow-band endoscopic imaging. J Biomed Opt. 2004;9(3):568–77. https://doi.org/10.1117/1.1695563.

11. Chiam KH, Shin SH, Choi KC, Leiria F, Militz M, Singh R. Current status of mucosal imaging with narrow-band imaging in the esophagus. Gut Liver. 2021;15(4):492–9. https://doi.org/10.5009/gnl20031.

12. Amano Y, Kushiyama Y, Ishihara S, Yuki T, Miyaoka Y, Yoshino N, Ishimura N, Fujishiro H, Adachi K, Maruyama R, Rumi MA, Kinoshita Y. Crystal violet chromoendoscopy with mucosal pit pattern diagnosis is useful for surveillance of short-segment Barrett's esophagus. Am J Gastroenterol. 2005;100(1):21–6. https://doi.org/10.1111/j.1572-0241.2005.40028.x.

13. Chedgy FJ, Subramaniam S, Kandiah K, Thayalasekaran S, Bhandari P. Acetic acid chromoendoscopy: improving neoplasia detection in Barrett's esophagus. World J Gastroenterol.

2016;22(25):5753–60. https://doi.org/10.3748/wjg.
v22.i25.5753.

14. Hoffman A, Kiesslich R, Bender A, Neurath MF, Nafe B, Herrmann G, Jung M. Acetic acid-guided biopsies after magnifying endoscopy compared with random biopsies in the detection of Barrett's esophagus: a prospective randomized trial with crossover design. Gastrointest Endosc. 2006;64(1):1–8. https://doi.org/10.1016/j.gie.2005.09.031.

15. Wang CH, Lee YC, Wang CP, Chen CC, Ko JY, Han ML, Chen TC, Lou PJ, Yang TL, Hsiao TY, Wu MS, Wang HP, Tseng PH. Use of transnasal endoscopy for screening of esophageal squamous cell carcinoma in high-risk patients: yield rate, completion rate, and safety. Dig Endosc. 2014;26(1):24–31. https://doi.org/10.1111/den.12053.

16. Atreya R, Neumann H, Neufert C, Waldner MJ, Billmeier U, Zopf Y, Willma M, App C, Munster T, Kessler H, Maas S, Gebhardt B, Heimke-Brinck R, Reuter E, Dorje F, Rau TT, Uter W, Wang TD, Kiesslich R, Vieth M, Hannappel E, Neurath MF. In vivo imaging using fluorescent antibodies to tumor necrosis factor predicts therapeutic response in Crohn's disease. Nat Med. 2014;20(3):313–8. https://doi.org/10.1038/nm.3462.

17. Lee JK, Enns R. Endoscopic mucosal resection in the setting of Barrett's esophagus. Can J Gastroenterol. 2007;21(3):151–4. https://doi.org/10.1155/2007/198728.

18. Qumseya BJ, David W, Wolfsen HC. Photodynamic therapy for Barrett's esophagus and esophageal carcinoma. Clinical endoscopy. 2013;46(1):30–7. https://doi.org/10.5946/ce.2013.46.1.30.

19. Mohan BP, Krishnamoorthi R, Ponnada S, Shakhatreh M, Jayaraj M, Garg R, Law J, Larsen M, Irani S, Ross A, Adler DG. Liquid nitrogen spray cryotherapy in treatment of Barrett's esophagus, where do we stand? A systematic review and meta-analysis. Dis Esophagus. 2019;32 (6). https://doi.org/10.1093/dote/doy130

20. Deprez PH. Barrett's esophagus: the advocacy for ESD. Endosc Int Open. 2016;4(6):E722-724. https://doi.org/10.1055/s-0042-109599.

21. Bazarbashi AN, McCarty TR, Dolan RD, Hathorn KE, Jajoo K, Thompson CC, Aihara H. S0361 endoscopic submucosal dissection vs endoscopic mucosal resection for the treatment of dysplastic Barrett's esophagus and adenocarcinoma. Official J Am Coll Gastroenterol ACG. 2020;115:S177–8. https://doi.org/10.14309/01.ajg.0000703492.28077.e1

22. Abe K, Goda K, Kanamori A, Suzuki T, Yamamiya A, Takimoto Y, Arisaka T, Hoshi K, Sugaya T, Majima Y, Tominaga K, Iijima M, Hirooka S, Yamagishi H, Irisawa A. Whole circumferential endoscopic submucosal dissection of superficial adenocarcinoma in long-segment Barrett's esophagus: a case report. World J Gastrointest Surg. 2021;13(10):1285–92. https://doi.org/10.4240/wjgs.v13.i10.1285.

23. Bechara R, Chen L, Chung W, Varma S. Salvage circumferential endoscopic submucosal dissection for refractory dysplastic Barrett's esophagus. VideoGIE. 2020;5(12):641–2. https://doi.org/10.1016/j.vgie.2020.07.005.

24. Lee L, Ronellenfitsch U, Hofstetter WL, Darling G, Gaiser T, Lippert C, Gilbert S, Seely AJ, Mulder DS, Ferri LE. Predicting lymph node metastases in early esophageal adenocarcinoma using a simple scoring system. J Am Coll Surg. 2013;217(2):191–9. https://doi.org/10.1016/j.jamcollsurg.2013.03.015.

25. Kaneshiro DK, Post JC, Rybicki L, Rice TW, Goldblum JR. Clinical significance of the duplicated muscularis mucosae in Barrett esophagus-related superficial adenocarcinoma. Am J Surg Pathol. 2011;35(5):697–700. https://doi.org/10.1097/PAS.0b013e3182159c4b.

26. Jiang KY, Huang H, Chen WY, Yan HJ, Wei ZT, Wang XW, Li HX, Zheng XY, Tian D. Risk factors for lymph node metastasis in T1 esophageal squamous cell carcinoma: a systematic review and meta-analysis. World J Gastroenterol. 2021;27(8):737–50. https://doi.org/10.3748/wjg.v27.i8.737.

27. Thakkar S, Kaul V. Endoscopic ultrasound stagingof esophageal cancer. Gastroenterol Hepatol (N Y). 2020;16(1):14–20.

28. Rice TW, Patil DT, Blackstone EH. 8th edition AJCC/UICC staging of cancers of the esophagus and esophagogastric junction: application to clinical practice. Ann Cardiothorac Surg. 2017;6(2):119–30. https://doi.org/10.21037/acs.2017.03.14.

29. Gamal GH. Does PET/CT give incremental staging information in cancer oesophagus compared to CECT? Egypt J Radiol Nucl Med. 2019;50(1):110. https://doi.org/10.1186/s43055-019-0114-8.

30. Lee WC, Lee TH, Jang JY, Lee JS, Cho JY, Lee JS, Jeon SR, Kim HG, Kim JO, Cho YK. Staging accuracy of endoscopic ultrasound performed by nonexpert endosonographers in patients with resectable esophageal squamous cell carcinoma: is it possible? Dis Esophagus. 2015;28(6):574–8. https://doi.org/10.1111/dote.12235.

31. Puli SR, Reddy JB, Bechtold ML, Antillon D, Ibdah JA, Antillon MR. Staging accuracy of esophageal cancer by endoscopic ultrasound: a meta-analysis and systematic review. World J Gastroenterol. 2008;14(10):1479–90. https://doi.org/10.3748/wjg.14.1479.

32. van Rossum PSN, Goense L, Meziani J, Reitsma JB, Siersema PD, Vleggaar FP, van Vulpen M, Meijer GJ, Ruurda JP, van Hillegersberg R. Endoscopic biopsy and EUS for the detection of pathologic complete response after neoadjuvant chemoradiotherapy in esophageal cancer: a systematic review and meta-analysis. Gastrointest Endosc. 2016;83(5):866–79. https://doi.org/10.1016/j.gie.2015.11.026.

33. Cazacu IM, Luzuriaga Chavez AA, Saftoiu A, Vilmann P, Bhutani MS. A quarter century of

EUS-FNA: progress, milestones, and future directions. Endosc Ultrasound. 2018;7(3):141–60. https://doi.org/10.4103/eus.eus_19_18.

34. Hihara J, Mukaida H, Hirabayashi N. Gastrointestinal stromal tumor of the esophagus: current issues of diagnosis, surgery and drug therapy. Transl Gastroenterol Hepatol. 2018;3(1).

35. Vazquez-Sequeiros E, Wiersema MJ, Clain JE, Norton ID, Levy MJ, Romero Y, Salomao D, Dierkhising R, Zinsmeister AR. Impact of lymph node staging on therapy of esophageal carcinoma. Gastroenterology. 2003;125(6):1626–35. https://doi.org/10.1053/j.gastro.2003.08.036.

36. Santos LM, Jacomelli M, Scordamaglio PR, Cardoso PFG, Figueiredo VR. Endobronchial ultrasound in esophageal cancer—when upper gastrointestinal endoscopy is not enough. J Bras Pneumol. 2019;45(3):e20180312. https://doi.org/10.1590/1806-3713/e20180312.

37. Fockens P, Manshanden CG, van Lanschot JJ, Obertop H, Tytgat GN. Prospective study on the value of endosonographic follow-up after surgery for esophageal carcinoma. Gastrointest Endosc. 1997;46(6):487–91. https://doi.org/10.1016/s0016-5107(97)70001-4.

38. Müller C, Kähler G, Scheele J. Endosonographic examination of gastrointestinal anastomoses with suspected locoregional tumor recurrence. Surg Endosc. 2000;14(1):45–50. https://doi.org/10.1007/s004649900009.

39. Wang AY, Hwang JH, Bhatt A, Draganov PV. AGA clinical practice update on surveillance after pathologically curative endoscopic submucosal dissection of early gastrointestinal neoplasia in the United States: commentary. Gastroenterology. 2021;161(6):2030–40.e2031. https://doi.org/10.1053/j.gastro.2021.08.058.

40. Spaander MC, Baron TH, Siersema PD, Fuccio L, Schumacher B, Escorsell À, Garcia-Pagán JC, Dumonceau JM, Conio M, de Ceglie A, Skowronek J, Nordsmark M, Seufferlein T, Van Gossum A, Hassan C, Repici A, Bruno MJ. Esophageal stenting for benign and malignant disease: European society of gastrointestinal endoscopy (ESGE) clinical guideline. Endoscopy. 2016;48(10):939–48. https://doi.org/10.1055/s-0042-114210.

41. Vermeulen BD, Siersema PD. Esophageal stenting in clinical practice: an overview. Curr Treat Options Gastroenterol. 2018;16(2):260–73. https://doi.org/10.1007/s11938-018-0181-3.

42. Ferguson MK. Esophageal perforation and caustic injury: management of perforated esophageal cancer. Dis Esophagus. 1997;10(2):90–4. https://doi.org/10.1093/dote/10.2.90.

43. Shi KD, Ji F. Prophylactic stenting for esophageal stricture prevention after endoscopic submucosal dissection. World J Gastroenterol. 2017;23(6):931–4. https://doi.org/10.3748/wjg.v23.i6.931.

44. Didden P, Reijm AN, Erler NS, Wolters LMM, Tang TJ, Ter Borg PCJ, Leeuwenburgh I, Bruno MJ, Spaander MCW. Fully vs. partially covered selfexpandable metal stent for palliation of malignant esophageal strictures: a randomized trial (the COPAC study). Endoscopy (2018);50(10):961–71. https://doi.org/10.1055/a-0620-8135.

45. Rafferty GP, Tham TC. Endoscopic placement of enteral feeding tubes. World J Gastrointest Endosc. 2010;2(5):155–64. https://doi.org/10.4253/wjge.v2.i5.155.

Radiologic Evaluation of Esophageal Cancer

Manuela Monrabal Lezama, Antonella Kovic, Emilia Martínez and Silvina De Luca

Abstract

Various methods are currently employed for esophageal cancer staging, including computed tomography (CT), positron emission tomography (PET), endoscopic ultrasound (EUS), magnetic resonance imaging (MRI), and histopathologic based staging, which encompasses endoscopic mucosal resection (EMR) and endoscopic submucosal dissection (ESD). However, no single modality can accurately stage every patient with esophageal cancer on its own. Given the crucial role of accurate staging in devising an optimal therapeutic approach, the use of a combination of these modalities is often necessary.

Keywords

Esophageal cancer · Radiology · CT · PET-CT · Endoscopic ultrasound

M. Monrabal Lezama
Department of Surgery, Hospital Alemán of Buenos Aires, 1640 Pueyrredón Av, Buenos Aires, Argentina
e-mail: mmonraballezama@hospitalaleman.com

A. Kovic · E. Martínez · S. De Luca (✉)
Department of Radiology, Hospital Alemán of Buenos Aires, Buenos Aires, Argentina
e-mail: sdeluca@hospitalaleman.com

E. Martínez
e-mail: emiliamartinez@hospitalaleman.com

Introduction

Esophageal cancer staging remains a complementary mix of multiple diagnostic modalities including computed tomography (CT), 18 FDG positron emission tomography (18 FDG PET), magnetic resonance imaging (MRI), endoscopic ultrasound (EUS) and esophagogastroduodenoscopy (EGD), being its approach multi-disciplinary and highly complex. As imaging remains the cornerstone of diagnosis, radiologists play an essential role in esophageal cancer staging [1].

Current treatment strategies range from organ preserving modalities to multimodality therapy combining surgery with chemotherapy with or without radiation [2, 3]. Organ sparing techniques, including endoscopic mucosal resection (EMR) and endoscopic submucosal resection (ESR) have shown optimal results in patients with node negative—T1a tumors (tumor confined to the mucosa), proving survival rates of 80–90% in properly selected cases [4].

Patients with deeper tumors such as T1b-T2 without clinical suspicion of nodal involvement are candidates for upfront radical surgical treatment, being esophagectomy with lymphadenectomy the pillar of curative intent therapy [5].

In cases of extended locally advanced disease and/or lymph node compromise (T3-N$^+$), several randomized studies have reported improved overall and disease-free survival with multimodality therapy, including chemotherapy with or

F. Schlottmann et al. (eds.), *Esophageal Cancer*,
https://doi.org/10.1007/978-3-031-39086-9_5

without radiation followed by radical surgery. In any case, a proper patient selection and accurate staging will help to determine the optimal therapy in order to achieve the best oncological outcome [2, 3, 6–9].

The globally used TNM classification system maintained by the American Joint Committee on Cancer (AJCC) and the Union for International Cancer Control (UICC) includes the depth of local invasion by the primary tumor (T), the extent of regional lymph node involvement (N), and the presence or absence of distant metastasis (M), providing a stage grouping on the basis of T, N, and M [10]. Furthermore, separate stage groupings are described for the two main histologic subtypes, squamous cell carcinoma (SCC) and adenocarcinoma (EAC).

For both EAC and SCC, T0 disease denotes high-grade dysplasia; T1 disease is divided into T1a and b and denotes absence or presence of invasion through the muscularis mucosa into the submucosa, respectively. T2 denotes invasion into the muscularis propria, T3 denotes invasion to the adventitia, and T4 denotes invasion into surrounding structures. This is further subdivided in T4a, defined as resectable disease (including diaphragm, pleura, and pericardium) and T4b, defined as unresectable (including trachea, aorta and, vertebral body).

Nodal disease is classified as N1 if fewer than three nodes are involved, as N2 if 3–6 nodes are involved, and N3 if 7 or more are involved. Any extra nodal metastases are classified as M1 [10] (Table 1).

The available techniques for accurate staging include both imaging and invasive studies. The aforementioned comprises mainly endoscopic ultrasound (EUS), CT and PET-CT. More invasive methods such as EMR, ESD or even laparoscopy can also help staging esophageal cancer [9].

This chapter provides a detailed review of the different imaging methods describing their applications, strengths and weaknesses for esophageal cancer staging. As no radiologic study will obtain the diagnosis and staging by itself, all of them should be considered as complimentary to one another. Consequently, the adequate combination of the studies will help obtaining an accurate staging.

Tumor "T" Staging

CT Scan and T Staging

CT remains the most commonly used study for preoperative T staging of esophageal cancer. CT scanners can provide volumetric data on the primary tumor, demonstrating an overall accuracy of 80% in the determination of T stage. However, as CT is unable to accurately differentiate the layers of the esophageal wall and the depth of tumor invasion, accuracy and specificity of the study decreases in early stages such as T1 and T2. Recently, multi-detector row CT with dynamic enhanced images has shown improved accuracy for T staging [8, 11, 12].

According to the literature, the accuracy of CT with respect to T-stage as compared to final histology is around 60% for T1 lesions and 75% for T3 lesions, acknowledging its lower specificity in earlier tumors [11, 12]. As proper staging of T1 against T2 tumors is required to consider a curative endoscopic treatment, these cases may be aided by EUS. On the other hand, CT scan seems to be more accurate on advanced tumors. For example, T3 stage is detected on multi-detector CT as periesophageal fat infiltration with 75% sensitivity and 78% specificity, and T4 stage is identified with loss of fat planes between the tumor and adjacent mediastinal structure with 75% sensitivity and 86% specificity (Fig. 1) [13].

Local invasion of tracheobronchial tree, aorta and/or heart can be assessed with almost 100% of sensitivity, however its specificity ranges from 52 to 97%. Loss of the fat plane between the esophagus and airway, visualization of a tracheoesophageal fistula and/or tumor contact>90° with the aorta represent very poor prognostic factors. Similarly, abutment of the tumor against the pericardium with associated pericardial effusion are concerning features (Fig. 2) [8, 12–15].

Table 1 AJCC 8th edition staging of esophageal cancer

	Clinical criteria
T stage	
Tx	Cannot be assessed
T0	High-grade dysplasia—confined by basement membrane
T1a	Invades lamina propria or muscularis mucosa
T1b	Invades into submucosa
T2	Invades muscularis propria
T3	Invades adventitia
T4a	Invades pleura, pericardium, azygous vein, diaphragm, peritoneum
T4b	Invades adjacent structures such as aorta and vertebral body
N stage	
NX	Cannot be assessed
N0	0 involved nodes
N1	1–2 involved regional nodes
N2	3–6 involved regional nodes
N3	7 or more involved regional nodes
M stage	
MX	Cannot be assessed
M0	No distant metastasis
M1	Distant metastasis
ADC Grade	
GX	Cannot be assessed
G1	Well differentiated
G2	Moderately differentiated
G3	Poorly differentiated
SCC Grade	
GX	Cannot be assessed
G1	Well differentiated
G2	Moderately differentiated
G3	Poorly differentiated
SCC Location	
LX	Cannot be assessed
Upper	Cervical esophagus to azygous vein
Middle	Lower border of azygous vein to inferior pulmonary vein
Lower	Inferior pulmonary vein to stomach

(continued)

Table 1 (continued)

Clinical (c) stage	T	N	M
ADC			
0	Tis	N0	M0
I	T1	N0	M0
IIA	T1	N1	M0
IIB	T2	0	0
III	T2 T3-4a	N1 N0-1	M0 M0
IVA	T1-4a T4b T1-4	N2 N0-2 N3	M0 M0 M0
IVB	T1-4	N0-3	M1
SCC			
0	Tis	N0	M0
I	T1	N0-1	M0
II	T2 T3	N0-1 N0	M0 M0
III	T3 T1-3	N1 N2	M0 M0
IVA	T4 T1-4	N0-2 N3	M0 M0
IVB	T1-4	N0-3	M1

ADC Adenocarcinoma, *SCC* Squamous cell carcinoma

Despite its high level of accuracy, diagnosis of T4 stage may represent a challenge in some cases, particularly in patients who had received surgery or radiotherapy or with cachexia due to the loss of fat planes [13].

MRI and "T" Staging

Currently, the use of magnetic resonance imaging (MRI) in patients with esophageal cancer is limited. This may be explained by the lack of uniform techniques for image acquisition and differences in image quality observed over time related to diverse MRI technologies. However, the quality of MRI continues to improve and is gaining ground for esophageal cancer staging, with encouraging results comparable with CT and EUS. Technical developments that diminish

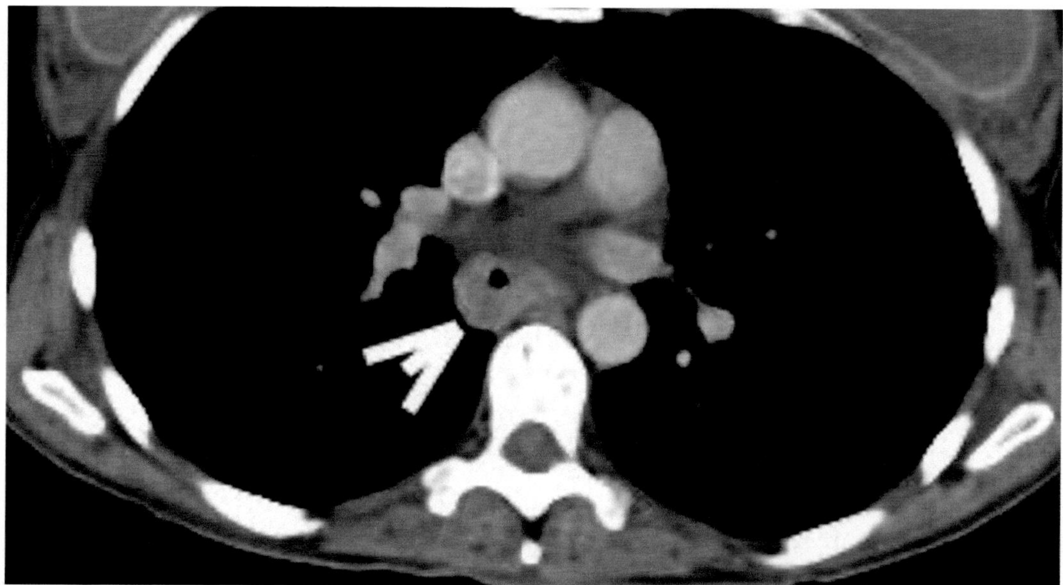

Fig. 1 CT scan showing esophageal tumor with intimal contact with the pericardium (T4a)

motion artifact and optimizes MRI image quality, such as application of high-resolution and ECG-triggered 1.5 T MRI are allowing this method to become increasingly used [16, 17].

With respect to T staging, a previous study showed that with the application of faster imaging sequence and ECG gated technique, accuracy of 1.5 T MRI was 33%, 58%, 96%, and 100% for T1, T2, T3 and T4 stage, respectively [18]. More recently, a study confirmed that high-resolution T2-weighted imaging (T2WI) provides meticulous imaging of the anatomical layers of the esophageal wall and surrounding tissues with an accuracy of 81% for T-staging (according to the signal intensity obtained in each esophageal layer) [19].

Overall, although the diagnostic value of MRI for T staging has significantly improved in recent years, further evidence and standardization of the technique are needed to broadly adopt this imaging method [17].

Endoscopic Ultrasound and "T" Staging

Endoscopic ultrasound (EUS) represents one of the preferred imaging modalities for the assessment of loco-regional disease in esophageal cancer. EUS has the ability to identify the depth of tumor invasion and pathologic regional lymphadenopathies. In addition, it has the possibility to obtain nodal biopsies with fine-needle aspiration (FNA) [8, 20–22].

According to its echogenicity, echoendoscopes can identify 5 layers of the esophageal wall: mucosa (first hyperechoic layer), muscularis mucosa (first hypoechoic layer), submucosa (second hyperechoic layer), muscularis propria (second hypoechoic layer), adventitia (esophageal) or serosa (gastric) (third hyperechoic layer) (Fig. 3).

The overall reported sensitivity and accuracy for assessing the T stage with EUS is 85–90%

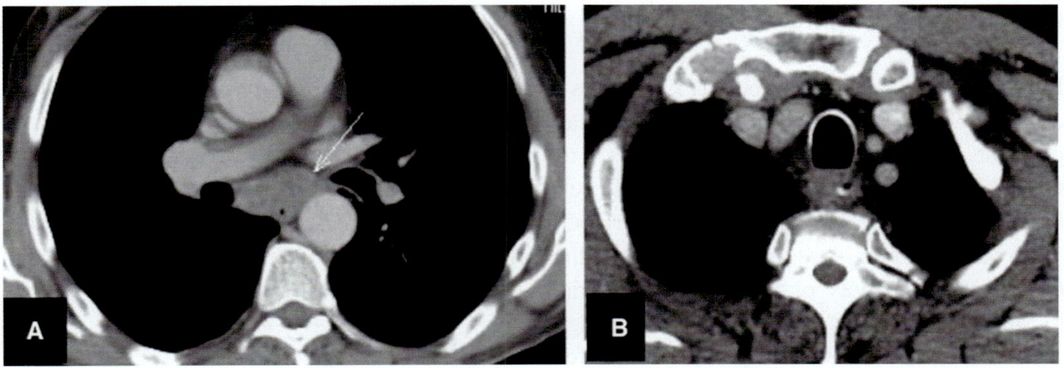

Fig. 2 CT scan showing esophageal tumor in direct contact with the aorta (A) and with the trachea (B)

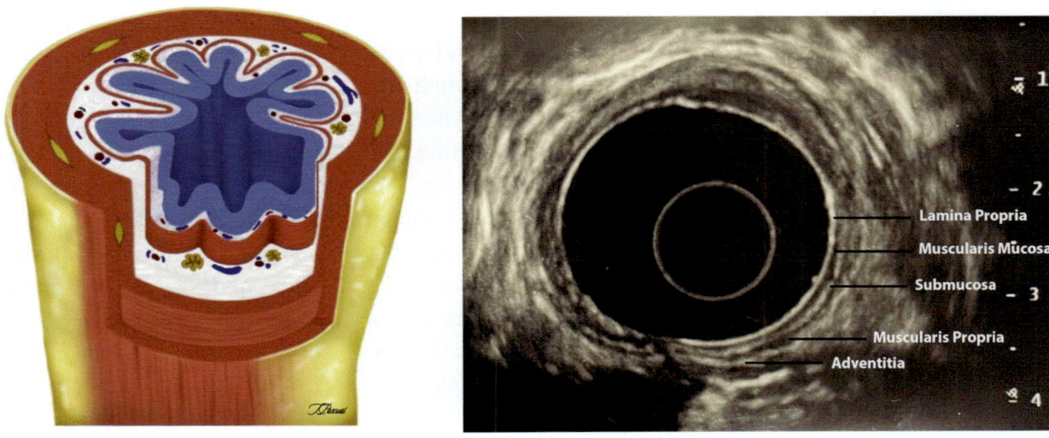

Fig. 3 Esophageal layers (Drawing by Tomás Pascual MD and Endoscopic Ultrasound Image from Stephen Gowing MD)

and 70–80%, respectively [23]. For early tumors, however, accuracy is decreased. Bianco et al. reported that EUS accurately staged 39% of T1a lesions and 70% of T1b lesions [24]. Similarly, another study reported that lesions diagnosed as cT1aN0 by EUS, turned out to be deeper or even pN1 in 15% of patients [25]. Shridhar and colleagues in a series of 1840 patients with T2N0M0 esophageal cancer (EAC or SCC) showed that clinical staging was accurate in only 30.7% of patients, describing tumor length > 3 cm and poor differentiation as risk factors for pathologic upstaging [26]. Likewise, Luu et al. reported understaging by EUS in 21% of patients with stage I or II (14% with unrecognized nodal disease). All these studies suggest that EMR or ESD might be necessary for accurate staging of early superficial tumors [27].

A previous study showed a significant increase in the utilization of neoadjuvant therapy in patients who underwent EUS staging as compared to those that only had a CT as staging modality (32.7% versus 15%). Consequently, an improved overall survival was seen in EUS-staged patients (58.9%) versus CT alone (47.7%) [28].

Overall, current data confirms that EUS is critical for adequate staging in most patients with esophageal cancer, mainly due to its ability to select patients for multimodal therapy and predict patient outcomes.

PET-CT and T Staging

Positron emission tomography (PET) plays a critical role in the staging of esophageal cancer. The study relies on the expression of the GLUT-1 glucose transporter on neoplastic cells for the uptake of fluorodeoxyglucose (FDG). Therefore, it provides information regarding the metabolic activity of the tumor in addition to anatomic features. Currently, PET images are often fused with CT images to more effectively localize sites of abnormal glucose uptake (PET-TC) (Figs. 4 and 5).

The majority of both esophageal squamous cell carcinoma (ESCC) and esophageal adenocarcinoma (EAC) are PET avid. ESCC, however, tends to be more PET avid and around 20% of EAC show little or no FDG avidity. Lack of avidity is more common in poorly differentiated tumors and signet cell lesions [29, 30].

With respect to differentiating between T stages, PET-CT cannot accurately differentiate the depth of invasion of the primary tumor, and thereby has a limited role in T staging. Given the relatively low resolution and detection threshold of the study, this study is less precise for early T1 disease and limited for differentiating between T1 or T2 lesions. Stage specific accuracy is thereby higher for T3 and T4 tumors. In addition, PET-TC provides valuable information regarding T stage in patients with obstructive tumors in whom endoscopy or EUS are not feasible [8, 29, 30] (Fig. 6).

Node "N" Staging

Currently, endoscopic ultrasound, CT and PET CT are commonly used to determine N stage. These modalities have low or moderate sensitivity and moderate-high specificity for assessment of lymph node status.

Lymph node involvement is critical for selecting patients for multimodal therapy. Regional lymph nodes include any paraesophageal lymph nodes from the cervical nodes to the celiac nodes. The N classification comprises N0 (no cancer-positive nodes), N1 (one or two cancer-positive nodes), N2 (three to six cancer-positive nodes), and N3 (seven or more cancer-positive nodes).

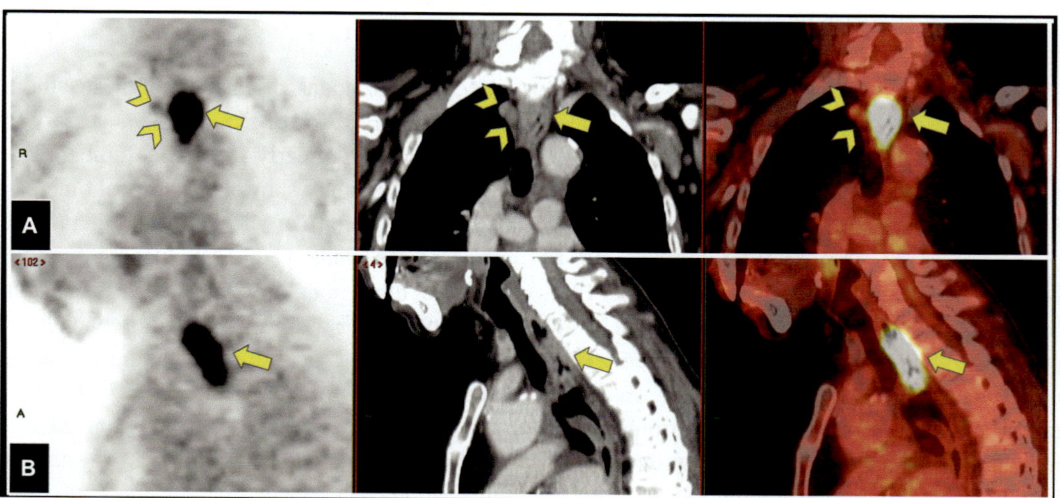

Fig. 4 Squamous cell carcinoma in upper third of the esophagus (T3N1M0). A) PET-CT coronal reconstruction demonstrates esophageal hypermetabolic wall thickening preserving peripheral fat (T3, arrow) and two hypermetabolic infracentimetric nodes to the right (N1, arrow heads). B) PET-CT sagittal reconstruction showing same findings

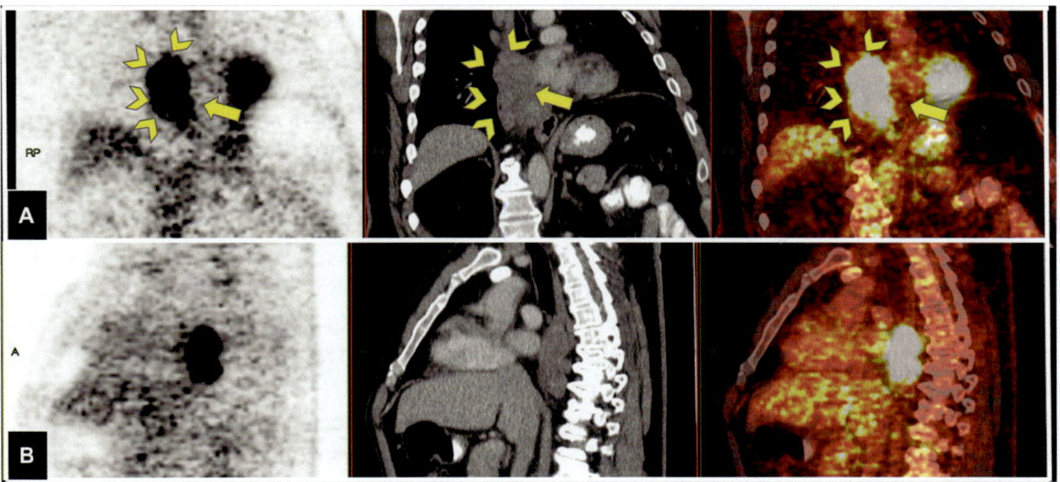

Fig. 5 Adenocarcinoma in lower third of the esophagus (T3N2M0). A) PET-CT coronal reconstruction demonstrates esophageal hypermetabolic wall thickening preserving peripheral fat (T3, arrow) and multiple regional hypermetabolic nodes (N2, arrow heads). B) PET-CT sagittal reconstruction showing same findings

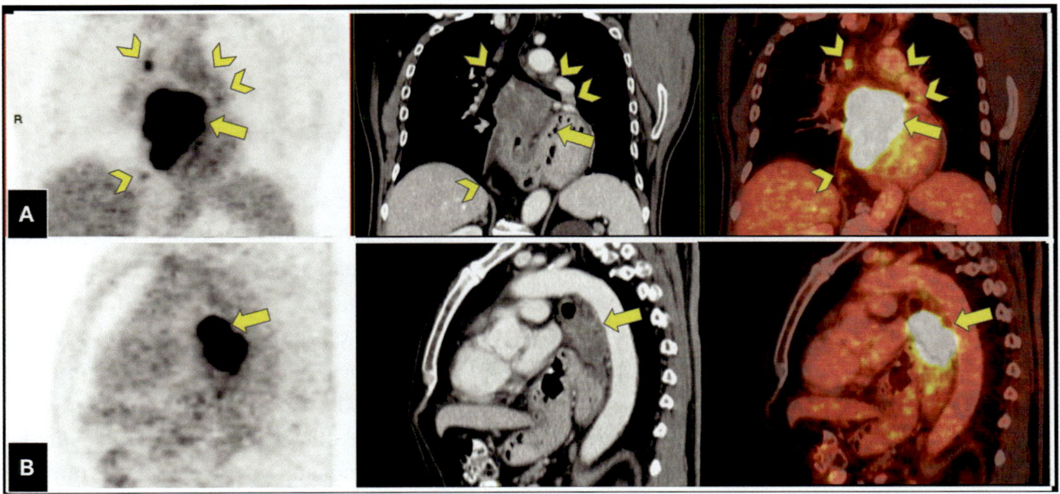

Fig. 6 Adenocarcinoma in middle third of the esophagus (T4N3M0). A) PET-CT coronal reconstruction demonstrates esophageal hypermetabolic wall thickening with periesophageal fat infiltration (T4, arrow) with a maximum SUV of 29.5 and multiple hypermetabolic mediastinal nodes (N3, arrow heads). B) PET-CT sagittal reconstruction showing same findings

CT Scan and N Staging

In CT scan, non-pathologic lymph nodes are usually smaller than 1 cm in short-axis diameter with a smooth well-defined border, uniform homogeneous attenuation, and a central fatty hilum [8].

The detection of metastatic lymph nodes with CT depends primarily on size criteria. In general, intrathoracic and abdominal lymph nodes greater than 1 cm in diameter are considered to be enlarged, and supraclavicular lymph nodes with a short axis greater than 5 mm are considered to be pathologic. However, most studies use the common size criteria of 1 cm to define a pathological lymph node [8, 9]. Sensitivity and specificity CT for detecting metastatic lymph nodes is somehow limited, with an overall accuracy reported of at best 66% in nodal staging [8, 9].

Unfortunately, even normal-sized lymph node might contain microscopic metastatic foci that are beyond the level of detection offered by CT. Moreover, the presence of reactive enlarged and inflammatory lymph nodes reduces the specificity of the study. Additionally, peritumoral nodes contacting directly with the mass can be indistinguishable from the primary tumor and may induce false-negative results [1, 12].

Luketich and colleagues reported a sensitivity and specificity of CT of the chest and abdomen for lymph node metastasis of 33% and 88%, respectively, proving to be inaccurate in more than 40% of patients [31].

MRI and N Staging

As mentioned above, MRI is not yet widely adopted for esophageal cancer staging. Studies exploring the effectiveness of MRI for N staging have shown heterogenous results. The estimated sensitivity and specificity currently range between 38%–70% and 67%–93%, respectively, owing this variation to diverse methods of image acquisition and threshold size for suspicious lymph nodes [30].

At present, MRI presents some drawbacks as compared to CT, such as higher cost and limited availability. Therefore, its use should be based on institutional experience or equivocal findings from CT.

Endoscopic Ultrasound and N Staging

Endoscopic ultrasound (EUS) is used to determine nodal involvement based on factors such as size, shape, borders, and internal characteristics of the nodes. Malignant lymph nodes are typically identified as round, hypoechoic with smooth borders that may be enlarged (> 10 mm) and are usually located near the tumor [1, 32]. The sensitivity and specificity of EUS range from 59.5%–100% to 40%–100%, respectively. However, more precise estimates have indicated that EUS can differentiate positive from negative nodes with a sensitivity and specificity of 85%–97% and 85%–96%, respectively, and an accuracy of 75%. Nonetheless, the false negative rate for EUS is 18%, while the false positive rate is 9% [8, 9, 20, 21, 31, 33].

Despite the accuracy of EUS, understaging of patients with micro metastatic disease is possible, [34]. FNA is a useful adjunct of the study for sampling suspicious nodes. Furthermore, EUS-CT has been shown to be more accurate than either modality alone for N staging, with EUS-CT even outperforming PET, as the sensitivity of combined EUS-CT was 83% compared to 22% for PET [27, 32].

PET-CT and N Staging

PET-CT is more sensitive than CT for detecting lymph node involvement because alterations in tissue metabolism measured by PET generally precede anatomic changes of affected nodes.

The uptake of the primary tumor, however, might sometimes hamper the identification of peri-lesional nodes.

Tumor metabolic activity might also predict the risk of lymphatic involvement. A previous study included patients with seemingly resectable esophageal cancer and analyzed their standardized uptake value (SUV) max on PET-CT with respect to pathologic stage and survival. Patients in the low SUV group (< 4.5) had earlier T stage tumors and lower incidence of nodal metastasis (8%). On the other hand, 48% of patients with SUV max > 4.5 had nodal involvement and this was correlated with poor survival [35].

Overall, one of the main benefits of PET-TC is its improved specificity in detecting lymph node involvement as compared to CT scan (mainly by detecting abnormal metabolic activity even in normal-sized lymph nodes). The PET SUV max of the primary tumor appears also to predict pathologic stage and overall survival. In addition, PET-CT it is a valuable tool to determine response to preoperative therapy (Fig. 7).

"M" Staging

The M classification designates M0 or M1 according to absence or presence of distant metastasis, respectively.

Distant metastases have been detected at initial presentation in 20–30% of patients with esophageal cancer and are most commonly reported in the liver (35%), lungs (20%), bones (9%), adrenal glands (5%), and, rarely, peritoneum and brain. CT, MRI and PET-CT are useful for determining the M status. EUS has limited value for assessing distant metastases because of the small field of view. This study can only detect distant metastases in direct contact with the upper gastrointestinal tract and ascites as an indirect sign of intraperitoneal metastases.

CT Scan and "M" Staging

CT imaging is highly effective in detecting distant metastases in organs such as the liver or lung. In particular, liver metastases are best seen in the portal venous phase as hypoattenuating

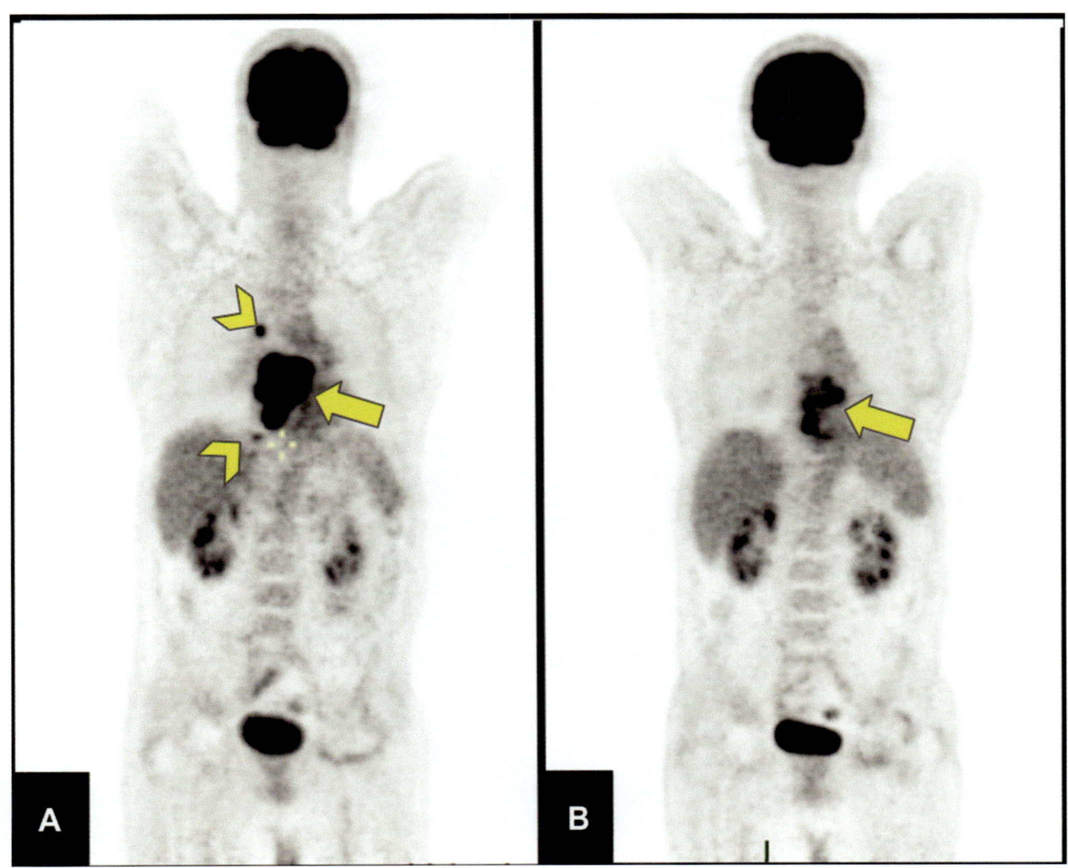

Fig. 7 PET-CT maximum intensity projection (MIP) maps showing tumor downsizing of a patient after neoadjuvant treatment. A) Baseline. Esophageal hypermetabolic wall thickening with periesophageal fat infiltration (T4) with a maximum SUV of 29, 5 and multiple hypermetabolic mediastinal nodes (N3). B) Restaging with partial response. Morphologic and metabolic reduction of the tumor (maximum SUV 8, 8, arrow) and nodal involvement

lesions. While metastatic lung nodules are usually round and smooth-bordered, they might be difficult to diagnose, specially in the absence of prior imaging. In such cases, biopsy by interventional radiology may be helpful.

Compared to PET, CT imaging has reduced sensitivity in detecting bone metastases. Additionally, CT has relatively poor accuracy in identifying peritoneal disease [1, 8, 9, 31, 36].

Accurate determination of M stage with complementary staging modalities such as PET-CT and even diagnostic laparoscopy is needed in some cases [8, 9, 37].

MRI and "M" Staging

Currently, there is scarce data evaluating the efficacy of MRI in detecting distant metastases. Consequently, the precise contribution of MRI for M staging remains uncertain.

PET-CT and "M" Staging

PET-CT is the most accurate imaging method to detect distant metastases. The study covers the entire body and its primary role is to detect distant sites of metastatic disease.

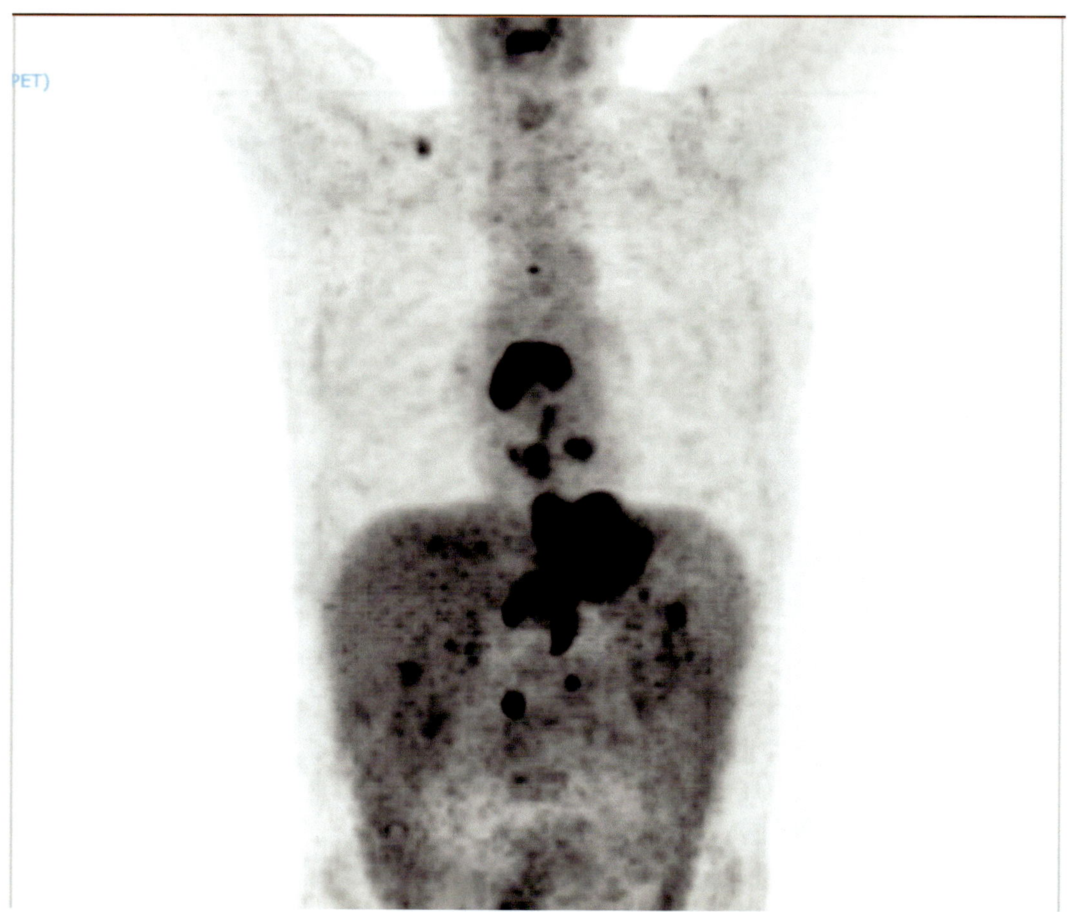

Fig. 8 PET-CT maximum intensity projection (MIP) map of a stage IV esophageal adenocarcinoma of the gastroesophagic junction. Esophageal hypermetabolic wall thickening with a maximum SUV of 22, 2 and multiple sites of distant metastases

Table 2 Performance characteristics of CT, MRI, CT-PET and EUS in the diagnostic workup of esophageal cancer

Modality	Sensitivity	Specificity	Accuracy
CT			
T1, 2, 3, 4	–	–	63%, 72.9%, 75.3%, 74.9% [8]
N	77.2%	78.3%	66.1–87% [8]
M	–	–	81% [8]
M peritoneum	58.8%	98.6%	
M peritoneum	66% [39]	[40]	
MRI			
T	–	–	81% [41]
T4b	86–100%	67–84%	75–87% [30]
N	25–62%	67–88% [30]	
M	–	–	–
CT-PET			
T 1/2	26–63% [8] 43% [25]	–	–
T 3/4	83–100% [8]	–	–
N	24–99%	46–98% [8]	
M	69–78%	–	82–88% [8]
EUS			
T	27.9%	90.9%	79.4% [21]
T1	81.6%	99.4%	66–97% GEJ
T2	81.4%	96.3%	85% [22]
T3	91.4%	94.4%	
T4	92.4%	97.4%	
T0/2vsT/34	79%	[33] 94%	
N	73%	77% [22]	57.1% [34]
w/o FNA	35.3%	90.9%	
w FNA	84.7%	84.6%	
N stage in uT1	96.7%	95.5%	
uT3	0%	90%	
	83%	55% [33]	

Obtained from Schlottmann et al. Esophageal Cancer: Diagnosis and Treatment (Springer, 2018)

PET-CT is superior to CT scan in identifying disease in liver and bones and it is also capable of detecting metastases in unusual locations (e.g. skeletal muscles, subcutaneous tissues, thyroid gland or pancreas). The detection of metastatic disease is critical during the initial evaluation of patients because it will direct patients to a palliative treatment pathway rather to an esophagectomy. During treatment, particularly after neoadjuvant therapy (chemotherapy or chemoradiotherapy), PET-CT is also valuable because it provides information regarding response but more importantly it can detect metastases that have developed since the induction therapy (Figs. 7 and 8) [38] (Table 2).

Conclusions

Effective management of esophageal cancer requires a precise staging. An accurate and thorough methodology during the staging process is indispensable for appropriate treatment selection. Each diagnostic method possesses its own distinct benefits and limitations that should be acknowledged when staging esophageal cancer patients.

References

1. Jayaprakasam VS, et al. Role of imaging in esophageal cancer management in 2020: update for radiologists. Am J Roentgenol. 2020;215:1–13.
2. van Hagen P, et al. Preoperative chemoradiotherapy for esophageal or junctional cancer. N Engl J Med. 2012;366(22):2074–84.
3. Cunningham D, et al. Perioperative chemotherapy versus surgery alone for resectable gastroesophageal cancer. N Engl J Med. 2006;355(1):11–20.
4. Cen P, et al. Value of endoscopic ultrasound staging in conjunction with the evaluation of lymphovascular invasion in identifying low-risk esophageal carcinoma. Cancer. 2008;112(3):503–10.
5. Mariette C, et al. Surgery alone versus chemoradiotherapy followed by surgery for stage I and II

esophageal cancer: final analysis of randomized controlled phase III trial FFCD 9901. J Clin Oncol. 2014;32(23):2416–22.

6. Natsugoe S, et al. Randomized controlled study on preoperative chemoradiotherapy followed by surgery versus surgery alone for esophageal squamous cell cancer in a single institution. Dis Esophagus. 2006;19(6):468–72.

7. Boonstra JJ, et al. Chemotherapy followed by surgery versus surgery alone in patients with resectable oesophageal squamous cell carcinoma: long-term results of a randomized controlled trial. BMC Cancer. 2011;11:181.

8. Hayes T, et al. Staging in esophageal and gastric cancers. Hematol Oncol Clin North Am. 2017;31(3):427–40.

9. Mehta K, et al. Minimally invasive staging of esophageal cancer. Ann Cardiothorac Surg. 2017;6(2):110–8.

10. Rice TW, Patil DT, Blackstone EH. 8th edition AJCC/UICC staging of cancers of the esophagus and esophagogastric junction: application to clinical practice. Ann Cardiothorac Surg. 2017;6(2):119–30.

11. Power SP, Moloney F, Twomey M, James K, O'Connor OJ, Maher MM. Computed tomography and patient risk: Facts, perceptions and uncertainties. World J Radiol. 2016;8(12):902–15.

12. Seevaratnam R, et al. How useful is preoperative imaging for tumor, node, metastasis (TNM) staging of gastric cancer? A meta-analysis. Gastric Cancer. 2012;15(Suppl 1):S3-18.

13. Elsherif SB, et al. Role of precision imaging in esophageal cancer. J Thorac Dis. 2020;12(9):5159–5176.

14. Quint LE, Bogot NR. Staging esophageal cancer. Cancer Imaging. 2008;8(Spec No A):S33–42.

15. Mukherjee P, et al. Imaging of the esophagus. In: Chawla A, editors. Thoracic imaging: basic to advanced. Singapore: Springer; 2019.

16. Guo J, et al. A prospective analysis of the diagnostic accuracy of 3 T MRI, CT and endoscopic ultrasound for preoperative T staging of potentially resectable esophageal cancer. Cancer Imaging. 2020;20(1):64.

17. Zhu Y, et al. The value of magnetic resonance imaging in esophageal carcinoma: tool or toy? Asia Pac J Clin Oncol. 2019;15(3):101–7.

18. Sakurada A, et al. Diagnostic performance of diffusion-weighted magnetic resonance imaging in esophageal cancer. Eur Radiol. 2009;19(6):1461–9.

19. Xing X, et al. Potential use of high-resolution T2-weighted MRI with histopathologic findings in staging esophageal cancer. Quant Imaging Med Surg. 2023;13(1):249–58.

20. Parry K, et al. Staging of adenocarcinoma of the gastroesophageal junction. Eur J Surg Oncol. 2016;42(3):400–6.

21. Bartel MJ, et al. Role of EUS in patients with suspected Barrett's esophagus with high-grade dysplasia or early esophageal adenocarcinoma: impact on endoscopic therapy. Gastrointest Endosc. 2017;86(2):292–8.

22. Barbour AP, et al. Endoscopic ultrasound predicts outcomes for patients with adenocarcinoma of the gastroesophageal junction. J Am Coll Surg. 2007;205(4):593–601.

23. Findlay JM, et al. Pragmatic staging of oesophageal cancer using decision theory involving selective endoscopic ultrasonography PET and laparoscopy. Br J Surg. 2015;102(12):1488–99.

24. Bianco V, et al. Evaluation of the accuracy of endoscopic ultrasound for stage I esophageal cancer. J Am Coll Surg. 219:S29.

25. Bergeron EJ, et al. Endoscopic ultrasound is inadequate to determine which T1/T2 esophageal tumors are candidates for endoluminal therapies. J Thorac Cardiovasc Surg. 2014;147:765–71.

26. Shridhar R, et al. Accuracy of endoscopic ultrasound staging for T2N0 esophageal cancer: a national cancer database analysis. J Gastrointest Oncol. 2018;9(5):887–93.

27. Luu C, et al. Endoscopic ultrasound staging for early esophageal cancer: are we denying patients neoadjuvant chemo-radiation? World J Gastroenterol. 2017;23(46):8193–9.

28. Harewood GC, et al. Assessment of clinical impact of endoscopic ultrasound on esophageal cancer. J Gastroenterol Hepatol. 2004;19(4):433–9.

29. Schmidt T, et al. Value of functional imaging by PET in esophageal cancer. J Natl Compr Cancer Netw. 2015;13(2):239–47.

30. van Rossum PS, et al. Imaging of oesophageal cancer with FDG-PET/CT and MRI. Clin Radiol. 2015;70(1):81–95.

31. Luketich JD, et al. Minimally invasive surgical staging for esophageal cancer. Surg Endosc. 2000;14(8):700–2.

32. DaVee T, et al. Is endoscopic ultrasound examination necessary in the management of esophageal cancer? World J Gastroenterol. 2017;23(5):751–62.

33. Puli SR, et al. Staging accuracy of esophageal cancer by endoscopic ultrasound: a meta-analysis and systematic review. World J Gastroenterol. 2008;14(10):1479–90.

34. Foley KG, et al. Accuracy of contemporary oesophageal cancer lymph node staging with radiological-pathological correlation. Clin Radiol. 2017;72(8):693 e1–693 e7

35. Rizk N, et al. Preoperative 18[F]-fluorodeoxyglucose positron emission tomography standardized uptake values predict survival after esophageal adenocarcinoma resection. Ann Thorac Surg. 2006;81(3):1076–81.

36. Nguyen NT, et al. Evaluation of minimally invasive surgical staging for esophageal cancer. Am J Surg. 2001;182(6):702–6.

37. Meyers BF, et al. The utility of positron emission tomography in staging of potentially operable carcinoma of the thoracic esophagus: results

of the American College of Surgeons Oncology Group Z0060 trial. J Thorac Cardiovasc Surg. 2007;133(3):738–45.

38. Raptis CA, et al. ACR appropriateness criteria® staging and follow-up of esophageal cancer. J Am Coll Radiol. 2022;19(11S):S462-S472.

39. de Graaf GW, et al. The role of staging laparoscopy in oesophagogastric cancers. Eur J Surg Oncol. 2007;33(8):988–92.

40. Leeman MF, et al. Multidetector computed tomography versus staging laparoscopy for the detection of peritoneal metastases in esophagogastric junctional and gastric cancer. Surg Laparosc Endosc Percutan Tech. 2017;27(5):369–74.

41. Riddell AM, et al. The appearances of oesophageal carcinoma demonstrated on high-resolution, T2-weighted MRI, with histopathological correlation. Eur Radiol. 2007;17(2):391–9.

Staging of Esophageal Cancer: Implications for Therapy

Camila Bras Harriott, Manuela Monrabal Lezama, Marco G. Patti and Francisco Schlottmann

Abstract

Different diagnostic tools are used for esophageal cancer staging. The clinical presentation of patients will guide the sequence and type of staging modalities. Currently, endoscopy, endoscopic ultrasound, computed tomography, and positron emission tomography are used for staging in most patients. Accurate staging ultimately helps defining the optimal treatment approach.

Keywords

Esophageal cancer · Staging · CT · PET-CT · Endoscopic ultrasound

C. Bras Harriott · M. Monrabal Lezama ·
F. Schlottmann (✉)
Department of Surgery, Hospital Alemán of
Buenos Aires, 1640 Pueyrredon Ave, Buenos Aires,
Argentina
e-mail: fschlottmann@hotmail.com

C. Bras Harriott
e-mail: cbrasharriott@hospitalaleman.com

M. Monrabal Lezama
e-mail: mmonraballezama@hospitalaleman.com

M. G. Patti
Department of Surgery, University of Virginia,
Charlottesville, VA, USA

F. Schlottmann
Department of Surgery, University of Illinois at Chicago,
Chicago, IL, USA

Introduction

Diagnostic and staging modalities have evolved over the past years. Current staging modalities include endoscopy, endoscopic ultrasound (EUS), computed tomography (CT), and positron emission tomography (PET). Endoscopic mucosal resection (EMR) and/or endoscopic submucosal resection (ESD) can also eventually help staging patients (histopathologic based staging). Accurate staging through the combination of all these methods is critical for appropriate treatment and follow up.

Esophageal cancer staging is defined by the American Joint Committee on Cancer (AJCC) staging system that establishes tumor-node-metastasis (TNM) and it is based on the most recent, 8th edition of the AJCC cancer staging manual for esophagus and esophagogastric junction cancers [1]. Table 1 shows the classifications based on the depth of invasion of the primary tumor (T), lymph node involvement (N), and extent of metastatic disease (M).

Non-anatomic factors also play a role in prognosis, including histologic subtype and tumor grade. Squamous cell carcinoma (SCC) carries a poorer stage specific prognosis, as compared to esophageal adenocarcinoma (EAC). Well and moderately differentiated tumors (G1-2) are associated with improved survival in both SCC and EAC, as compared to poorly differentiated tumors. For SCC,

Table 1 Definitions for T, N, M. AJCC 8th edition staging of esophageal cancer

T	Primary tumor
TX	Primary tumor cannot be assessed
T0	No evidence of primary tumor
TIS	High-grade dysplasia, defined as malignant cells confined to the epithelium by the basement membrane
T1	Tumor invades the lamina propria, muscularis mucosae, or submucosa
T1a	Tumor invades the lamina propria or muscularis mucosae
T1b	Tumor invades the submucosa
T2	Tumor invades the muscularis propria
T3	Tumor invades adventitia
T4	Tumor invades adjacent structures
T4a	Tumor invades the pleura, pericardium, azygos vein, diaphragm or peritoneum
T4b	Tumor invades other adjacent structures, such as the aorta, vertebral body or airway
N	Regional lymph nodes
NX	Regional lymph nodes cannot be assessed
N0	No regional lymph node metastasis
N1	Metastasis in one or two regional lymph nodes
N2	Metastasis in three to six regional lymph nodes
N3	Metastasis in seven or more regional lymph nodes
M	Distant metastasis
M0	No distant metastasis
M1	Distant metastasis
G	Histologic grade
GX	Grade cannot be assessed
G1	Well differentiated
G2	Moderately differentiated
G3	Poorly differentiated, undifferentiated

prognosis is also affected by tumor location, with upper and middle third tumors carrying worse prognosis than tumors of the distal third of the esophagus [1, 2]. Table 2 shows the different clinical staging for EAC and SCC.

Overview of Staging Modalities

The esophagus crosses the neck, thorax and abdomen and is surrounded by important organs and structures (Fig. 1). Lymphatic drainage is

Table 2 Clinical staging for esophageal adenocarcinoma (EAC) and esophageal squamous cell carcinoma (ESCC). AJCC 8th edition staging of esophageal cancer

	T	N	M
EAC			
STAGE 0	Tis	N0	M0
STAGE I	T1	N0	M0
STAGE IIa	T1	N1	M0
STAGE IIb	T2	N0	M0
STAGE III	T2	N1	M0
	T3	N0-1	M0
	T4a	N0-1	M0
STAGE IVa	T1-T4a	N2	M0
	T4b	N0-2	M0
	Any T	N3	M0
STAGE IVb	Any T	Any N	M1
ESCC			
STAGE 0	Tis	N0	M0
STAGE I	T1	N0-1	M0
STAGE II	T2	N0-1	M0
	T3	N0	M0
STAGE III	T3	N1	M0
	T1-T3	N2	M0
STAGE IVa	T4	N0-2	M0
	Any T	N3	M0
STAGE IVb	Any T	Any N	M1

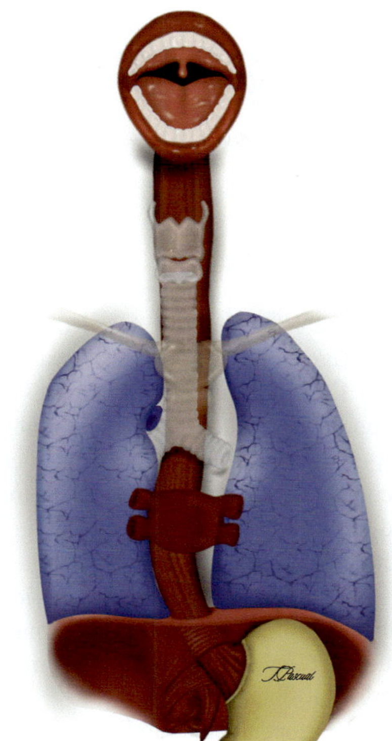

Fig. 1 Esophageal anatomy (Drawing by Tomás Pascual MD)

abundant and somehow erratic (Fig. 2). Staging modalities should be wisely used to determine location, locoregional invasion and potential sites of distant metastases.

Endoscopy

Endoscopy helps to determine the location of the tumor and to obtain tissue sample for histopathologic assessment. The location of the tumor relative to the teeth and esophagogastric junction, the length of the tumor, the degree of obstruction and the extent of circumferential involvement should be carefully assessed to define the treatment planning. For suspected early staged tumors, an endoscopic resection provides more accurate information on the depth of tumor invasion. Endoscopic mucosal

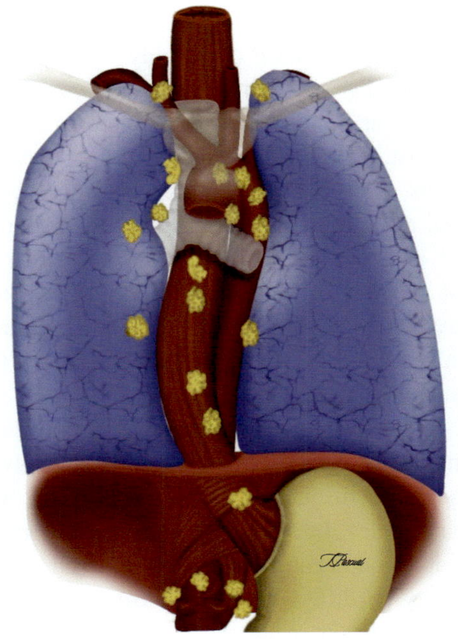

Fig. 2 Regional lymph node stations of the esophagus (Drawing by Tomás Pascual MD)

resection (EMR) and endoscopic submucosal dissection (ESD) can be used to accurately stage and even treat early tumors [3].

EUS

Locoregional staging with EUS provides the most accurate cT staging because is the only method capable of delineating all the layers of the esophageal wall. For early tumors, however, the EUS is limited for distinguishing the extension to the mucosa (T1a) or submucosa (T1b) [4, 5]. For this reason, in these cases an endoscopic resection (EMR or ESD) might be needed for accurate staging [3, 6].

Pathological periesophageal, perigastric or mediastinal lymph nodes can also be identified with this method. The addition of fine-needle aspiration (FNA) of suspected nodes might also help for nodal staging.

Operator dependency and impossibility to perform the study in obstructive tumors are the main limitations of EUS.

CT Scan

CT scan is the most commonly employed staging modality at the time of diagnosis. A CT scan of chest and abdomen with oral and endovenous contrast should be performed. For advanced stages (i.e. obstructed tumors causing dysphagia), a CT scan should be promptly performed. For early asymptomatic tumors, the study will not be able to accurately assess the depth of invasion through the layers of the esophageal wall (EUS plays a more important role in these patients) [7, 8].

Regarding nodal staging, CT scan provides limited information because reactive lymph nodes are difficult to differentiate from metastatic nodes. In addition, peritumoral metastatic lymph nodes can be missed due to the impossibility to differentiate them from the primary tumor. Distant metastases in liver or lungs are well assessed with a high sensitivity [9]. Bone, central nervous system or other infrequent sites of metastasis might be harder to diagnose [7].

PET-CT

This imaging modality is the best method for detecting distant metastases as it is more sensitive than CT alone. SCC tends to be more PET avid than EAC. Furthermore, poorly differentiated EAC or signet ring lesions are more likely to demonstrate low or no PET avidity [10].

In patients with early staged disease, PET-CT has limited value. The study cannot differentiate the depth of invasion of the primary tumor and there is a high likelihood that early (Tis, T1) lesions will be missed given the resolution of this modality [10, 11].

Laparoscopy

The principal role of staging laparoscopy is to identify peritoneal metastases [12]. It is recommended for patients with locally advanced esophagogastric junction tumors, particularly Siewert III tumors. Staging laparoscopy is critical in these patients to ensure that a curative intent surgery is possible and to spare palliative patients the morbidity of an unnecessary operation [13].

Staging and Treatment Algorithm

The appropriate diagnostic workup depends on patient presentation as to suspect early, moderate or advanced stage. In patients who present asymptomatic and the lesion is discovered incidentally or in the context of surveillance for gastroesophageal reflux, early disease is likely to be found. In these cases, EUS (with FNA if necessary) is used to determine T and N stage, combined with CT to rule out occult metastases.

In patients presenting with dysphagia, locally advanced disease is suspected and PET-CT serves as an appropriate starting point. Patients

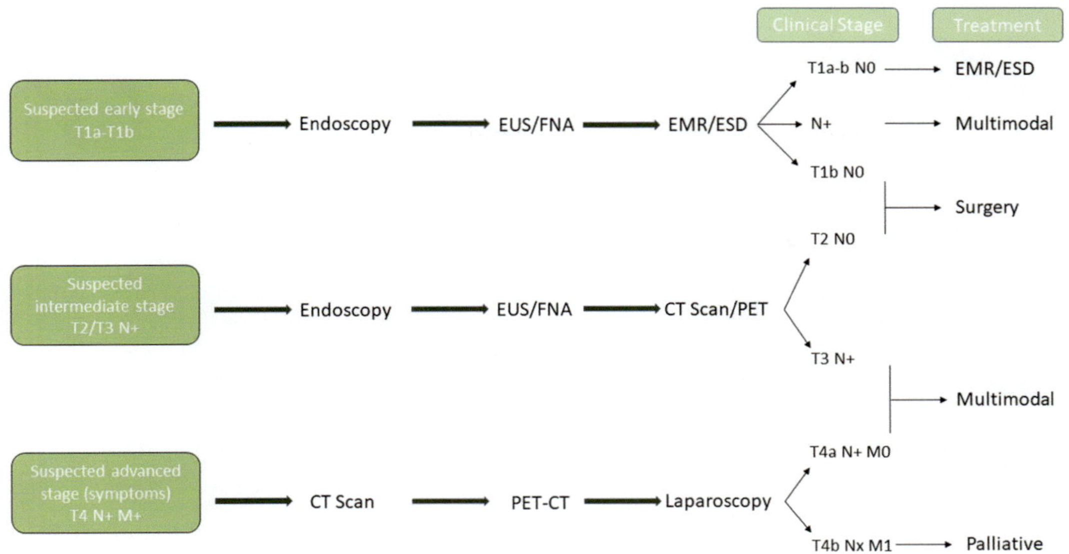

Fig. 3 Staging and treatment algorithm for esophageal cancer. EUS: endoscopic ultrasound. FNA: fine needle aspiration. CT: computed tomography. PET: positron emission tomography. EMR: endoscopic mucosal resection ESD: endoscopic submucosal dissection

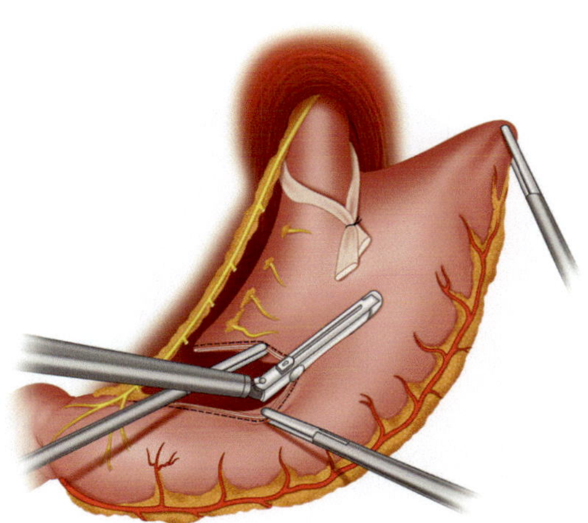

Fig. 4 Creation of gastric conduit

found to be free of occult metastases or node negative should proceed to endoscopy and EUS to further characterize the T stage and obtain tissue for diagnosis.

Patients with bulky abdominal nodal disease, particularly those with esophagogastric junction adenocarcinoma Siewert III, should undergo diagnostic laparoscopy to rule out peritoneal metastasis and further assess resectability (Fig. 3).

For most patients with locally advanced esophageal cancer, minimally invasive esophagectomy remains the cornerstone of curative treatment (Figs. 4, 5, 6, 7, and 8).

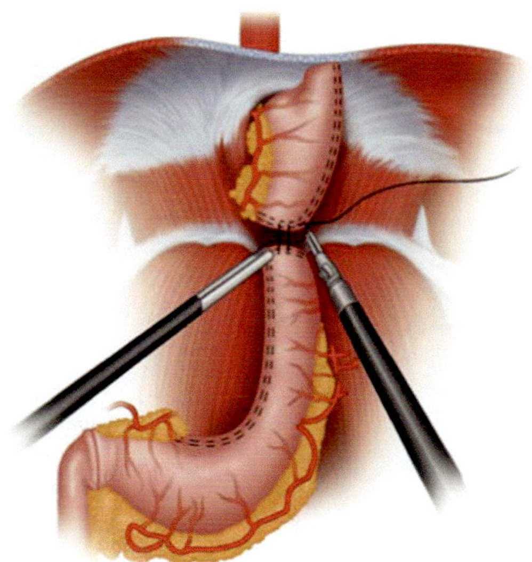

Fig. 5 The gastric conduit will be pulled up to chest

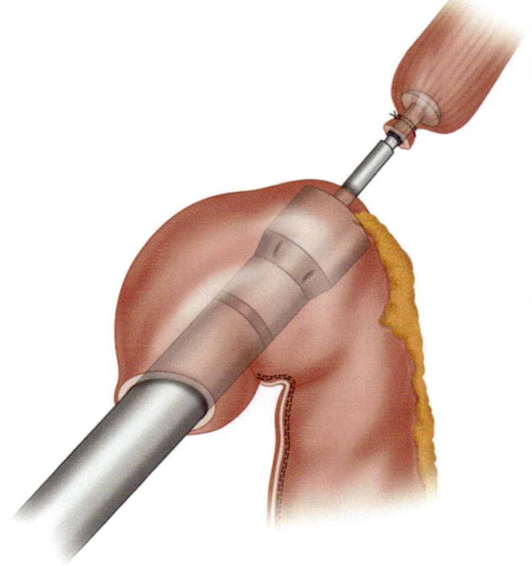

Fig. 7 Esophagogastric anastomosis with circular stapler

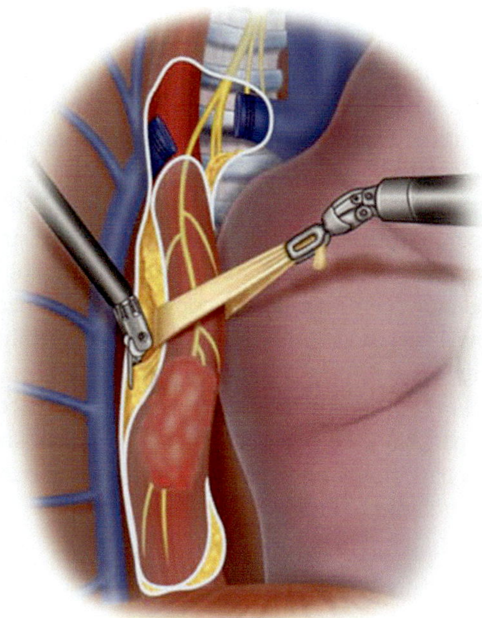

Fig. 6 Dissection of intrathoracic esophagus

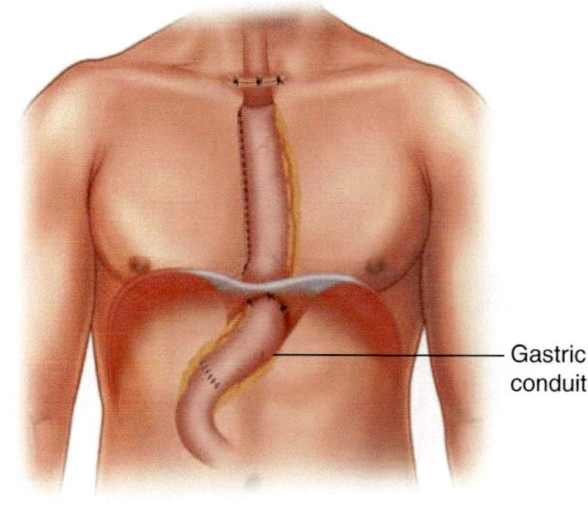

Fig. 8 Final anatomy after reconstruction with gastric conduit

Conflicts of Interest The authors have no conflicts of interest.

References

1. Rice TW, Patil DT, Blackstone EH. 8th edition AJCC/UICC staging of cancers of the esophagus and esophagogastric junction: application to clinical practice. Ann Cardiothorac Surg. 2017;6(2):119–30.
2. Siewert JR, Ott K. Are squamous and adenocarcinomas of the esophagus the same disease? Semin Radiat Oncol. 2007;17:38–44.
3. Ning B, Abdelfatah MM, Othman MO. Endoscopic submucosal dissection and endoscopic mucosal resection for early stage esophageal cancer. Ann Cardiothorac Surg. 2017;6(2):88–98.
4. Kutup A, Link BC, Schurr PG, et al. Quality control of endoscopic ultrasound in preoperative staging of esophageal cancer. Endoscopy. 2007;39:715–9.
5. Pech O, Günter E, Dusemund F, et al. Accuracy of endoscopic ultrasound in preoperative staging of esophageal cancer: results from a referral center for early esophageal cancer. Endoscopy. 2010;42:456–61.
6. Choi J, Kim SG, Kim JS, Jung HC, Song IS. Comparison of endoscopic ultrasonography (EUS), positron emission tomography (PET), and computed tomography (CT) in the preoperative locoregional staging of resectable esophageal cancer. Surg Endosc. 2010;24(6):1380–6.
7. Hayes T, et al. Staging in esophageal and gastric cancers. Hematol Oncol Clin North Am. 2017;31(3):427–40.
8. Erasmus JJ, Munden RF. The role of integrated computed tomography positron-emission tomography in esophageal cancer: staging and assessment of therapeutic response. Semin Radiat Oncol. 2007;17(1):29–37.
9. Berry MF. Esophageal cancer: staging system and guidelines for staging and treatment. J Thorac Dis. 2014;6 Suppl 3(Suppl 3):S289–97.
10. Schmidt T, et al. Value of functional imaging by PET in esophageal cancer. J Natl Compr Cancer Netw. 2015;13(2):239–47.
11. Van Rossum PSN, van Lier ALHMW, Lips IM, Meijer GJ, Reerink O, van Vulpen M, Lam MGEH, van Hillegersberg R, Ruurda JP. Imaging of oesophageal cancer with FDG-PET/CT and MRI. Clin Radiol. 2015;70(1):81–95.
12. Nguyen NT, et al. Evaluation of minimally invasive surgical staging for esophageal cancer. Am J Surg. 2001;182(6):702–6.
13. de Graaf GW, et al. The role of staging laparoscopy in oesophagogastric cancers. Eur J Surg Oncol. 2007;33(8):988–92.

Endoscopic Management of Early Esophageal Cancer

Noel E. Donlon and Lorenzo Ferri

Abstract

Although esophagectomy is an effective treatment of early esophageal cancer, due to high rates of morbidity and potential mortality, and also, importantly, the potentially reduced quality of life, endoscopic therapy represents a favorable approach where appropriate. Endoscopic resection therapies have been successfully applied to selected patients with early tumors of the esophagus with equivalent oncological outcomes. This chapter will address the selection of tumors appropriate for endoscopic resection and review the technical approaches and outcomes of the two main technical approaches, including Endoscopic Mucosal Resection (EMR) and Endoscopic Submucosal Dissection (ESD).

N. E. Donlon (✉)
Department of Surgery, St James's Hospital, Trinity College Dublin, Dublin, Ireland
e-mail: donlonn@tcd.ie

L. Ferri
Division of Thoracic and Upper Gastrointestinal Surgery, Montreal General Hospital—McGill University Health Center, Montreal, QC, Canada
e-mail: lorenzo.ferri@mcgill.ca

Keywords

Esophageal cancer · Early esophageal cancer · EMR · ESD

Introduction

Esophageal cancer has exponentially increased annually in the contemporary era, with a shift in anatomical and histological subtype from esophageal squamous cell carcinoma to adenocarcinoma in North America and Western Europe [1]. Although the overall 5-year relative survival rate is only approximately 20%, patients with early-stage disease have a better chance of survival, and cure rates of successfully treated early esophageal cancer approach 90%.

The conventional treatment of localized disease consists of esophagectomy, open initially and currently minimally invasively. Although traditional surgical resection is an effective treatment of early esophageal cancer, due to high rates of morbidity 50–60%, and potential mortality of 1–3%, and also, importantly, the potentially reduced quality of life, endoscopic therapy represents a favorable approach where appropriate [2]. Indeed, endoscopic resection therapies have been successfully applied to selected patients with early tumors of the esophagus with equivalent oncological outcomes. This chapter will address the selection of tumors appropriate

for endoscopic resection and review the technical approaches and outcomes of the two main technical approaches, including Endoscopic Mucosal Resection (EMR) and Endoscopic Submucosal Dissection (ESD).

Selecting the Appropriate Tumors for Endoscopic Resection

To justify an organ-sparing endoscopic resection approach for cure, two main criteria must be met: (1) negligible rate of occult lymph node metastasis and (2) ability to resect the lesion completely en bloc with negative margins, particularly the deep margin. Staging investigations are often required to eliminate clinically apparent regional/distant disease, including cross-sectional imaging, endoscopic ultrasound, and PET scans.

There is an exponentially increased incidence of nodal disease with advancing T stage. Consequently, it is essential to appropriately stage the patient ab initio to delineate patients suitable for endotherapy versus those necessitating a formal resection. The esophageal wall comprises four layers, with the mucosa being the most superficial layer. The mucosa encompasses the epithelium, lamina propria, and muscularis mucosa. Immediately beyond is the submucosa, which is made of connective tissue, including blood vessels, lymphatics, and Meissner's plexus. The submucosa connects the mucosa to the muscularis propria, made of inner circular and outer longitudinal muscle layers along with the Auerbach plexus. The deepest level comprised of connective tissue is called the adventitia.

The incidence of nodal metastases directly correlates to the subclassification of T1a and T1b disease, with invasion confined to the epithelium (m1), laminal propria (m2), or muscularis propria (m3) for T1a disease, and lesions infiltrating the submucosa (T1b) can be further categorized into sm1 (inner third), sm2 (middle third) and sm3 (outer third) (Table 1 and Fig. 1).

For decades, oncological surgical resection was the conventional curative therapy for malignancies of the esophagus. Endoscopic therapy of early carcinomas is now increasingly established as the gold standard, with the main challenge still to diagnose and carry out endoscopic therapy in good time before metastasis. It is also important to note that tumors over 2 cm with adverse features of tumor biology, such as poor differentiation, have higher incidences of metastases, with late diagnosis still common due to the indolent nature of the disease. Some scoring algorithms have been devised as simple metrics to predict those at risk of lymph node metastasis (LNM) to aid decision-making in patients with T1 esophageal adenocarcinoma undergoing endoscopic resection [3].

Table 1 Incidence of lymph node metastases by depth of invasion into mucosa and submucosal layers (from Araki et al., Endo et al., Westerterp et al., Leers et al., Bollschweiler et al., and Leers et al.)

Tumors	Depth of invasion (AJCC staging)	Rate of lymph node metastasis adenocarcinoma %	Rate of lymph node metastasis squamous cell cancer %
Mucosal M1	Limited to the epithelial layer (Tis)	0	0
M2	Invades the lamina propria (T1a)	0	0
M3	Invades into, but not through, the muscularis mucosae (T1a)	0–6	0–8
Submucosal SM1	Penetrates the shallowest one-third of the submucosa (T1b)	0–22	8–33
SM2	Penetrates into the intermediate one-third of the submucosa (T1b)	0–35	17–30
SM3	Penetrates the deepest one-third of the submucosa (T1b)	26–78	36–69

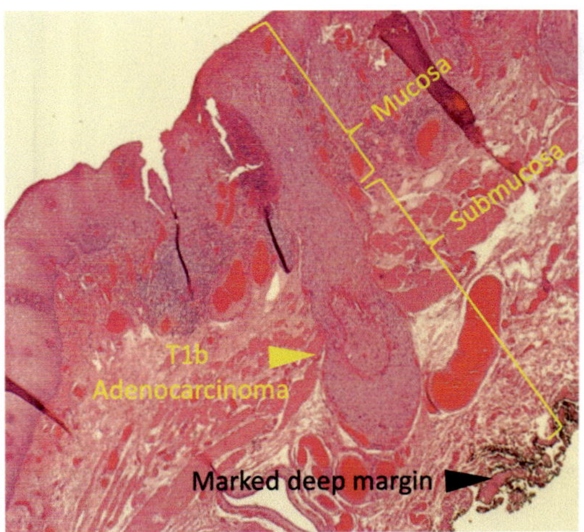

Fig. 1 Risk of nodal metastases increases exponentially with submucosal invasion

Diagnostic and Staging Work-Up

To facilitate patient stratification, pre-treatment evaluation of esophageal cancer consists of locoregional staging and evaluation for distant metastases. Locoregional staging assesses both the degree of extension of the tumor into the esophageal wall and the nodal status. As already alluded to, as tumor depth progresses, so does the risk of LNM. From older surgical series, the rate of LNM in treatment-naive resected esophageal adenocarcinoma ranges between 0 and 7%. Most series have a clinically negligible rate of regional disease on pathology for pathology T1a tumors [4]. In comparison, this risk increases to up to 27% for T1b adenocarcinoma.

The Society of Thoracic Surgeons has published guidelines on staging patients with esophageal cancer [5]. Fluorodeoxyglucose (FDG) positron-emission tomography (PET) scans can improve overall staging by detecting metastatic disease in up to 15–20% of patients and should complement conventional CT imaging to identify metastatic disease [6]. In addition, FDG-PET has also been shown to have prognostic value that can be applied to patient management and aid in developing emerging therapies.

EUS aids locoregional staging and can guide treatment planning of esophageal cancer in the absence of distant metastases. In early esophageal cancer, T staging may help select appropriate cases for minimally invasive treatment using EMR and ESD techniques. Puli and colleagues reported the sensitivity and specificity of EUS for staging esophageal cancer to be 81.6 and 99.4% in T1 tumors [7]. The specificity and the sensitivity for identifying lymph node disease are better when EUS is combined with fine-needle aspiration (FNA) or fine needle biopsy (FNB) compared to EUS alone [8].

There are occasions where additional studies may be worthwhile before therapies are initiated, such as bronchoscopy considered for tumors in the upper and middle esophagus to rule out airway invasion. Although staging laparoscopy has been suggested for locally advanced esophagogastric junction adenocarcinoma, in early esophageal disease, the risk of peritoneal involvement is nominal, and thus this diagnostic test can be avoided.

Chromoendoscopy and advanced endoscopic imaging techniques have the potential to improve the workup of patients with early esophageal neoplastic lesions. It involves using dye stains such as Lugol's iodine for squamous cell cancer, acetic acid for Barrett's esophagus, and Narrow Band Imaging (NBI), enabling detailed lesion assessment and extent (Figs. 2 and 3).

Lugol's solution highlights glycogen-rich nonkeratinized squamous epithelium. An abnormal staining pattern is present in conditions that deplete glycogen in squamous cells, including dysplastic and early neoplastic lesions. Lugol's iodine has a sensitivity of 91–100% and a specificity of 40–95% for detecting squamous neoplasia in the esophagus.

Acetic acid improves the diagnostic yield for identifying Barrett's esophagus specialized columnar epithelium in comparison to random biopsies (57% vs. 26%, $P = 0.12$) [9, 10].

NBI has been combined with magnification endoscopy to predict the invasion depth of superficial squamous cell cancer [11]. Lugol's chromoendoscopy is a simple technique in which the liquid is sprayed into the mucosa

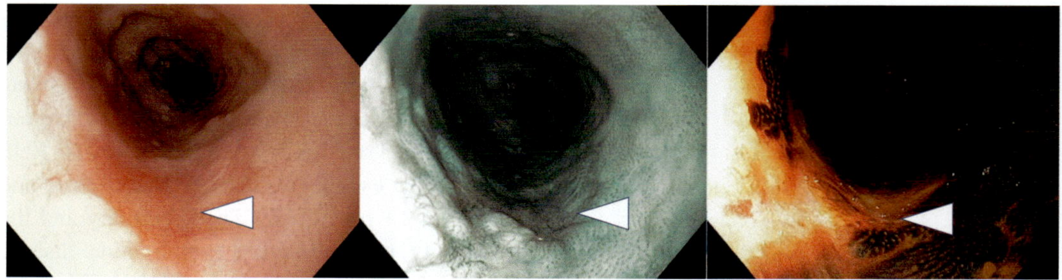

Fig. 2 Mid esophageal squamous cell carcinoma under white light, NBI, and Lugol's Iodine

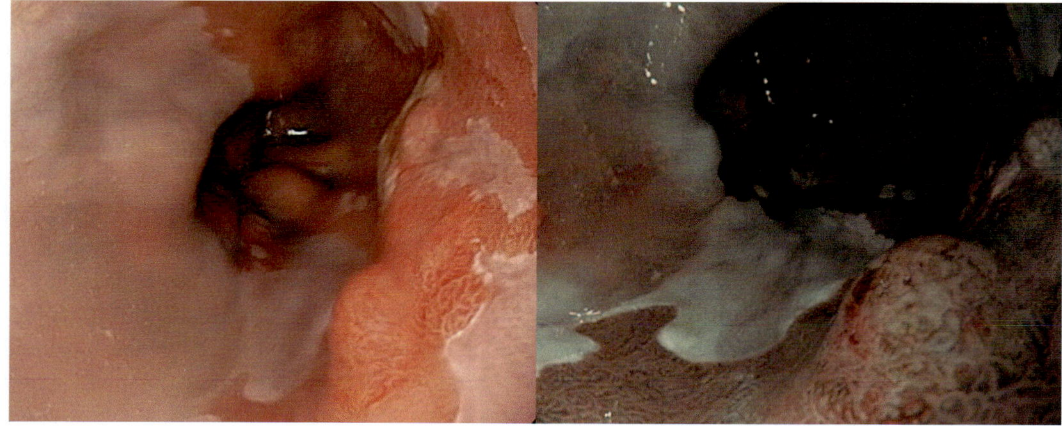

Fig. 3 Esophageal adenocarcinoma in field of Barrett's esophagus under white light and NBI

through an injection spray catheter via the endoscope's working channel. The iodine-potassium iodide forms a dark brown complex with the physiological squamous epithelium, which allows the delineation of dysplastic carcinoma cells that do not stain, and this helps with the sometimes-difficult differentiation from healthy tissue, which is essential for R0 resection. NBI can also enhance the mucosa and the underlying vascular pattern, providing greater convenience for evaluation.

Endoscopic Mucosal Resection (EMR)

Endoscopic mucosal resection (EMR) is a technique that was originally pioneered and introduced in 1978 in Japan for early gastric cancer [12]. In the contemporary era, endoscopic techniques have replaced the traditional process of esophagectomy as the preferred treatment modality for high-grade dysplastic Barrett's, intramucosal cancer [13], and in cases of early invasive cancer, with the decision influenced by the risk of LNM.

"Early carcinoma of the esophagus" is not uniformly defined and refers in the following to in situ and T1 tumors in non-metastatic disease. Notwithstanding higher cure rates are achieved with esophagectomy, the decision on treatment strategy must be borne in mind with the significant treatment-related morbidity and mortality, even in very experienced high volume tertiary referral centers, between 2 and 7% and up to 20% in others [14, 15]. In addition to this, high-risk cardiovascular patients may not be able to tolerate the anesthesia or esophagectomy itself, leaving very few options available for these patients.

Curative endoscopic resection for mucosal carcinomas is possible in adenocarcinoma, analogous to early squamous cell carcinoma. Consequently, endoscopic resection has evolved to become the first-line therapy for managing superficial early esophageal neoplasia. The term *superficial*, however, is in some ways confusing, because it is not directly related to histology or invasiveness of a GI cancer but simply describes the endoscopic appearance of a lesion, which looks to be restricted to *superficial* layers of the GI tract. EMR is an established simpler and faster technique compared to endoscopic submucosal dissection (ESD) but is limited by its inability to resect large lesions en bloc. In essence, piecemeal EMR of large lesions includes a high rate of recurrence and arduous tissue specimen histologic evaluation for accurate staging and margin assessment for R0 resections.

There is a significant risk of leaving disease behind with up to 30% local recurrence with EMR of lesions > 1 cm [16]. Alternatively, ESD, on the other hand, is technically more complex, and traditionally has been associated with a higher rate of adverse events but facilitates en bloc resection regardless of lesion size, reducing risk for recurrence and facilitating precise histologic staging. Ultimately, the optimal endoscopic technique should be selected based on organ location, type of neoplastic lesion, and local expertise. The role of ESD has expanded in Eastern regions beyond squamous cell lesions in the esophagus and gastric cancer to include superficial Barrett's esophagus (BE). However, there is controversy in Western regions over the use of ESD for BE. Thus, focusing on practical considerations for formulating the most appropriate endoscopic resection approach for each patient must be applied.

Although there are several approaches for EMR, we prefer the band ligation technique (Fig. 4). After a lesion is sucked into the overtube, a rubber band is released to form a pseudopolyp. Once the ligation device is detached, the pseudopolyp is removed at the base with a diathermy snare under or above the rubber band. The standard multi-bander ligation devices necessitate the removal of the endoscope to disassemble the ligation device and reintroduce the endoscope to remove the pseudopolyp with a standard polypectomy snare. Although some endoscopists recommend a prior submucosal

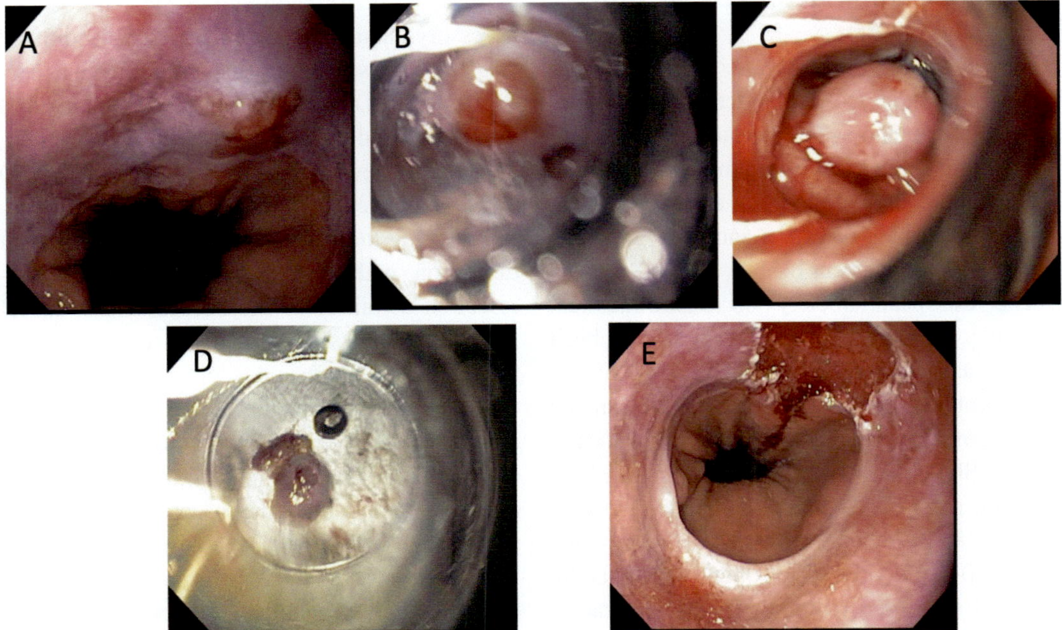

Fig. 4 Steps of endoscopic mucosal resection (EMR) of an early esophageal adenocarcinoma

injection to facilitate elevation of the mucosa [17], we have found that this is not necessary in the vast majority of cases and do not perform this technical step routinely. The specimen is then fixed for the pathologist. For larger lesions, several sequential EMRs are required, complicating accurate pathological assessment of mucosal margin status.

The recommendation for endoscopic resection for m1 to m3 adenocarcinoma remains steadfast and is made based on patient factors and the risk of metastatic disease with high-risk disease or poor prognostic factors such as adverse biology [17, 18]. In the case of sm1 carcinomas, a deep infiltration of $<500\,\mu m$ is required for endoscopic resection, otherwise, there is a borderline case between surgical and endoscopic therapy [19]. The Japan Esophageal Society provides primary endoscopic resection for m1/m2 carcinomas. In the case of m3 carcinomas, the general condition essentially determines whether surgical, endoscopic, or radio/chemotherapy is indicated. The recommendations apply regardless of the histopathological typing/grading [20].

Endoscopic Submucosal Dissection (ESD)

Endoscopic submucosal dissection (ESD) was developed in Japan as an alternative to the limitations of the well-established modality of EMR for the curative treatment for early GI cancer facilitating en bloc resection and, therefore, histopathologic assessment [21].

The European Society of Gastrointestinal Endoscopy (ESGE) guidelines which have been updated as of June 2022 advocate ESD as the first option for superficial esophageal squamous cell carcinoma (SCC) with a series of 15 studies on ESD for superficial SCC finding en bloc resection rates of 83–100%, complete resection rates of 78–100%, and low rates of local recurrence of 0–2.6% [22]. Consequently, ESD is the preferred treatment modality for M1 (intraepithelial) and M2 (invasion into the lamina propria) disease.

To ensure the correct patient cohort is selected, tumor morphology should be employed to predict tumor depth. Paris classification lesions 0-IIa, 0-IIb, and 0-IIc are typically intramucosal and the Japan Esophageal Society guidelines have advocated Paris 0-II lesions with m1–m2 invasion and $<2/3$ circumferential extent as absolute indications for endoscopic resection. The rationale for this recommendation is based on the negligible risk of LNM for M1 and M2 disease as well as the morbidity and mortality of esophagectomy.

The role of ESD in Barrett's esophagus-related adenocarcinoma is limited due to the high efficacy of EMR. Endoscopic ablation of Barrett's esophagus is a gold standard treatment for patients with high-grade dysplasia in the absence of visible lesions. Endoscopic resection is the treatment of choice for patients with visible or flat neoplasia. EMR is a technically limited resection as it is piecemeal resection which hinders determination of negative margins. A systematic review compared outcomes of ESD and EMR and there were no significant differences in local recurrence rates, positive margins, lymph node positivity, complications, or patients requiring surgery [23, 24].

ESD is performed with a standard, single accessory-channel endoscope. Carbon dioxide is used for insufflation. Special equipment necessary for ESD is a transparent cap, submucosal injection needle and solutions, ESD knives, coagulation devices, and endoclips. Typical ESD is accomplished in a stepwise manner, including marking the lesion, incision and submucosal dissection with simultaneous hemostasis. Pre-resection definition of the border of esophageal neoplasms is essential to avoid compromising the margins. Chromoendoscopy or NBI, as illustrated above, can be useful for pre-procedural assessment. An argon plasma coagulation (APC) or ESD knife using a soft coagulation current can be applied to mark the resection borders with dots around the lesion (Fig. 5). This should be at least 1 mm away from the margin of the invasive component of the tumor. If resecting early cancer within a field of Barrett's esophagus, it is not necessary to resect all of the flat columnar

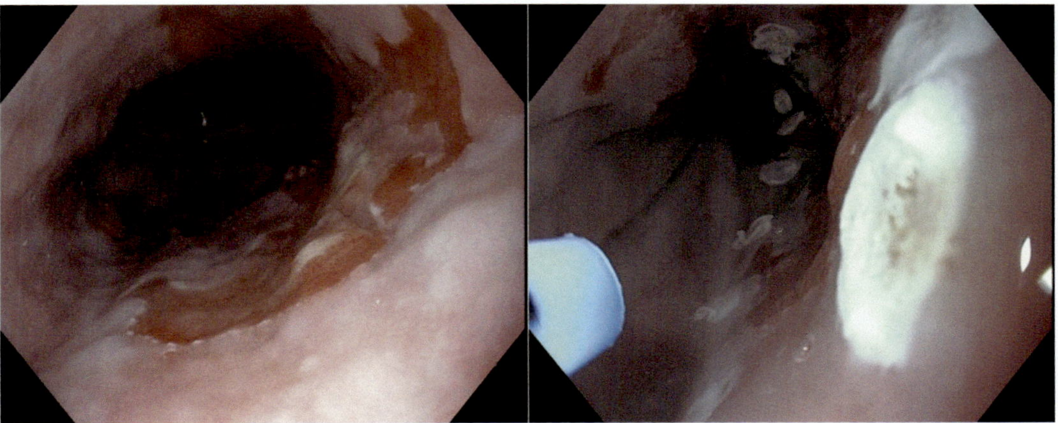

Fig. 5 Marking margins of resection with argon plasma coagulation (APC)/dual knife in a patient with C4M5 Barrett's in a cT1b lesion

mucosa, which can be addressed by subsequent ablative therapies at a separate setting.

After the resection borders are marked, an injectable liquid can be injected beneath the mucosa and submucosa off of the muscularis propria by an injection needle through the endoscopic channel to create a cushion. Although several elevating liquids have been proposed, such as hyaluronic acid, we have generally used cheaper options, such as glycerol 10% or a readily available intravenous starched-based volume expander (Fig. 6).

A circumferential incision is made along the marginal markings. For esophageal ESDs we usually mark the distal extent of the lesion first to define the end point (Fig. 7), followed by the proximal incision (Fig. 8). Then, the mucosal incision is imitated with an uncovered needle knife or a short blunt-tip knife prior to generating a submucosal tunnel.

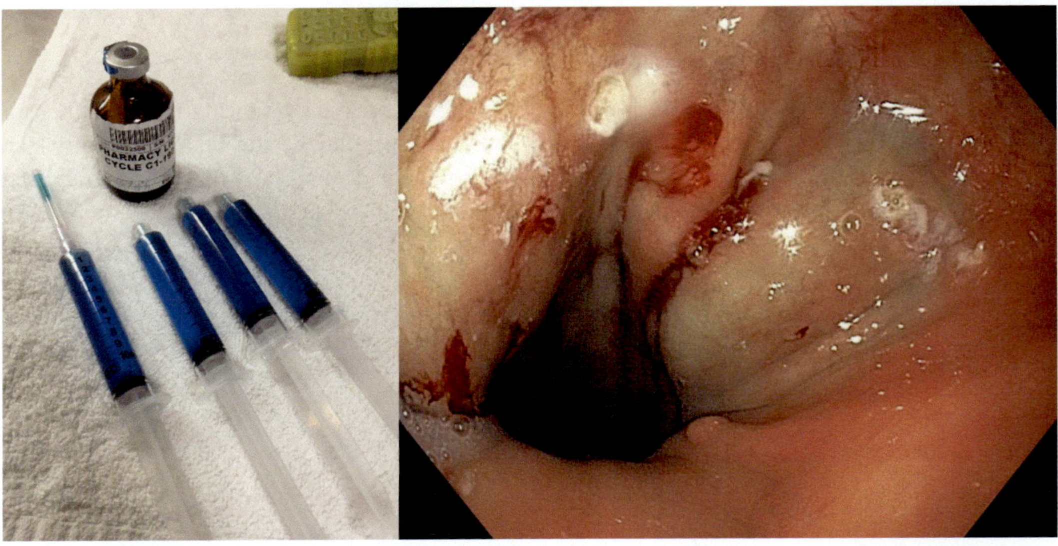

Fig. 6 Submucosa injected with Glycerol 10% (displayed) or commercially available intravenous starch volume expander

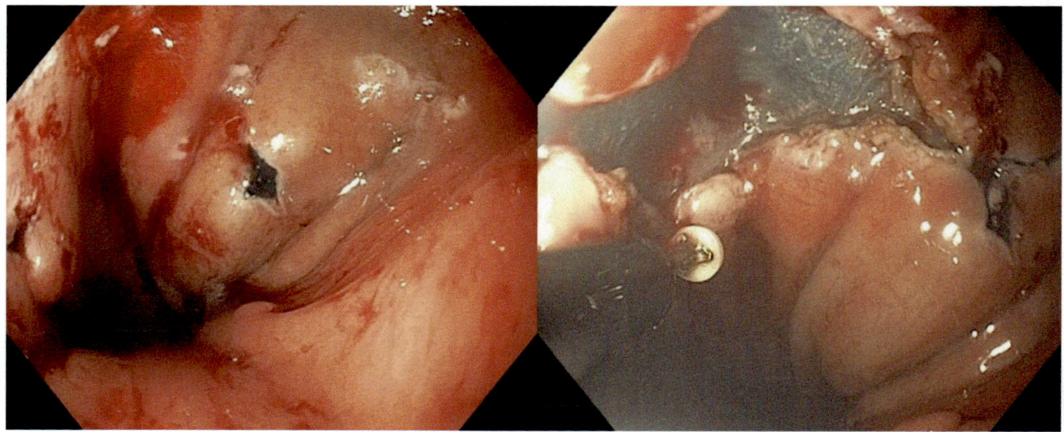

Fig. 7 Initiating the distal margin mucosal incision

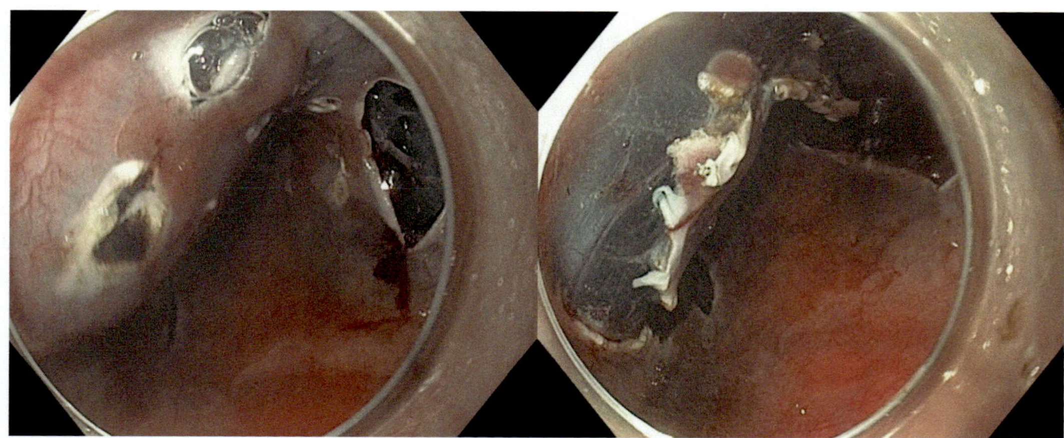

Fig. 8 Identifying and defining the proximal margin

Starting at the proximal cut, we begin a submucosal tunnel to cut the distal mucosal margin (Fig. 9). The entire lesion is stripped or peeled from the muscularis propria by ESD knives in the submucosal space. During this step, the submucosal injection needle and ESD knives are used interchangeably to lift the lesion and dissect the submucosal tissue (Fig. 10).

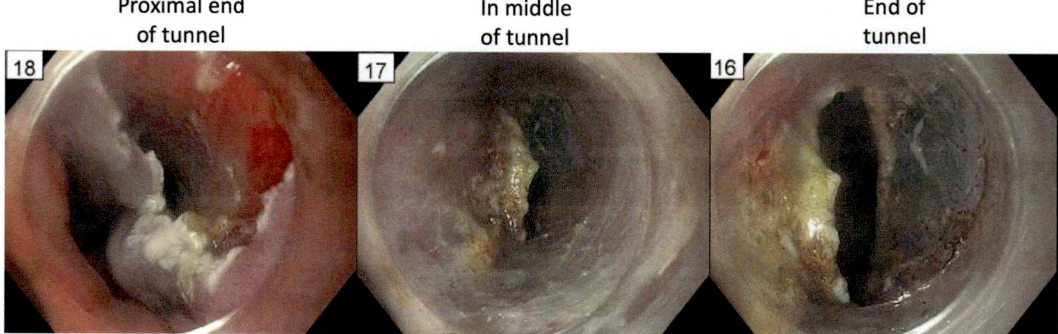

Fig. 9 Sequential imaging of the submucosal tunnel during dissection from proximal to end of the tunnel

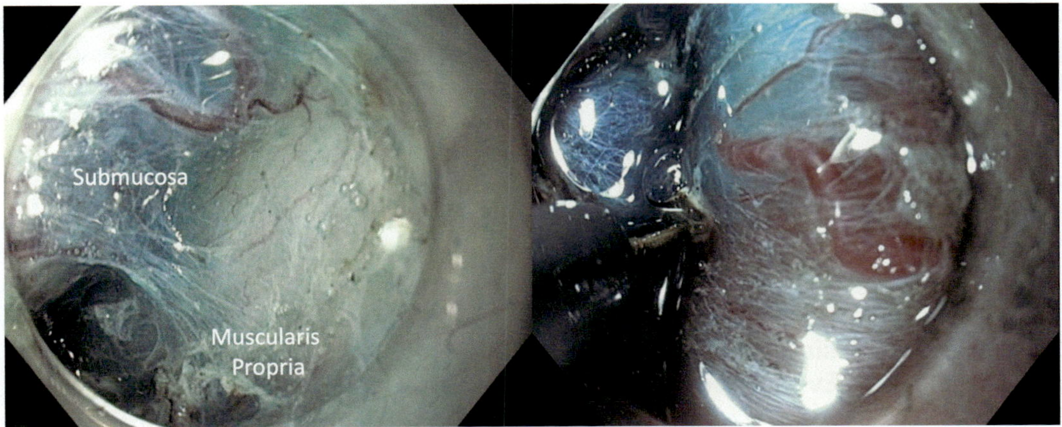

Fig. 10 Submucosal dissection lifting mucosa/submucosal (blue) off of the muscularis propria with the distal cap and dissection submucosa-MP junction with IT2 or Dual knife

EMR/ESD Complications

Bleeding

A potential complication of ESD is bleeding, which can occur during the procedure or as a delayed phenomenon. Therefore, meticulous and prophylactic coagulation and prompt identification and treatment are essential for successful patient outcomes, with various tools available to do so. All ESD knives have at least a limited capacity for hemostasis on small bleeding points. The ball tip knives typically have improved hemostatic efficiency compared with standard needle knives [25]. Hybrid knives have been demonstrated to reduce the need for hemostatic devices and regular hemostasis compared with conventional knives [26]. It is important to balance the use of these coagulation devices with potential thermal injury.

For larger vessels and associated bleeds, specific hemostatic devices may be necessary. The Coagrasper (Olympus, Tokyo, Japan) is a monopolar forceps which is commonly used during ESD. Clips are not widely used for bleeding intraprocedural as they can interfere with continued dissection. They are thus reserved for uncontrolled bleeding or at the end of dissection.

Perforation

There is also an increased risk of perforation with ESD compared to EMR. Risk estimates range from 0 to 6.9% in esophageal ESD, and 2.4 to 9.6% in gastric ESD [27, 28]. Perforation may be visualized as a definite defect during the procedure or delayed after the procedure is diagnosed clinically or on radiograph or CT demonstrating pneumoperitoneum.

The use of conservative decompression with nasogastric or nasoduodenal tubes to divert gastrointestinal fluid and nutritional support during healing post-repair is also advocated for the successful management of these complications. A chest drain may also be warranted for pneumothoraxes or defects in the pleura resulting in effusions. Small defects of approximately 1 cm can generally be treated by through the scope clips, while over-the-scope clips may be considered for holes less than 2 cm [29], and fully covered self-expanding metallic stents are always a salvage option.

Strictures

Strictures are common after any esophageal resection, with the phenomenon more frequently encountered post esophageal ESD than other

GI tract areas. Esophageal strictures occur in patients who undergo more than a 75% circumference ESD resection of the esophagus. The multimodal treatment of strictures includes one or more sessions of endoscopic balloon dilatation which may be combined with local injection of steroids (triamcinolone, betamethasone) or implantation of a temporal esophageal stent.

Specimen Processing and Histological Evaluation

After specimen retrieval, it is placed on the cork board and orientated. After fixation and sectioning, it is essential to critically assess pathology for (*a*) mucosal and deep margins, and (*b*) histological features predicting occult lymph node metastasis to provide a consistent and accurate diagnosis (Fig. 11).

Several factors, such as maintenance of proper orientation, meticulous macroscopic examination, accurate mapping of the lesion, and appropriate morphologic diagnosis are the main concerns. It is important to mention that the maintenance of orientation is crucial in slicing, histological analysis, and reporting. The factors relevant to prognosis and further treatment decisions, include histologic type, the size of the lesion, depth of invasion, association conditions (ulcer/scar), lymphovascular/venous invasion, and cut margin status (horizontal and vertical), which should always be carefully evaluated and reported.

After careful analysis by an appropriately experienced pathologist and discussion at the tumor board, any cases with positive margins should be considered for an esophagectomy [30]. There is no robust data available on surveillance endoscopy for such cases [31, 32]. However, mitigating circumstances such as those who are heavily co-morbid may be more appropriately managed with a watch and wait approach.

Conclusions

Endoscopic resection of early esophageal cancer is a feasible and safe treatment strategy in appropriately selected early esophageal lesions. EMR and ESD are acceptable endoscopic treatment modalities for these early esophageal cancer lesions. ESD requires technical expertise but is associated with higher rates of en bloc, R0, and curative resections and lower recurrence

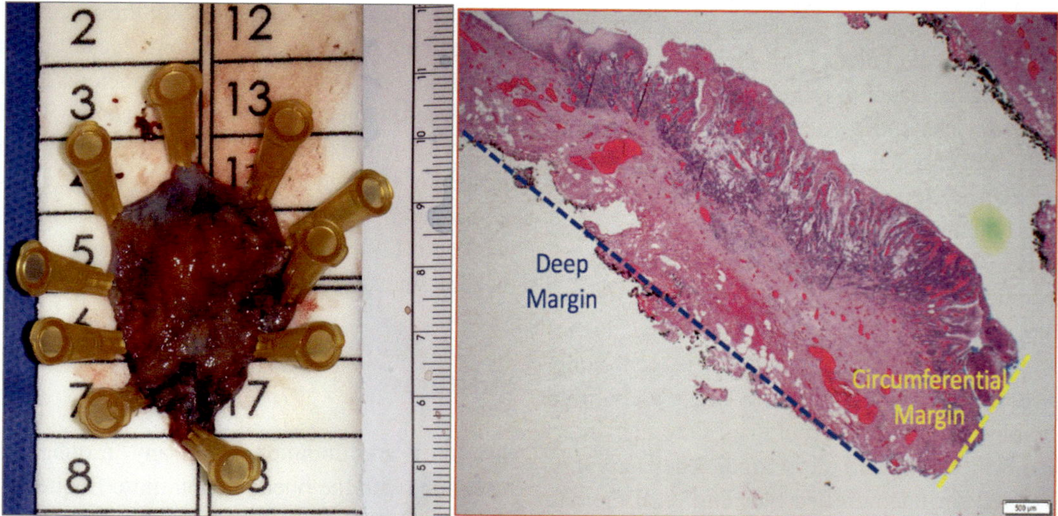

Fig. 11 Orientating the specimen of an early esophago-gastric junctional tumor with histological analysis for assessment of deep and circumferential (mucosal) margins

rates compared to EMR. It is paramount to ensure sufficient training and institutional support for obtaining safe and high-quality resections. Ultimately, the choice of resection technique is made individually and not least depending on the circumstances of the treating center. Hybrid techniques are being evaluated to provide an optimal approach to combine the advantages of ESD and EMR.

References

1. Brown LM, Devesa SS, Chow WH. Incidence of adenocarcinoma of the esophagus among white Americans by sex, stage, and age. J Natl Cancer Inst. 2008;100(16):1184–7.
2. Zheng H, Kang N, Huang Y, Zhao Y, Zhang R. Endoscopic resection versus esophagectomy for early esophageal cancer: a meta-analysis. Transl Cancer Res. 2021;10(6):2653–62.
3. Lee L, Ronellenfitsch U, Hofstetter WL, Darling G, Gaiser T, Lippert C, et al. Predicting lymph node metastases in early esophageal adenocarcinoma using a simple scoring system. J Am Coll Surg. 2013;217(2):191–9.
4. Barbour AP, Jones M, Brown I, Gotley DC, Martin I, Thomas J, et al. Risk stratification for early esophageal adenocarcinoma: analysis of lymphatic spread and prognostic factors. Ann Surg Oncol. 2010;17(9):2494–502.
5. Varghese TK Jr, Hofstetter WL, Rizk NP, Low DE, Darling GE, Watson TJ, et al. The society of thoracic surgeons guidelines on the diagnosis and staging of patients with esophageal cancer. Ann Thorac Surg. 2013;96(1):346–56.
6. Yang GY, Wagner TD, Jobe BA, Thomas CR. The role of positron emission tomography in esophageal cancer. Gastrointest Cancer Res. 2008;2(1):3–9.
7. Puli SR, Reddy JB, Bechtold ML, Antillon D, Ibdah JA, Antillon MR. Staging accuracy of esophageal cancer by endoscopic ultrasound: a meta-analysis and systematic review. World J Gastroenterol. 2008;14(10):1479–90.
8. Facciorusso A, Crinò SF, Muscatiello N, Gkolfakis P, Samanta J, Londoño Castillo J, et al. Endoscopic ultrasound fine-needle biopsy versus fine-needle aspiration for tissue sampling of abdominal lymph nodes: a propensity score matched multicenter comparative study. Cancers (Basel). 2021;13(17).
9. Dawsey SM, Fleischer DE, Wang GQ, Zhou B, Kidwell JA, Lu N, et al. Mucosal iodine staining improves endoscopic visualization of squamous dysplasia and squamous cell carcinoma of the esophagus in Linxian China. Cancer. 1998;83(2):220–31.
10. Hoffman A, Korczynski O, Tresch A, Hansen T, Rahman F, Goetz M, et al. Acetic acid compared with i-scan imaging for detecting Barrett's esophagus: a randomized, comparative trial. Gastrointest Endosc. 2014;79(1):46–54.
11. Inoue H, Kaga M, Ikeda H, Sato C, Sato H, Minami H, et al. Magnification endoscopy in esophageal squamous cell carcinoma: a review of the intrapapillary capillary loop classification. Ann Gastroenterol. 2015;28(1):41–8.
12. Faivre J, Bory R, Moulinier B. Benign tumors of oesophagus: value of endoscopy. Endoscopy. 1978;10(4):264–8.
13. Westerterp M, Koppert LB, Buskens CJ, Tilanus HW, ten Kate FJ, Bergman JJ, et al. Outcome of surgical treatment for early adenocarcinoma of the esophagus or gastro-esophageal junction. Virchows Arch. 2005;446(5):497–504.
14. Birkmeyer JD, Siewers AE, Finlayson EV, Stukel TA, Lucas FL, Batista I, et al. Hospital volume and surgical mortality in the United States. N Engl J Med. 2002;346(15):1128–37.
15. Heitmiller RF, Redmond M, Hamilton SR. Barrett's esophagus with high-grade dysplasia. An indication for prophylactic esophagectomy. Ann Surg. 1996;224(1):66–71.
16. Nelson DB, Dhupar R, Katkhuda R, Correa A, Goltsov A, Maru D, et al. Outcomes after endoscopic mucosal resection or esophagectomy for submucosal esophageal adenocarcinoma. J Thorac Cardiovasc Surg. 2018;156(1):406-13.e3.
17. Gockel I, Hoffmeister A. Endoscopic or surgical resection for gastro-esophageal cancer. Dtsch Arztebl Int. 2018;115(31–32):513–9.
18. Donlon NE, Elliott JA, Donohoe CL, Murphy CF, Nugent T, Moran B, et al. Adverse biology in adenocarcinoma of the esophagus and esophagogastric junction impacts survival and response to neoadjuvant therapy independent of anatomic subtype. Ann Surg. 2020;272(5):814–9.
19. Hoeppner J, Plum PS, Buhr H, Gockel I, Lorenz D, Ghadimi M, et al. Surgical treatment of esophageal cancer-indicators for quality in diagnostics and treatment. Chirurg. 2021;92(4):350–60.
20. Lian J, Chen S, Zhang Y, Qiu F. A meta-analysis of endoscopic submucosal dissection and EMR for early gastric cancer. Gastrointest Endosc. 2012;76(4):763–70.
21. Ono H, Kondo H, Gotoda T, Shirao K, Yamaguchi H, Saito D, et al. Endoscopic mucosal resection for treatment of early gastric cancer. Gut. 2001;48(2):225–9.
22. Pimentel-Nunes P, Libânio D, Bastiaansen BAJ, Bhandari P, Bisschops R, Bourke MJ, et al. Endoscopic submucosal dissection for superficial gastrointestinal lesions: European society of gastrointestinal endoscopy (ESGE) guideline—update 2022. Endoscopy. 2022;54(6):591–622.

23. Sgourakis G, Gockel I, Lang H. Endoscopic and surgical resection of T1a/T1b esophageal neoplasms: a systematic review. World J Gastroenterol. 2013;19(9):1424–37.
24. Pan L, Liu X, Wang W, Zhu L, Yu W, Lv W, et al. The influence of different treatment strategies on the long-term prognosis of T1 stage esophageal cancer patients. Front Oncol. 2021;11:700088.
25. Harlow C, Sivananthan A, Ayaru L, Patel K, Darzi A, Patel N. Endoscopic submucosal dissection: an update on tools and accessories. Ther Adv Gastrointest Endosc. 2020;13:2631774520957220.
26. Huang R, Yan H, Ren G, Pan Y, Zhang L, Liu Z, et al. Comparison of o-type hybridknife to conventional knife in endoscopic submucosal dissection for gastric mucosal lesions. Medicine (Baltimore). 2016;95(13):e3148.
27. Noguchi M, Yano T, Kato T, Kadota T, Imajoh M, Morimoto H, et al. Risk factors for intraoperative perforation during endoscopic submucosal dissection of superficial esophageal squamous cell carcinoma. World J Gastroenterol. 2017;23(3):478–85.
28. Ding X, Luo H, Duan H. Risk factors for perforation of gastric endoscopic submucosal dissection: a systematic review and meta-analysis. Eur J Gastroenterol Hepatol. 2019;31(12):1481–8.
29. Paspatis GA, Arvanitakis M, Dumonceau JM, Barthet M, Saunders B, Turino SY, et al. Diagnosis and management of iatrogenic endoscopic perforations: European society of gastrointestinal endoscopy (ESGE) position statement—update 2020. Endoscopy. 2020;52(9):792–810.
30. Wang WP, Ni PZ, Yang JL, Wu JC, Yang YS, Chen LQ. Esophagectomy after endoscopic submucosal dissection for esophageal carcinoma. J Thorac Dis. 2018;10(6):3253–61.
31. Wang AY, Hwang JH, Bhatt A, Draganov PV. AGA clinical practice update on surveillance after pathologically curative endoscopic submucosal dissection of early gastrointestinal neoplasia in the United States: commentary. Gastroenterology. 2021;161(6):2030–40.
32. Parikh MP, Thota PN, Raja S, Murthy S, Ahmad U, Gupta NM, et al. Outcomes of endoscopic submucosal dissection in esophageal adenocarcinoma staged T1bN0 by endoscopic ultrasound in non-surgical patients. J Gastrointest Oncol. 2019;10(2):362–6.

Multimodal Therapy for Locally Advanced Esophageal Cancer

James Tankel and Lorenzo Ferri

Abstract

The differences in EAC and ESCC as diseases processes has been highlighted by the advancements in neoadjuvant treatment regimens. In our opinion, these two diseases entities should be treated differently. It is clear that chemotherapy or chemoradiotherapy should be given before surgery; however, perioperative systemic regimens have taken over the landscape for patients with EAC in many centers around the world. Although significant regional differences exist, the data suggest that for EAC docetaxel-based therapy given in a perioperative fashion followed by en bloc surgical should be considered the standard of care for this histological subtype. Successful identification of the agent, and patients, who will benefit from immunotherapy or biological agents to the neoadjuvant setting will likely influence future recommendations. For patients with locally advanced ESCC, nCRT followed by surgery seems to be the best treatment option available. The addition of adjuvant checkpoint inhibition in the presence of residual disease seems to be the best augment for this approach. However, significant regional differences exist in this setting as well with docetaxel-based therapy emerging as a viable alternative based on several trials. Finally, selective surgery after induction chemoradiation is also on the horizon for both ESCC and EAC and future studies may provide a foundation for treating certain patients definitively.

Keywords

Esophageal cancer · Neoadjuvant therapy · Chemotherapy · Immunotherapy

Introduction

Early experiences with neoadjuvant treatment of esophageal cancer were marred by high levels of toxicity, treatment related mortality and marginal survival benefits. However, drastic improvements in neoadjuvant chemotherapy (nCT) and chemoradiotherapy (nCRT) regimens has led to multiple randomized studies demonstrating the survival benefit of this approach compared with upfront surgery. However, the ideal regimen has yet to be elucidated and treatment paradigms are likely to change in the face of immunotherapy, the role of which has yet to be clearly defined.

Although a transthoracic en bloc esophagogastrectomy with extended lymphadenectomy forms the cornerstone of the management of patients with esophageal cancer, the nature of surgical intervention is beyond the scope of this

J. Tankel · L. Ferri (✉)
Division of Thoracic and Upper Gastrointestinal Surgery, Montreal General Hospital, McGill University Health Centre, 1650 Cedar Avenue, Montreal, QC, Canada
e-mail: Lorenzo.Ferri@mcgill.ca

chapter. Rather, we will present the evidence base on which neoadjuvant treatment decisions should be made and highlight ongoing studies that may alter the way locally advanced esophageal cancer is managed in the future.

could be elucidated when compared to upfront surgery [2]. Therefore, nRT should not be used in treating locally advanced esophageal cancer and we suggest that radiation as a monotherapy should be offered in the palliative setting only.

Neoadjuvant Radiotherapy

Historic studies published in the 1950's explored the role of neoadjuvant radiotherapy (nRT) for locally advanced esophageal squamous cell carcinoma (ESCC). Summarized by a Cochrane review, the addition of nRT engendered little benefit over surgery alone with a 5-year overall survival of just 6–10% [1]. However, the dose of radiotherapy given in these early studies was considerably lower than modern regimens and was not combined with concurrent chemotherapy. Nevertheless, even when a higher radiation dose of 40 Gy was used, no sustained survival benefit

Neoadjuvant Chemoradiotherapy or Upfront Surgery

By combining systemic chemotherapy with radiotherapy micrometastatic disease lying beyond the radiation field is treated. In addition, several chemotherapy agents act as radiosensitizers including 5FU, cisplatin and paclitaxel. Finally, ESCC seems more sensitive to the effects of radiotherapy making this an attractive treatment option for this histological subtype.

A summary of recent randomized trials of nCRT versus upfront surgery is presented in Table 1. Early studies demonstrated that higher

Table 1 Selection of randomized studies that compare neoadjuvant chemoradiotherapy with surgery

Trial	Year	Histology	Neoadjuvant regimen	N	Survival outcomes
Le Prise [4]	1994	ESCC	Cisplatin, 5 FU, 20 Gy	Sx 45 nCRT 41	3 year overall survival 14% 19%
Walsh [6]	1996	EAC	Cisplatin, 5 FU, 40 Gy	Sx 55 nCRT 58	3 year overall survival 6% 32%*
Burmeister [5]	2005	EAC/ESCC	Cisplatin, 5 FU, 35 Gy	Sx 128 nCRT 128	Median survival (months) 19.3 22.2
Cao [2]	2009	ESCC	Cisplatin, mitomycin, 5 FU, 40 Gy	Sx 118 nCRT 118	3 year overall survival 53.4% 73.3%*
CROSS [7]	2012	EAC/ESCC	Carboplatin, paclitaxel, 41.4 Gy	Sx 188 nCRT 178	Median survival (months) 24.0 49.4*
Mariette [11]	2014	ESCC	Cisplatin, 5 FU, 45 Gy	Sx 97 nCRT 98	Median survival (months) 31.8 41.2
Yang [10]	2018	ESCC	Vinorelbine, cisplatin, 40 Gy	Sx 227 nCRT 224	Median survival (months) 66.1 100.1*

Sx Upfront surgery, *nCRT* Neoadjuvant chemoradiotherapy, *EAC* esophageal adenocarcinoma, *ESCC* esophageal squamous cell carcinoma, * statistically significant difference

doses of ionizing radiation are associated with greater treatment toxicity. In one study of nCRT based upon 64.8Gy, 9% of patients died due to treatment related complications [3]. Therefore, finding the balance between toxicity and therapeutic benefit is a common theme throughout older studies of nCRT as lower doses of radiotherapy failed to engender a survival benefit. In the study by La Prise, only 20Gy of external beam radiotherapy was used and although downstaging of the primary lesion was found, the rate of pathological complete response was low and the R0 resection rate not improved [4]. Overall survival was also no better among recipients of nCRT. Conversely, in a study by Burmeister in which 35Gy of radiotherapy was utilized, although significant pathological improvement with nCRT was demonstrated, this was not associated with a survival benefit [5] (Tables 2 and 3).

These studies either included solely, or predominantly, patients with ESCC. The study by Walsh et al. randomized 113 patients with locally advanced esophageal adenocarcinoma (EAC) to be treated either with neoadjuvant 5FU, cisplatin and 40Gy of radiation or surgery alone [6]. Pathological complete response occurred in 25% of patients treated with nCRT, and 42% had metastatic lymph nodes compared to 82% treated with upfront surgery ($p<0.001$). The 3-year overall survival was 32% versus 6% respectively. Limitations of this study concern

Table 2 Selection of randomized trials that compare neoadjuvant chemotherapy with surgery

Trial	Year	Histology	Neoadjuvant chemotherapy regimen	N	Survival outcomes
Kelsen [15]	1998	EAC, ESCC	Cisplatin, 5 FU	Sx 213 nCT 227	Median survival (months): 16.1 14.9
MRC OEO2 [18]	2002	EAC, ESCC	Cisplatin, 5 FU	Sx 402 nCT 400	Median survival (months) 13.3 16.8
MAGIC [19]	2006	EAC	Epirubicin, Cisplatin, 5 FU	Sx 253 nCT 250	5-year overall survival: 23% 36%*
Schuhmacher [17]	2010	EAC	Cisplatin, 5 FU	Sx 72 nCT 72	Median survival (months): 52.3 64.6
Boonstra [24]	2011	ESCC	Cisplatin, etoposide	Sx 84 nCT 85	Median survival (months): 12.0 16.0*
FNCLCC/FFCD [20]	2011	EAC	Cisplatin, 5 FU	Sx 111 nCT 113	5 year overall survival: 24% 38%*

Sx upfront surgery, *nCT* neoadjuvant chemotherapy, *EAC* esophageal adenocarcinoma, *ESCC* esophageal squamous cell carcinoma, * statistically significant difference

Table 3 A selection of studies comparing neoadjuvant chemotherapy with neoadjuvant chemoradiotherapy

Name	Year	Histology	Neoadjuvant regimen	N	Survival outcomes
Cao [2]	2009	ESCC	nCT—Cisplatin, mitomycin, 5FU nCRT—Cisplatin, mitomycin, 5FU, 40Gy	237	3 year overall survival 57.1% 73.3%*
Klevebro [29]	2016	EAC/ESCC	nCT—Cisplatin, 5FU nCRT- Cisplatin, 5FU, 40Gy	181	3 year overall survival 49% 47%
Stahl [28]	2017	EAC	nCT—Cisplatin, leucovorin, 5FU nCRT—Cisplatin, leucovorin, 5FU, etoposide, 50Gy	119	3 year overall survival 27.7% 47.4%*
Reynolds [30]	2021	EAC	nCT—Epirubicin, cisplatin/oxaliplatin, 5FU/capecitabine or 5FU, leucovorin, oxaliplatin, docetaxel nCRT—Carboplatin, paclitaxel, 41.4Gy	377	3 year estimated survival: 57% 56%
Wang [27]	2021	ESCC	nCT—Cisplatin, paclitaxel nCRT—Cisplatin, paclitaxel, 40Gy	264	1 year overall survival 82.6% 87.1%

nCT neoadjuvant chemotherapy, *nCRT* neoadjuvant chemoradiotherapy, *EAC* esophageal adenocarcinoma, *ESCC* esophageal squamous cell carcinoma, * statistically significant difference

the poor surgical technique with studies of the same era incorporating a greater number of oncological resections describing better survival outcomes following upfront surgery.

Considering the heterogenicity of data, the seminal CROSS study aimed to provide greater clarity regarding the role of nCRT in treating esophageal cancer [7]. By demonstrating a survival benefit following systemic paclitaxel and carboplatin in conjunction with 41.4 Gy of concurrent radiation versus surgery alone, this trial was responsible for establishing nCRT as the standard of care for both ESCC and EAC in the Western world. Pathological complete response was found in 25% of patients with EAC and 49% in patients with ESCC. Furthermore, nCRT was associated with greater rates of R0 resection (92% vs. 69%) and fewer metastatic lymph nodes (31% vs. 75%). This translated into a significantly lower incidence of locoregional recurrence in patients allocated to the trimodality arm (22% vs. 38%, hazard ratio 0.45, 95% CI 0.3–0.66, $p \leq 0.001$). Long-term follow up of the original cohort supports the durability of this benefit but highlighted that the median survival was higher among ESCC patients compared to EAC patients (81.6 months vs. just 43.2 months) [8]. This demonstrates how the differing histology is affected by the neoadjuvant treatment modality which ultimately impacts survival.

Beyond the histological subtype, the surgical approach utilized after nCRT also affects survival outcomes. Whilst a persistent benefit of nCRT for patients who underwent a trans-hiatal resection has been shown, for those treated with a transthoracic esophagectomy this benefit appears limited [9]. This suggests, albeit controversially, that additional local therapy may not be needed if the surgical approach includes an en bloc esophagectomy.

Considering the data of the more recent NEOCRTEC5010 study, the role and safety of nCRT becomes somewhat clearer [10]. Of the 451 patients with locally advanced but resectable ESCC randomized to receive vinorelbine, cisplatin and 40Gy of concurrent radiotherapy an improvement in median overall survival was found (100.1 months vs. 66.5 months, $p = 0.002$) with a similar incidence of postoperative complications compared to the upfront surgery arm.

With regards to disease recurrence, when comparing nCRT with surgery alone the former seems to provide better local disease control. Conversely, distal relapse rates in the CROSS study were similar between the trimodality and upfront surgery arms. However, patients with ESCC may derive an attenuate systemic benefit in comparison to patients with EAC following treatment with nCRT. A subset analysis of the CROSS cohort suggested that some systemic benefit may be derived from nCRT at 5 years among patients with ESCC. Furthermore, in the NEOCRETC5010 study, recipients of trimodality care also had lower distal disease recurrence in comparison to those treated with surgical monotherapy.

In summary, when comparing nCRT with surgery alone, the former is associated with a significantly higher pathologic complete response rate, reduction in lymph node disease burden, improved rates of R0 resection and improved local and distal disease control. Each of these factors correlate with improved survival and highlights the excellent local disease control achieved with nCRT. Considering that nCRT has a less impressive impact on EAC in terms of these metrics, we suggest that trimodality therapy be reserved for those with ESCC.

Can Neoadjuvant Chemoradiotherapy Be Used in Early Esophageal Cancer?

In the French FFCD9901 study, Mariette et al. randomized 195 patients with stage I and II esophageal cancer to receive nCRT or upfront surgery [11]. The standard of surgical resection was high with all patients receiving a transthoracic two-field lymphadenectomy. Impressive pathological downstaging was noted in those treated with nCRT which translated into a lower rate of locoregional recurrence (28.6% vs. 44.3%, $p = 0.002$). However, no difference was observed in terms of distal disease relapse (22.5% vs. 28.9% $p = 0.31$) or survival (median overall survival 31.8 vs. 41.1 months). In hospital mortality was significantly higher in patients receiving nCRT (11.1% vs. 3.4% $p = 0.049$). These results suggest that the oncologic benefit of nCRT in patients with locally advanced esophageal cancer is not maintained in patients with earlier stage disease. Data is conflicting as a survival benefit was found in a retrospective study of 382 patients with cT3N0 ESCC and EAC amalgamated from more than 30 European centers (38.4 vs. 29.9 months, $p = 0.007$) [12].

The sensitivity of ESCC to radiotherapy has led some to question whether surgery improves survival in the setting of early disease in this specific histological subtype. In a large registry study, a survival benefit was only noted in patients with stage IIA and above [13]. Similarly, JCOG0502 trial with randomized patients with cT1bN0 ESCC to either definitive chemoradiotherapy or upfront surgery found similar survival in the surgery and non-surgery groups (86.5 and 85.5% respectively) [14]. More data regarding the benefit of surgery after chemoradiation will be provided by several ongoing trials including the NEEDS and SANO trials.

The Benefit of Neoadjuvant and Perioperative Chemotherapy

Effective systemic chemotherapy has several benefits. By treating micrometastatic disease, survivability is improved. Dysphagia is also reduced affording patients a better nutritional intake before surgery. Furthermore, non-resectable lesions may be down-staged and rendered resectable. Finally, the administration of nCT provides an opportunity to observe the clinical efficacy of the drug regimen being used. Whilst this has a prognostic benefit, alternate treatment strategies can be initiated depending on treatment response and, rarely, futile surgery avoided in the presence of disease progression during nCT.

Early data including mixed histologies failed to show a survival benefit of nCT versus upfront surgery [15]. However, it seems that patients who responded to nCT had significantly better survival than those who did not response (response vs. no response HR 2.83 1.84–4.35 $p<0.001$). Similar data exists for patients with ESCC found to have a pathological response to nCT (median survival 20 months vs. 6 months $p=0.008$) [16].

With regards to EAC, the European EORTC 40,954 study, found that nCT was associated with a lower incidence of lymph node metastases (61.4% vs. 76.5%, $p=0.018$) and higher rate of R0 resection (81.9% vs. 66.7%, $p=0.036$). Nevertheless, there was no survival difference noted between the treatment arms [17]. However, few esophageal cancers were included and the study was based on an outdated triplet therapy regimen (cisplatin, 5FU and leucovorin).

Building on these results, the Medicine Research Council OEO2 study included patients with both EAC and ESCC and gave preoperative cisplatin and 5FU [18]. Preoperative systemic treatment was associated with significant pathological downstaging and, in comparison to those treated with surgery alone, the five-year survival increased significantly from 17 to 23% (HR 0.79 95%CI 0.67–0.93 $p=0.004$). This study was responsible for firmly establishing the role of nCT for locally advanced esophagogastric cancer in the United Kingdom. Of note, histological subtype did not affect the pathological response to perioperative treatment and no long-term survival differences between ESCC and EAC were noted.

Reflecting on these benefits, the British MAGIC [19] and French FNLCC/FFCD [20] trials were performed to assess the role of perioperative chemotherapy versus upfront surgery. In the former perioperative epirubicin, cisplatin and 5FU was found to be particularly effective in patients with EAC. Whilst esophageal lesions were underrepresented in the study, perioperative chemotherapy was associated with an improvement in the rate of R0 resections (79.3% vs. 70.3% $p=0.03$), smaller tumours and fewer metastatic lymph nodes. Improved overall survival was also noted in those receiving systemic treatment with a 5-year survival of 36.3% versus 23% (HR 0.75 95CI (0.6–0.93 $p=0.009$). This improvement was despite only 55% of patients being able to receive the adjuvant part of their systemic treatment.

Due to the poor patient tolerance of the adjuvant arm of the perioperative regimens described above, efforts shifted to identifying regimens that may be less toxic with an equivalent, or even better, oncological profile. Based on the observation that metastatic gastric cancer could be effectively treated with to docetaxel-based triplet therapy and acceptable toxicity, our center was one of the first to explore the role of docetaxel, cisplatin and 5FU (DCF) in the perioperative setting [21]. An investigator-initiated phase II single-arm trial was undertaken for patients with EAC and, despite a heavy tumour burden, an exceptional 5-year survival of over 50% was found. The subsequent landmark study by Al Batran formalized the use of FLOT (5FU, leucovorin, oxaliplatin and docetaxel) as the standard of care for perioperative chemotherapy for the treatment of gastro-esophageal adenocarcinoma [22]. In the FLOT4 trial, 716 patients were randomized to receive either FLOT or the ECF regimen given in the MAGIC trial. With an equivalent toxicity profile and incidence of postoperative complications, the median overall survival improved from 35 to 50 months in patients treated with FLOT. Real world data has confirmed these results and whilst true esophageal adenocarcinomas were excluded from these studies, a recently published multicentre observational cohort study demonstrated excellent results of FLOT in patients with esophageal cancer with a 5-year overall survival of 60% [23].

The role of perioperative chemotherapy (cisplatin and etoposide) was also explored in the setting of ESCC by Boontra [24]. Pathological complete response occurred in just 7% of patients although no difference in the R0 resection rate or number of metastatic lymph nodes was found between the treatment arms. Nevertheless, a significant survival advantage in patients receiving perioperative chemotherapy was noted (median overall survival 16 months vs. 12 months). The survival advantage of neoadjuvant cisplatin and 5FU was also demonstrated in the JCOG9907 trial [25]. In this study, neoadjuvant as opposed to adjuvant chemotherapy was associated with an increase in 5-year overall survival by 12–55%.

Similar to EAC, the addition of docetaxel to nCT regimens for ESCC is also being explored. Preliminary results from the NeXT trial suggest that neoadjuvant DCF significantly improves survival in comparison CF alone in patients with ESCC (3-year overall survival 62.6% vs. 72.1%) [26].

In summary, neoadjuvant and perioperative regimens are safe and have been clear demonstration of a survival advantage for both ESCC and EAC in comparison to surgery alone. Older treatments have made way for docetaxel-based therapies which have demonstrated excellent oncological profiles. As such, docetaxel-based triplet therapy can be considered acceptable standards of care for both of these histological subtypes of esophageal cancer.

Neoadjuvant Chemotherapy or Chemoradiotherapy

Data comparing nCRT with nCT for patients with ESCC varies. A randomized trial showed fewer cancer related deaths among patients with ESCC patients who received nCRT (40Gy, paclitaxel, cisplatin) in comparison to nCT (paclitaxel and cisplatin) [27]. However, there was no difference in overall survival when comparing both treatment arms (3-year overall 64% vs. 55%). An additional randomized 4 arm study (nCT, nCRT, upfront sugery, nRT) found that all neoadjuvant regimens had similar survival outcomes at 5 years [2]. The NeXT trial, by Kato et al. also failed to find a difference in survival outcomes among patients allocated to the nCT and nCRT arms despite progression free survival being longer in the latter [26].

Data comparing nCT with nCRT in patients with adenocarcinoma is available from several randomized trials. The PreOperative therapy in Esophagogastric adenocarcinoma Trial (POET) study randomized 119 patients with Siewert I-III adenocarcinoma to receive wither nCT or nCRT [28]. Survival among recipients of nCRT was higher (5-year overall survival or 39.5% vs. 24.4%). Whilst the results may suggest that nCRT is superior to nCT in terms of survival, the survival in the nCT arm is lower when compared with modern neoadjuvant regimens. The surgical approach may be the cause of this outcome as only 47% of patients in the nCT arm underwent thransthoracic esophagectomy.

The NeoRes study randomized 181 patients with EAC and ESCC [29]. Whilst pathological complete response rate and incidence of R0 resections was higher in the nCRT arm irrespective of histological type, survival was similar between the two arms. Whilst the long-term data supports the non-inferiority of nCT, it should be noted that the study protocol used a dose of radiotherapy below that which is commonly used (40 Gy) and a non-standard of care chemotherapy regimen (cisplatin, 5FU).

The NeoAEGIS study aims to address these limitations [30]. In total, 362 patients with adenocarcinoma of the esophagus and esophagogastric junction were randomized to receive either the CROSS or MAGIC regimens. The recently released results also failed to show inferiority of either regimen with a 3-year overall survival of 57% versus 55% respectively (HR 1.03, 95% CI 0.77–1.38). Only 15% of patients in the nCT arm received FLOT and considering the superiority of this regimen over ECF, it may be that the nCT arms survival outcomes were underpowered. The results of the ESOPEC study, that compares FLOT versus CROSS, are eagerly awaited, as are the results from the TOPGEAR and RACE studies which also compare ECF with CROSS.

Pending the release of this data, a retrospective analysis of 2367 patients of 11,167 EAC and 2,367 ESCC patients found that overall survival was similar when comparing nCT with nCRT (37% vs. 36%, $p = 0.123$) [31]. However, when stratified by histological subtype, patients with ESCC fared significantly better in terms of survival after being treated with nCRT (5-year overall survival 45% vs. 38%, $p = 0.026$).

It is noteworthy that survival following pathological complete response is inferior when achieved following nCRT as compared with nCT (odds ratio 2.50, 95% CI 1.25–4.99) [32]. This highlights the fundamental role of effective systemic disease control in disease survival. Therefore, the current data supports an approach that nCT is not inferior to nCRT for the treatment of EAC. With regards to ESCC, whilst nCRT achieves local control compared to nCT, it seems that equivalent survival can be achieved with nCT. As such, both modalities are accepted standards of care.

Safety of Neoadjuvant Chemotherapy and Chemoradiotherapy

Data regarding this topic also varies with morbidity and mortality improving significantly in comparison to historical studies. The postoperative mortality of 10.2% in the study by Stahl is considerably higher than the 1% of more recent studies, even in patients who received neoadjuvant therapy [28]. For example, in recent retrospective multi-institutional study of 2944 patients, nCRT was not associated with an increased risk of anastomotic leak or pneumonia, although was associated with an increased risk of chylothorax, cardiovascular complications and thromboembolic events [33]. Similarly, in a randomized trial of minimally invasive esophagectomy following nCT or nCRT in patients with ESCC, the incidence of morbidity and mortality was the same irrespective the neoadjuvant treatment received (morbidity following nCRT and nCT 47.4% vs. 42.6% and mortality 3.5% vs. 2.2%, respectively) [34].

Conversely, whilst safety data from the NeoAEGIS trial was similar, significantly more patients treated with nCRT had Clavien Dindo grade III complications and above (30% vs. 17%, $p = 0.05$) as well as a higher mean comprehensive complication index [30].

Immunotherapy and Biological Agents

Whilst several studies have demonstrated the efficacy of either immunotherapy or biological agents for patients with advanced or metastatic esophageal cancer, the role of these agents in the neoadjuvant setting has yet to be established. Using neoadjuvant trastuzamab in patients with Her2 + EAC after nCRT failed to improve survival [35]. Moreover, the incidence of treatment related deaths in the trastuzamab arm were twice as high as those who didn't receive this treatment (6% vs. 3%).

Multiple other trials exploring the role novel agents including neoadjuvant Pembrolizumab and Avelumab are ongoing. Preliminary data suggests that neoadjuvant Pembrolizumab and Nivolumab increase pathological response to neoadjuvant therapy [36, 37]. However, the potential impact that this may have on survival has not yet been described. Similarly, in the single-armed ESONICT-2 trial, neoadjuvant toripalimab was added to docetaxel and cisplatin in patients with ESCC. Major pathological response occurred in 41.7% however survival data is also yet to be presented [38].

There is a clear paucity of data regarding survival outcomes in patients treated with neoadjuvant immunotherapy. Emerging data from prospective trials will fill this void and shape treatment outcomes going forward. As such, no treatment recommendations with regards to neoadjuvant immunotherapy and biological agents can currently be made.

Completion of Chemotherapy

For patients with adenocarcinoma, the perioperative regimen presented in the FLOT4 trial involves 4 preoperative and 4 postoperative cycles. Evidence suggests that irrespective of the degree of response to the initial 4 cycles, a survival benefit is derived by completion of the systemic therapy [39]. In the patient who did not receive neoadjuvant therapy, systemic chemotherapy can be given in keeping with the CLASSIC study (capecitabine/oxaliplatin) [40]. We strongly try to avoid irradiation following esophagogastrectomy as this is often highly toxic. Only in the presence of a positive proximal or distal margin is this considered. If nCRT was given, then no protocol for completion of therapy exists.

For patients with ESCC treated with nCT, completion of systemic therapy is recommended. If nCRT is utilized, no formal

guidelines exist regarding the provision of additional therapy although practice varies between institutions based on retrospective data the suggests a survival benefit if residual disease is present [41]. The Checkmate 577 study randomized 532 patients with both ESCC and EAC with residual disease after nCRT and surgical resection to receive nivolumab or placebo. A significant improvement in disease free survival was noted (22.4 vs. 11.0 months, HR 0.69, 95% CI 0.56–0.86) [42]. Whilst these benefits were attenuated among patients with ESCC, this landscape is changing and recommendations may change as more evidence becomes available.

References

1. Arnott SJ, Duncan W, Gignoux M, Hansen HS, Launois B, Nygaard K, Parmar MK, Rousell A, Spilopoulos G, Stewart G, Tierney JF, Wang M, Rhugang Z, Oeosphageal Cancer Collaborative Group. Preoperative radiotherapy for esophageal carcinoma. Cochrane Database Syst Rev. 2005;2005(4):CD001799. https://doi.org/10.1002/14651858.CD001799.pub2. PMID: 16235286; PMCID: PMC8407511.

2. Cao XF, He XT, Ji L, Xiao J, Lv J. Effects of neoadjuvant radiochemotherapy on pathological staging and prognosis for locally advanced esophageal squamous cell carcinoma. Dis Esophagus. 2009;22(6):477–81. https://doi.org/10.1111/j.1442-2050.2008.00910.x. PMID: 19703071.

3. Minsky BD, Neuberg D, Kelsen DP, Pisansky TM, Ginsberg RJ, Pajak T, Salter M, Benson AB 3rd. Final report of Intergroup Trial 0122 (ECOG PE-289, RTOG 90–12): Phase II trial of neoadjuvant chemotherapy plus concurrent chemotherapy and high-dose radiation for squamous cell carcinoma of the esophagus. Int J Radiat Oncol Biol Phys. 1999;43(3):517–23. https://doi.org/10.1016/s0360-3016(98)00463-5. PMID: 10078631.

4. Le Prise E, Etienne PL, Meunier B, Maddern G, Ben Hassel M, Gedouin D, Boutin D, Campion JP, Launois B. A randomized study of chemotherapy, radiation therapy, and surgery versus surgery for localized squamous cell carcinoma of the esophagus. Cancer. 1994;73(7):1779–84. https://doi.org/10.1002/1097-0142(19940401)73:7<1779::aid-cncr2820730702>3.0.co;2-t. PMID: 8137201.

5. Burmeister BH, Smithers BM, Gebski V, Fitzgerald L, Simes RJ, Devitt P, Ackland S, Gotley DC, Joseph D, Millar J, North J, Walpole ET, Denham JW, Trans-Tasman Radiation Oncology Group, Australasian Gastro-Intestinal Trials Group. Surgery

alone versus chemoradiotherapy followed by surgery for resectable cancer of the oesophagus: a randomised controlled phase III trial. Lancet Oncol 2005;6(9):659–68. https://doi.org/10.1016/S1470-2045(05)70288-6. PMID: 16129366; Walsh TN, Noonan N, Hollywood D, Kelly A, Keeling N, Hennessy TP. A comparison of multimodal therapy and surgery for esophageal adenocarcinoma. N Engl J Med. 1996;335(7):462–7. https://doi.org/10.1056/NEJM199608153350702. Erratum in: N Engl J Med 1999 Jul 29;341(5):384. PMID: 8672151.

6. Walsh TN, Noonan N, Hollywood D, Kelly A, Keeling N, Hennessy TP. A comparison of multimodal therapy and surgery for esophageal adenocarcinoma. N Engl J Med. 1996;335(7):462–7. https://doi.org/10.1056/NEJM199608153350702.Erratum.In:NEnglJMed1999;341(5):384. PMID: 8672151.

7. van Hagen P, Hulshof MC, van Lanschot JJ, Steyerberg EW, van Berge Henegouwen MI, Wijnhoven BP, Richel DJ, Nieuwenhuijzen GA, Hospers GA, Bonenkamp JJ, Cuesta MA, Blaisse RJ, Busch OR, ten Kate FJ, Creemers GJ, Punt CJ, Plukker JT, Verheul HM, Spillenaar Bilgen EJ, van Dekken H, van der Sangen MJ, Rozema T, Biermann K, Beukema JC, Piet AH, van Rij CM, Reinders JG, Tilanus HW, van der Gaast A, CROSS Group. Preoperative chemoradiotherapy for esophageal or junctional cancer. N Engl J Med. 2012;366(22):2074–84. https://doi.org/10.1056/NEJMoa1112088. PMID: 22646630.

8. Shapiro J, van Lanschot J, Hulshof M, van Hagen P, van Berge HM, Wijnhoven BPL, et al. Neoadjuvant chemoradiotherapy plus surgery versus surgery alone for oesophageal or junctional cancer (CROSS): long-term results of a randomised controlled trial. Lancet Oncol. 2015;16:1090–8. https://doi.org/10.1016/S1470-2045(15)00040-6.

9. Noordman BJ, van Klaveren D, van Berge Henegouwen MI, Wijnhoven BPL, Gisbertz SS, Lagarde SM, van der Gaast A, Hulshof MCCM, Biermann K, Steyerberg EW, van Lanschot JJB; also on behalf of the CROSS-Study Group. Impact of surgical approach on long-term survival in esophageal adenocarcinoma patients with or without neoadjuvant chemoradiotherapy. Ann Surg. 2018;267(5):892–897. https://doi.org/10.1097/SLA.0000000000002240. PMID: 28350565.

10. Yang H, Liu H, Chen Y, Zhu C, Fang W, Yu Z, Mao W, Xiang J, Han Y, Chen Z, Yang H, Wang J, Pang Q, Zheng X, Yang H, Li T, Lordick F, D'Journo XB, Cerfolio RJ, Korst RJ, Novoa NM, Swanson SJ, Brunelli A, Ismail M, Fernando HC, Zhang X, Li Q, Wang G, Chen B, Mao T, Kong M, Guo X, Lin T, Liu M, Fu J, AME Thoracic Surgery Collaborative Group. Neoadjuvant chemoradiotherapy followed by surgery versus surgery alone for locally advanced squamous cell carcinoma of the esophagus (NEOCRTEC5010): a Phase III multicenter, randomized, open-label clinical trial. J Clin Oncol. 2018;36(27):2796–2803. https://doi.org/10.1200/JCO.2018.79.1483. Epub 2018 Aug 8. PMID: 30089078; PMCID: PMC6145832.

11. Mariette C, Dahan L, Mornex F, Maillard E, Thomas P, Meunier B, Boige V, Pezet D, Robb WB, Le Brun-Ly V, et al. Surgery alone versus chemoradiotherapy followed by surgery for Stage I and II esophageal cancer: final analysis of randomized controlled Phase III Trial FFCD 9901. J Clin Oncol. 2014;32:2416–22. https://doi.org/10.1200/JCO.2013.53.6532.

12. Mantziari S, Gronnier C, Renaud F, Duhamel A, Théreaux J, Brigand C, Carrère N, Lefevre JH, Pasquer A, Demartines N, Collet D, Meunier B, Mariette C, on behalf of the FREGAT working group—FRENCH—AFC. Survival benefit of neoadjuvant treatment in clinical T3N0M0 esophageal cancer: results from a retrospective multicenter European study. Ann Surg. 2017;266(5):805–813. https://doi.org/10.1097/SLA.0000000000002402

13. Yen YC, Chang JH, Lin WC, Chiou JF, Chang YC, Chang CL, Hsu HL, Chow JM, Yuan KS, Wu ATH, Wu SY. Effectiveness of esophagectomy in patients with thoracic esophageal squamous cell carcinoma receiving definitive radiotherapy or concurrent chemoradiotherapy through intensity-modulated radiation therapy techniques. Cancer. 2017;123(11):2043–53. https://doi.org/10.1002/cncr.30565. Epub 2017 Feb 2 PMID: 28152166.

14. Kato K, Igaki H, Ito Y, et al. Parallel-group controlled trial of esophagectomy versus chemoradiotherapy in patients with clinical stage I esophageal carcinoma (JCOG0502). J Clin Oncol. 2019;37(4)7. https://doi.org/10.1200/jco.2019.37.4_suppl.7.

15. Kelsen DP, Ginsberg R, Pajak TF, Sheahan DG, Gunderson L, Mortimer J, Estes N, Haller DG, Ajani J, Kocha W, Minsky BD, Roth JA. Chemotherapy followed by surgery compared with surgery alone for localized esophageal cancer. N Engl J Med. 1998;339(27):1979–84. https://doi.org/10.1056/NEJM199812313392704. PMID: 9869669.

16. Ancona E, Ruol A, Santi S, Merigliano S, Sileni VC, Koussis H, Zaninotto G, Bonavina L, Peracchia A. Only pathologic complete response to neoadjuvant chemotherapy improves significantly the long term survival of patients with resectable esophageal squamous cell carcinoma. Cancer. 2001;91:2165–74. https://doi.org/10.1002/1097-0142(20010601)91:11<2165::AID-CNCR1245>3.3.CO;2-8.

17. Schuhmacher C, Gretschel S, Lordick F, Reichardt P, Hohenberger W, Eisenberger CF, Haag C, Mauer ME, Hasan B, Welch J, Ott K, Hoelscher A, Schneider PM, Bechstein W, Wilke H, Lutz MP, Nordlinger B, Van Cutsem E, Siewert JR, Schlag PM. Neoadjuvant chemotherapy compared with surgery alone for locally advanced cancer of the stomach and cardia: European Organisation for Research

and Treatment of Cancer randomized trial 40954. J Clin Oncol. 2010;28(35):5210–8. https://doi.org/10.1200/JCO.2009.26.6114. Epub 2010 Nov 8. PMID: 21060024; PMCID: PMC3020693.

18. Girling DJ, Bancewicz J, Clark PI, et al. Surgical resection with or without preoperative chemotherapy in oesophageal cancer: a randomised controlled trial. Lancet. 2002;366(22):2074–84. https://doi.org/10.1016/S0140-6736(02)08651-8.

19. Cunningham D, Allum WH, Stenning SP, et al. Perioperative chemotherapy versus surgery alone for resectable gastroesophageal cancer. N Engl J Med. 2006;355(1):11–20. https://doi.org/10.1056/nejmoa055531.

20. Ychou M, Boige V, Pignon JP, Conroy T, Bouché O, Lebreton G, Ducourtieux M, Bedenne L, Fabre JM, Saint-Aubert B, Genève J, Lasser P, Rougier P. Perioperative chemotherapy compared with surgery alone for resectable gastroesophageal adenocarcinoma: an FNCLCC and FFCD multicenter phase III trial. J Clin Oncol. 2011;29(13):1715–21. https://doi.org/10.1200/JCO.2010.33.0597. Epub 2011 Mar 28 PMID: 21444866.

21. Ferri LE, Ades S, Alcindor T, et al. Perioperative docetaxel, cisplatin, and 5-fluorouracil (DCF) for locally advanced esophageal and gastric adenocarcinoma: A multicenter phase II trial. Ann Oncol. 2012;23(6):1512–7. https://doi.org/10.1093/annonc/mdr465.

22. Al-Batran SE, Homann N, Pauligk C, et al. Perioperative chemotherapy with fluorouracil plus leucovorin, oxaliplatin, and docetaxel versus fluorouracil or capecitabine plus cisplatin and epirubicin for locally advanced, resectable gastric or gastro-oesophageal junction adenocarcinoma (FLOT4): a randomised pahse II/III trian. Lancet. 2019;393(10184):1948–57. https://doi.org/10.1016/S0140-6736(18)32557-1.

23. Donlon NE, Kammili A, Roopnarinesingh R, et al. FLOT-regimen chemotherapy and transthoracic en bloc resection for esophageal and junctional adenocarcinoma. Ann Surg. 2021;274(5):814–20. https://doi.org/10.1097/SLA.0000000000005097.

24. Boonstra JJ, Kok TC, Wijnhoven BPL, et al. Chemotherapy followed by surgery versus surgery alone in patients with resectable oesophageal squamous cell carcinoma: Long-term results of a randomized controlled trial. BMC Cancer. 2011;16(9):1090–8. https://doi.org/10.1186/1471-2407-11-181.

25. Ando N, Kato H, Igaki H, Shinoda M, Ozawa S, Shimizu H, Nakamura T, Yabusaki HAN, Kurita A, Ikeda K, Kanda T, Tsujinaka T, Nakamura K, Fukuda H. A randomized trial comparing postoperative adjuvant chemotherapy with cisplatin and 5-fluorouracil versus preoperative chemotherapy for localized advanced squamous cell carcinoma of the thoracic esophagus (JCOG9907). Ann Surg Oncol. 2012;19:68–74.

26. Kato K, Ito Y, Daiko H, et al. A randomized controlled phase III trial comparing two chemotherapy regimen and chemoradiotherapy regimen as neoadjuvant treatment for locally advanced esophageal cancer, JCOG1109 NExT study. J Clin Oncol. 2022;40(4)238. https://doi.org/10.1200/JCO.2022.40.4_suppl.238.

27. Wang H, Tang H, Fang Y, Tan L, Yin J, Shen Y, Zeng Z, Zhu J, Hou Y, Du M, Jiao J, Jiang H, Gong L, Li Z, Liu J, Xie D, Li W, Lian C, Zhao Q, Chen C, Zheng B, Liao Y, Li K, Li H, Wu H, Dai L, Chen KN. Morbidity and mortality of patients who underwent minimally invasive esophagectomy after neoadjuvant chemoradiotherapy vs neoadjuvant chemotherapy for locally advanced esophageal squamous cell carcinoma: a randomized clinical trial. JAMA Surg. 2021;156(5):444–51. https://doi.org/10.1001/jamasurg.2021.0133.PMID:33729467; PMCID:PMC7970392.

28. Stahl M, Walz MK, Riera-Knorrenschild J, et al. Preoperative chemotherapy versus chemoradiotherapy in locally advanced adenocarcinomas of the oesophagogastric junction (POET): long-term results of a controlled randomised trial. Eur J Cancer. 2017;81:183–90. https://doi.org/10.1016/j.ejca.2017.04.027.

29. Klevebro F, Alexandersson von Döbeln G, Wang N, Johnsen G, Jacobsen AB, Friesland S, Hatlevoll I, Glenjen NI, Lind P, Tsai JA, Lundell L, Nilsson M. A randomized clinical trial of neoadjuvant chemotherapy versus neoadjuvant chemoradiotherapy for cancer of the oesophagus or gastro-oesophageal junction. Ann Oncol. 2016;27(4):660–7. https://doi.org/10.1093/annonc/mdw010. Epub 2016 Jan 17. PMID: 26782957.

30. Reynolds J V., Preston SR, O'Neill B, et al. Neo-AEGIS (neoadjuvant trial in adenocarcinoma of the esophagus and esophago-gastric junction international study): preliminary results of phase III RCT of CROSS versus perioperative chemotherapy (modified MAGIC or FLOT protocol). (NCT01726452). J Clin Oncol. 2021;39(15)4004. https://doi.org/10.1200/jco.2021.39.15_suppl.4004.

31. Kamarajah SK, Phillips AW, Ferri L, Hofstetter WL, Markar SR. Neoadjuvant chemoradiotherapy or chemotherapy alone for oesophageal cancer: population-based cohort study. Br J Surg. 2021;108(4):403–11. https://doi.org/10.1093/bjs/znaa121. PMID: 33755097.

32. Cools-Lartigue J, Markar S, Mueller C, Hofstetter W, Nilsson M, Ilonen I, Soderstrom H, Rasanen J, Gisbertz S, Hanna GB, Elliott J, Reynolds J, Kisiel A, Griffiths E, Van Berge HM, Ferri L. An international cohort study of prognosis associated with pathologically complete response following neoadjuvant chemotherapy versus chemoradiotherapy of surgical treated esophageal adenocarcinoma. Ann Surg. 2022;276(5):799–805. https://doi.org/10.1097/

SLA.0000000000005619. Epub 2022 Jul 21 PMID: 35861351.

33. Gronnier C, Tréchot B, Duhamel A, Mabrut JY, Bail JP, Carrere N, Lefevre JH, Brigand C, Vaillant JC, Adham M, Msika S, Demartines N, El Nakadi I, Piessen G, Meunier B, Collet D, Mariette C, FREGAT Working Group-FRENCH-AFC, Luc G, Cabau M, Jougon J, Badic B, Lozach P, Cappeliez S, Lebreton G, Alves A, Flamein R, Pezet D, Pipitone F, Iuga BS, Contival N, Pappalardo E, Mantziari S, Hec F, Vanderbeken M, Tessier W, Briez N, Fredon F, Gainant A, Mathonnet M, Bigourdan JM, Mezoughi S, Ducerf C, Baulieux J, Pasquer A, Baraket O, Poncet G, Vaudoyer D, Enfer J, Villeneuve L, Glehen O, Coste T, Fabre JM, Marchal F, Frisoni R, Ayav A, Brunaud L, Bresler L, Cohen C, Aze O, Venissac N, Pop D, Mouroux J, Donici I, Prudhomme M, Felli E, Lisunfui S, Seman M, Petit GG, Karoui M, Tresallet C, Ménégaux F, Hannoun L, Malgras B, Lantuas D, Pautrat K, Pocard M, Valleur P. Impact of neoadjuvant chemoradiotherapy on postoperative outcomes after esophageal cancer resection: results of a European multicenter study. Ann Surg. 2014;260(5):764–70; discussion 770–1. https://doi.org/10.1097/SLA.0000000000000955. PMID: 25379847.

34. Wang H, Tang H, Fang Y, Tan L, Yin J, Shen Y, Zeng Z, Zhu J, Hou Y, Du M, Jiao J, Jiang H, Gong L, Li Z, Liu J, Xie D, Li W, Lian C, Zhao Q, Chen C, Zheng B, Liao Y, Li K, Li H, Wu H, Dai L, Chen KN. Morbidity and mortality of patients who underwent minimally invasive esophagectomy after neoadjuvant chemoradiotherapy vs neoadjuvant chemotherapy for locally advanced esophageal squamous cell carcinoma: a randomized clinical trial. JAMA Surg. 2021;156(5):444–451. https://doi.org/10.1001/jamasurg.2021.0133. PMID: 33729467; PMCID: PMC7970392.Wang DB, Zhang X, Han HL, Xu YJ, Sun DQ, Shi ZL. Neoadjuvant chemoradiotherapy could improve survival outcomes for esophageal carcinoma: a meta-analysis. Dig Dis Sci. 2012;57(12):3226–33. https://doi.org/10.1007/s10620-012-2263-8. Epub 2012 Jun 14. PMID: 22695886.

35. Safran HP, Winter K, Ilson DH, et al. Trastuzumab with trimodality treatment for oesophageal adenocarcinoma with HER2 overexpression (NRG Oncology/RTOG 1010): a multicentre, randomised, phase 3 trial. Lancet Oncol. 2022;23(2):259–69. https://doi.org/10.1016/S1470-2045(21)00718-X.

36. Shah MA, Almhanna K, Iqbal S, et al. Multicenter, randomized phase II study of neoadjuvant pembrolizumab plus chemotherapy and chemoradiotherapy in esophageal adenocarcinoma (EAC). J Clin Oncol. 2021;39(15):4005. https://doi.org/10.1200/jco.2021.39.15_suppl.4005.

37. Shen D, Chen Q, Wu J, Li J, Tao K, Jiang Y. The safety and efficacy of neoadjuvant PD-1 inhibitor with chemotherapy for locally advanced esophageal squamous cell carcinoma. J Gastrointest Oncol. 2021;12(1):1–10. https://doi.org/10.21037/JGO-20-599.

38. Park SY, Hong MH, Kim HR, et al. The feasibility and safety of radical esophagectomy in patients receiving neoadjuvant chemoradiotherapy with pembrolizumab for esophageal squamous cell carcinoma. J Thorac Dis. 2020;12(11):6426–34. https://doi.org/10.21037/jtd-20-1088.

39. Stüben BO, Stuhlfelder J, Kemper M, Tachezy M, Ghadban T, Izbicki JR, Bokemeyer C, Sinn M, Karstens KF, Reeh M. Completion of FLOT therapy, regardless of tumor regression, significantly improves overall survival in patients with esophageal adenocarcinoma. Cancers (Basel). 2022;14(4):1084. https://doi.org/10.3390/cancers14041084.PMID:35205833;PMCID: PMC8870232.

40. Bang YJ, Kim YW, Yang HK, Chung HC, Park YK, Lee KH, Lee KW, Kim YH, Noh SI, Cho JY, Mok YJ, Kim YH, Ji J, Yeh TS, Button P, Sirzén F, Noh SH, CLASSIC trial investigators. Adjuvant capecitabine and oxaliplatin for gastric cancer after D2 gastrectomy (CLASSIC): a phase 3 open-label, randomised controlled trial. Lancet. 2012;379(9813):315–21. https://doi.org/10.1016/S0140-6736(11)61873-4. Epub 2012 Jan 7. PMID: 22226517.

41. Mokdad AA, Yopp AC, Polanco PM, Mansour JC, Reznik SI, Heitjan DF, Choti MA, Minter RR, Wang SC, Porembka MR. Adjuvant chemotherapy vs postoperative observation following preoperative chemoradiotherapy and resection in gastroesophageal cancer: a propensity score-matched analysis. JAMA Oncol. 2018;4(1):31–8. https://doi.org/10.1001/jamaoncol.2017.2805.PMID:28975352;PMCID: PMC5833647.

42. Kelly RJ, Ajani JA, Kuzdzal J, Zander T, Van Cutsem E, Piessen G, Mendez G, Feliciano J, Motoyama S, Lièvre A, Uronis H, Elimova E, Grootscholten C, Geboes K, Zafar S, Snow S, Ko AH, Feeney K, Schenker M, Kocon P, Zhang J, Zhu L, Lei M, Singh P, Kondo K, Cleary JM, Moehler M, CheckMate 577 Investigators. Adjuvant Nivolumab in resected esophageal or gastroesophageal junction cancer. N Engl J Med. 2021;384(13):1191–1203. https://doi.org/10.1056/NEJMoa2032125. Erratum in: N Engl J Med. 2023 Feb 16;388(7):672. PMID: 33789008.

Definitive Chemoradiotherapy for Esophageal Cancer

Ailén Martiarena, Mercedes Tamburelli
and Javier Castillo

Abstract

Esophagectomy is associated with significant morbidity and mortality, especially in small volume centers. Current data suggest that definitive chemoradiotherapy (dCRT) is at least equivalent to trimodality therapy in terms of long-term survival for patients with esophageal squamous cell carcinoma (ESCC). Frail patients with ESCC who are not fit for surgery should receive dCRT. For those who are considered fit for esophagectomy, decision between dCRT and trimodality therapy should be taken on a case-by-case basis. The use of dCRT in patients with esophageal adenocarcinoma is not supported by data.

Keywords

Esophageal cancer · Definitive chemoradiotherapy · Squamous cell carcinoma

A. Martiarena · M. Tamburelli · J. Castillo (✉)
Department of Medical Oncology, Hospital Alemán of Buenos Aires, Buenos Aires, Argentina
e-mail: jcastillo@hospitalaleman.com

M. Tamburelli
e-mail: mtamburelli@hospitalaleman.com

Introduction

Management of patients with esophageal cancer is challenging and requires a multimodal approach. Endoscopic or surgical treatment is recommended for carcinoma in situ and stage IA esophageal cancer. For locally advanced disease, surgical treatment with perioperative chemotherapy or preoperative chemoradiotherapy is recommended for most patients who are fit for surgery.

Definitive chemoradiotherapy (dCRT) is a reasonable option for poor surgical candidates, and might even have comparable results in those with locally-advanced non-metastatic esophageal squamous cell carcinoma (ESCC), as compared to multimodality therapy. Esophagectomy is associated with significant morbidity (e.g. pulmonary complications, anastomotic dehiscence, cardiac arrhythmias) and mortality, especially in small volume centers. While dCRT also presents toxicity and side effects, this approach is less invasive than surgical resection and might result in reduced mortality and shorter hospital stay. Therefore, current NCCN and ESMO guidelines include dCRT as a treatment option for esophageal cancer patients [1, 2].

Most studies on dCRT for esophageal cancer include ESCC patients. These patients often have many comorbidities, which increase the risk for postoperative complications. Even in experienced centers surgical mortality is high

(1–7%) after an esophagectomy [3]. For this reason, it is important to weigh risks and benefits before deciding therapy.

The RTOG 85-01 trial established dCRT as standard non-operative therapy for localized esophageal cancer [4]. More recent investigations identified prognostic factors for long term survival. For instance, a population-based study showed survival rates at 2 years of 29 and 17% in patients with ESCC and esophageal adenocarcinoma (EAC), respectively, showing histology as an independent prognostic factor after dCRT [5]. In other study, the 3-year survival of ESCC patients dropped down from 42% in stage I to 25 and 16% in stage II and III, respectively [6]. Initial T-category and response to dCRT (evaluated by PET-TC and biopsy) are also prognostic factors for long term survival after dCRT [7, 8].

Definitive CRT Versus RT Alone

The addition of cisplatin-based chemotherapy to RT has significantly improved survival over RT alone [4, 9–11]. Unfortunately, available data are almost exclusively in patients with ESCC, and none of the trials have performed adequate pretreatment staging to reliably correlate outcome with locoregional tumor extent. Based on the results of the phase III RTOG 85-01trial, the standard therapy for patients with localized esophageal cancer selected for non-surgical treatment is dCRT [4]. In this trial (ESCC, n = 106 and EAC, n = 15), patients were randomly assigned to receive four cycles of fluorouracil (5-FU 1000 mg/m^2 per day, days 1–4, weeks 1 and 5] plus cisplatin [75 mg/m^2 day 1 of weeks 1 and 5]) with radiation therapy (50 Gy in 25 fractions over five weeks) delivered concurrently with the first cycle of chemotherapy or to radiation therapy alone (64 Gy in 32 fractions over 6.5 weeks). The study showed a significant survival advantage in patients with the combined modality and was finished prematurely, when an interim analysis showed a significant survival advantage for CRT (5-year overall survival 26% vs. 0%). Despite this benefit, the

incidence of local/regional failure was 47% at 12 months.

Subsequent randomized studies confirmed these findings and showed survival rates of 35–40% at 2 years and around 20% at 5 years after dCRT [12–14]. The issue of the unacceptably high locoregional failure rate was addressed in the INT 0123 trial [14]. In this trial, 236 patients with non-metastatic ESCC or EAC who received dCRT (RTOG 85-01-scheme) were randomly assigned to one of two different RT doses: 50.4 Gy (28 fractions over 5.5 weeks) or 64.8 Gy (36 fractions over 7 weeks). After a 2-year follow-up, locoregional control was moderately improved by 52–56% (not significant) in the high-dose group, but there was a trend towards worse overall survival (OS) (31% vs. 40%). High-dose RT was significantly more toxic, and during radiotherapy, 11 deaths were observed in the high-dose arm vs. 2 deaths in the low-dose arm ($p < 0.01$). Interestingly, 7 of the 11 deaths occurred at total doses ≤ 50.4 Gy. During subsequent follow-up, 13 non-index cancer-related deaths were observed in the high-dose arm vs. 3 in the low-dose arm ($P < 0.01$). The results of INT 0123 are still inconclusive and do not exclude a benefit of radiation with doses higher than 50.4 Gy in conventional fractionation. In addition, this study was conducted between 1995 and 1999 (i.e. before the era of 3D-CRT).

At present, 50.4 Gy of RT plus concurrent cisplatin and FU remains the standard approach.

In most trials, improved locoregional tumor control was associated with higher total radiation doses, concurrent chemotherapy, lower tumor volume and SCC histology [15, 16]. In locally advanced esophageal cancer, however, improved locoregional tumor control after higher radiation doses does not appear to translate into improved OS. Long-term (5-year) locoregional control rates after radiotherapy and CRT vary between 32 and 75%.

Overall, the optimal radiation dose remains elusive. Investigators in Japan and China consider total doses of 59.4–66 Gy in 30–33 fractions to be standard radiation therapy [17, 18]. Modern radiation techniques such as intensity-modulated radiation (IMRT) and volumetric modulated arc therapy (VMAT), which use simultaneous integrated boost radiotherapy, have shown to significantly decrease the radiation dose to critical organs such as the heart and lungs [19, 20].

Excellent results have been reported in a phase II trial (n = 60) in which modern technologies were used to deliver 66 Gy in 30 fractions in combination with 2 cycles of cisplatin and 5-FU [21]. A Chinese trial suggested that definitive CRT using the combination of IMRT plus concurrent cisplatin plus docetaxel improves local control and prolongs survival over IMRT alone, but with more prominent side effects [22].

Definitive CRT: Which Chemotherapy?

Several study groups have investigated CRT with different combinations of cisplatin and 5-FU in order to decrease toxicity and improve compliance, and potentially improve treatment efficacy.

The RTOG 85-01 trial established two cycles of cisplatin and 5-FU combined with radiotherapy followed by another two cycles of chemotherapy alone for standard CRT in esophageal cancer. However, the toxicity of this treatment was relatively high. In the study, 20% of patients had life-threatening side effects and 2% died from treatment-related toxicity. In a subsequent RTOG study (94-05, INT 0123) with the same regimen, more than 70% of patients developed side effects of grade 3 or higher [4, 12].

A sequential phase II/III study (PRODIGE 5/ACCORD17) involving 267 patients compared FOLFOX4 chemotherapy scheduled for 6 cycles, 3 of them combined with RT 50 Gy, with the standard RTOG regimen. The relative dose intensity of 5-FU and platinum was comparable in both treatment groups, as well as the percentage of patients with premature discontinuation of chemotherapy and overall toxicity. Similar progression-free survival (median survival 20.2 vs. 17.5 months), OS (3-year survival rate 19.9% vs. 26.9%, HR = 0.94, $P = 0.70$) and

clinical complete response rates (44% vs. 43%) were also observed. However, fewer toxic deaths occurred in the FOLFOX4 group compared to dCRT with cisplatin and 5-FU (1% vs. 6%) [17].

In Europe, the CROSS regimen with weekly carboplatin and paclitaxel chemotherapy scheduled in preoperative combined CRT gained wide acceptance due to its very good tolerability and sparked interest in investigating taxane-based chemotherapy for dCRT [23]. A group from the Netherlands reported their experience with the adaptation of the CROSS regimen for dCRT [19]. Patients with locally advanced esophageal or junctional cancer who had received dCRT at a total dose of 46.8–70 Gy combined with four cycles of cisplatin and 5-FU (RTOG 8501 regimen) or with 5–6 weekly applications of carboplatin (AUC 2) and Paclitaxel (50 mg/m^2) were analyzed. Overall survival was similar in both groups (cisplatin/FU: median OS 16.1 months, carboplatin/paclitaxel: median OS 13.8 months, $P = 0.97$). However, the probability of completing planned dCRT was significantly higher in the carboplatin/paclitaxel group (82% vs. 57%, $P = 0.01$) and treatment-related mortality was lower (1.8% vs. 4.3%).

A propensity-matched analysis compared survival of dCRT with either cisplatin/5-fluorouracil (PF group) or docetaxel/cisplatin (DP group). PF group patients received two cycles of cisplatin (60 mg/m^2) and 5-fluorouracil (300 mg/m^2) at 4-week intervals during radiotherapy. DP group patients received a concurrent three-weekly schedule of docetaxel (60 mg/m^2) and cisplatin (80 mg/m^2) or cisplatin (25 mg/m^2) and docetaxel (25 mg/m^2) weekly. A significant improvement in progression-free survival and OS in favor of DP regimen was observed. It is unclear, however, if the results were related to the inclusion of a taxane in the experimental group or to the reduced dose of cisplatin and the unusual dose of 5-FU in the so-called standard group of this analysis [20].

The SCOPE1 study investigated the role of adding the epidermal growth factor receptor (EGFR) inhibitor cetuximab to dCRT in resectable esophageal cancer. Treatment consisted of induction chemotherapy (two cycles of cisplatin and capecitabine) followed by CRT (50 Gy combined with two cycles of cisplatin and capecitabine) with or without weekly cetuximab. The study was stopped prematurely; OS was significantly worse in the cetuximab group (2-year OS 41.3% vs. 56.0%, HR = 1.45 (1.01–2.09), $P = 0.04$) and subgroup analysis favored CRT alone, particularly in patients with ESCC [24]. Thus, EGFR inhibition combined with dCRT cannot be recommended in unselected patients with esophageal cancer.

Overall, carboplatin/paclitaxel might be an alternative chemotherapy in dCRT. Further studies comparing standard dCRT and dCRT including weekly carboplatin/paclitaxel are needed.

Definitive CRT Versus Surgery Alone

A Japanese study compared results between esophagectomy and dCRT (RT 50–60 Gy with cisplatin and 5-FU) in patients with T1bN0M0 ESCC (n = 173). The 5-year survival was similar in both groups (77.7% vs. 68.6%, $p = 0.12$). Treatment-related mortality was 0%. Progression-free survival, however, was significantly improved in patients undergoing esophagectomy [25].

Another study compared esophageal cancer patients receiving dCRT (n-173), surgery alone (n = 126) or neoadjuvant chemotherapy followed by surgery (n = 118). Patients deemed unsuitable for surgery or with bulky local disease received dCRT. Overall 2-year survival rates were 44.3, 56.2 and 42.4% ($p = 0.42$) [26].

A study from China randomized patients with ESCC of the mid- or lower thoracic esophagus to dCRT (n = 36) or esophagectomy (n = 45). The overall 5-year survival favored dCRT but this was not statiscally significant (50% vs. 29.4%, $p = 0.147$). A trend to improved 5-year survival with dCRT was noted in patients with node-positive disease (47.4% vs. 11.8%, $P = 0.06$) [27].

A previous meta-analysis included 6 randomized studies comparing dCRT with either surgery alone (3 studies) or surgery plus induction

therapy (3 studies). Most patients had thoracic ESCC (810/929). Local tumor progression was more common in patients receiving dCRT ($P < 0.001$) and distant metastases were more often in patients undergoing surgery ($P = 0.06$). Overall survival was equivalent between dCRT and surgery. The study suggests that dCRT is equivalent to surgery (with or without preoperative therapy) in patients with locally advanced ESCC [28].

Definitive CRT Versus Trimodality Therapy

The addition of surgery increases morbidity and mortality, but at the same time it might also favor local control of the disease.

A German study included patients with locally advanced ESCC and randomized 172 patients to induction chemotherapy followed by chemoradiotheray (40 Gy) and surgery or induction chemotherapy followed by dCRT (at least 65 Gy). This study reported equivalent OS in both groups with a 2-year survival rate of 39.9% vs. 35.4% ($p = 0.007$), and an updated long-term survival at 10 years of 19.2% vs. 12.2% ($p = 0.36$) [12, 29]. Although the addition of surgery significantly increased treatment-related mortality (12.8% vs. 3.5%, $p = 0.03$), local tumor progression was significantly worse after dCRT (at 2 years 63.3% vs. 40.7%, $p = 0.003$).

The FFCD 9102 trial included resectable T3N0-1M0 esophageal cancer patients (88.8% ESCC) and randomized those who had response to induction CRT (46 Gy/4.5 weeks or 30 Gy/4 weeks combined with cisplatin and 5-FU) to either surgery or further CRT (total radiation dose of 66 Gy or 45 Gy). The rate of early death was significantly higher after surgery (3-month mortality 9.3% vs. 0.8%, $p = 0.002$). Two-year survival rate was similar in both groups (34% vs. 40%, $p = 0.90$) [13]. These results suggested that in patients with locally advanced ESCC who respond to chemoradiation, there is no benefit for the addition of surgery compared to continuing with additional chemoradiation.

A Cochrane database systemic review compared non-surgical versus surgical treatment for esophageal cancer [30]. Long-term mortality was similar between chemoradiotherapy and surgery (HR 0.88, 95% CI 0.76–1.03; 602 participants; four studies; low quality evidence). In addition, there was no difference in long-term recurrence between non-surgical treatment and surgery (HR 0.96, 95% CI 0.80–1.16; 349 participants; two studies; low quality evidence). The study concluded that dCRT is at least equivalent to surgery in short- and long-term survival in patients with ESCC who are fit for surgery and are responsive to induction chemoradiotherapy. There is uncertainty in the comparison of dCRT versus surgery for patients with EAC [30].

Conclusions

Current data suggest that dCRT is at least equivalent to trimodality therapy in terms of long-term survival for patients with ESCC. Frail patients with ESCC who are not fit for surgery should receive dCRT. For those who are considered fit for esophagectomy, decision between dCRT and trimodality therapy should be taken on a case-by-case basis. The use of dCRT in patients with EAC is not supported by data.

References

1. Esophageal and Esophagogastric Junction Cancers. NCCN clinical practice guidelines in oncology version 2. 2023. www.nccn.org.
2. Oesophageal Cancer. ESMO Clinical Practice Guideline for diagnosis, treatment and follow-up. 2022.
3. Messager M, de Steur WO, van Sandick JW, et al. Variations among 5 European countries for curative treatment of resectable oesophageal and gastric cancer: a survey from the EURECCA Upper GI Group (European Registration of Cancer Care). Eur J Surg Oncol 2016;42:116–22.
4. Cooper JS, Guo MD, Herskovic A, et al. Chemoradiotherapy of locally advanced esophageal cancer: long-term follow-up of a prospective randomized trial (RTOG 85–01). Radiation Therapy Oncology Group. JAMA. 1999;281:1623.
5. Smit JK, Muijs CT, Burgerhof JG, et al. Survival after definitive (chemo)radiotherapy in esophageal cancer patients: a population-based study in the north-East Netherlands. Ann Surg Oncol. 2013;20:1985–92.
6. Chen HS, Hung WH, Ko JL, et al. Impact of treatment modalities on survival of patients with locoregional esophageal squamous-cell carcinoma in Taiwan. Medicine (Baltimore). 2016;95:e3018.
7. Lin SH, Wang J, Allen PK, et al. A nomogram that predicts pathologic complete response to neoadjuvant chemoradiation also predicts survival outcomes after definitive chemoradiation for esophageal cancer. J Gastrointest Oncol. 2015;6:45–52.
8. Amini A, Ajani J, Komaki R, et al. Factors associated with local-regional failure after definitive chemoradiation for locally advanced esophageal cancer. Ann Surg Oncol. 2014;21:306–14.
9. Chan KKW, Saluja R, Delos Santos K, et al. Neoadjuvant treatments for locally advanced, resectable esophageal cancer: a network meta-analysis. Int J Cancer. 2018;143:430.
10. Herskovic A, Martz K, al-Sarraf M, et al. Combined chemotherapy and radiotherapy compared with radiotherapy alone in patients with cancer of the esophagus. N Engl J Med 1992;326:1593.
11. Wong R, Malthaner R. Combined chemotherapy and radiotherapy (without surgery) compared with radiotherapy alone in localized carcinoma of the esophagus. Cochrane Database Syst Rev 2001;CD002092.
12. Stahl M, Wilke H, Lehmann N, et al. Long-term results of a phase III study investigating chemoradiation with and without surgery in locally advanced squamous cell carcinoma (LA-SCC) of the esophagus. J Clin Oncol. 2008;26:431–6. https://doi.org/10.1200/jco.2008.26.15_suppl.4530.
13. Bedenne L, Michel P, Bouché O, et al. Chemoradiation followed by surgery compared with chemoradiation alone in squamous cancer of the esophagus: FFCD 9102. J Clin Oncol. 2007;25:1160–8.
14. Minsky BD, Pajak TF, Ginsberg RJ, et al. INT 0123 (radiation therapy oncology group 94–05) phase III trial of combined-modality therapy for esophageal cancer: high dose versus standard-dose radiation therapy. J Clin Oncol. 2002;20:1167–74.
15. Crehange G, Maingon P, Peignaux K, et al. Phase III trial of protracted compared with split-course chemoradiation for esophageal carcinoma: federation Francophone de Cancerologie Digestive 9102. J Clin Oncol. 2007;25:4895–901. https://doi.org/10.1200/JCO.2007.12.3471.
16. Shridhar R, Almhanna K, Meredith KL, et al. Radiation therapy and esophageal cancer. Cancer Control. 2013;20:97–110.
17. Conroy T, Galais MP, Raoul JL, et al. Definitive chemoradiotherapy with FOLFOX versus fluorouracil and cisplatin in patients with oesophageal

cancer (PRODIGE5/ACCORD17): final results of a randomised, phase 2/3 trial. Lancet Oncol. 2014;15:305–14.

18. Akutsu Y, Matsubara H. Chemoradiotherapy and surgery for T4 esophageal cancer in Japan. Surg Today. 2015;45:1360–5.

19. Honing J, Smit JK, Muijs CT, et al. A comparison of carboplatin and paclitaxel with cisplatinum and 5-fluorouracil in definitive chemoradiation in esophageal cancer patients. Ann Oncol. 2014;25:638–43.

20. Zhang P, Xi M, Li QQ, et al. Concurrent cisplatin and 5-fluorouracil versus concurrent cisplatin and docetaxel with radiotherapy for esophageal squamous cell carcinoma: a propensity score-matched analysis. Oncotarget. 2016;7:44686–94.

21. Chen J, Guo H, Zhai T, et al. Radiation dose escalation by simultaneous modulated accelerated radiotherapy combined with chemotherapy for esophageal cancer: a phase II study. Oncotarget. 2016;7:22711–9.

22. Ji FZ, Zhu WG, Yu CH, et al. A randomized controlled trial of intensity-modulated radiation therapy plus docetaxel and cisplatin versus simple intensity-modulated radiation therapy in II–III stage esophageal carcinoma. Zhonghua Wei Chang Wai Ke Za Zhi. 2013;16:842.

23. Honing J, Smit JK, Muijs CT, et al. A comparison of carboplatin and paclitaxel with cisplatin and 5-fluorouracil in definitive chemoradiation in esophageal cancer patients. Ann Oncol. 2014;25:638.

24. Crosby T, Hurt CN, Falk S, et al. Chemoradiotherapy with or without cetuximab in patients with oesophageal cancer (SCOPE1): a multicentre, phase 2/3 randomised trial. Lancet Oncol. 2013;14:627–37.

25. Motoori M, Yano M, Ishihara R, et al. Comparison between radical esophagectomy and definitive chemoradiotherapy in patients with clinical T1bN0M0 esophageal cancer. Ann Surg Oncol. 2012;19:2135–41.

26. Morgan MA, Lewis WG, Casbard A, et al. Stage-for-stage comparison of definitive chemoradiotherapy, surgery alone and neoadjuvant chemotherapy for oesophageal carcinoma. Br J Surg. 2009;96:1300–7.

27. Teoh AY, Chiu PW, Yeung WK, et al. Long-term survival outcomes after definitive chemoradiation versus surgery in patients with resectable squamous carcinoma of the esophagus: results from a randomized controlled trial. Ann Oncol. 2013;24:165–71.

28. Pöttgen C, Stuschke M. Radiotherapy versus surgery within multimodality protocols for esophageal cancer—a meta-analysis of the randomized trials. Cancer Treat Rev. 2012;38:599–604.

29. Stahl M, Stuschke M, Lehmann N, et al. Chemoradiation with and without surgery in patients with locally advanced squamous cell carcinoma of the esophagus. J Clin Oncol. 2005;23:2310–7.

30. Best LM, Mughal M, Gurusamy KS. Non-surgical versus surgical treatment for oesophageal cancer. Cochrane Database Syst Rev. 2016;3:CD011498.

Immunotherapy in Esophageal Cancer

Federico Esteso and Berenice Freile

Abstract

This chapter provides an overview of the latest advances in the use of immunotherapy for the treatment of esophageal cancer. This chapter highlights the biology and the potential role of identifying biomarkers of response, and offers a comprehensive overview of the clinical trials that have evaluated the use of immunotherapy in different settings of the treatment of esophageal cancer.

Keywords

Esophageal cancer · Immunotherapy · Targeted agents · Precision medicine

Introduction

Esophageal cancer is the 6th malignant tumor in incidence and the 5th leading cause of cancer-related mortality worldwide [1]. Esophageal and gastric cancer are often grouped together in systemic therapy clinical trials, given their similarities in underlying risk factors, biology, and overlapping management strategies. The two main esophageal cancer histologic subtypes include esophageal squamous cell carcinoma (ESCC) and esophageal adenocarcinoma (EAC). ESCC and EAC are two completely different diseases, with different risk factors, molecular profiles and prognosis. Although being historically treated as the same entity, current data suggest that both diseases should be considered separately.

While surgery remains the mainstay for the treatment of esophageal cancer, neoadjuvant chemoradiotherapy (nCRT) or perioperative chemotherapy have significantly improved survival compared to surgery alone in patients with locally advanced disease [2, 3]. However, despite all the available treatments, survival remains poor. Therefore, it is necessary to explore novel and effective treatments to improve survival. Luckily, the management of esophageal cancer has experienced changes during the last decades due to the deeper knowledge of its biology [4]. Consequently, the type of systemic therapy now depends on multiple variables such as tumor location, histology, and several biomarkers (e.g. microsatellite instability (MSI), HER2, and programmed death-1 ligand (PD-L1) expression) [5].

The results of recent clinical trials have shown benefits with regards to the use of immunotherapy and targeted therapy. The rationale to develop immunotherapy comes from the recognized link between esophageal cancer and

F. Esteso (✉) · B. Freile
Medical Oncology, Instituto Alexander Fleming, Buenos Aires, Argentina
e-mail: festeso@alexanderfleming.org

precursor chronic inflammatory lesions and high mutational rates [6]. The main risk factors for ESCC tumorigenesis are smoking and alcohol consumption, whereas chronic gastroesophageal reflux and obesity are risk factors for EAC [7].

Immunity and Microenvironment of Esophageal Cancer

Understanding the Complex Tumor Environment

One of the established hallmarks of cancer is the escape or evasion of the immune system [8]. This capacity to escape immunologic surveillance is related to the disruption of tumor microenvironment (TME), which as we known, has a complex composition (i.e. immune cells, fibroblasts, endothelial cells and extracellular matrix). Once the balance of the TME is disrupted, the tumor can develop by blocking apoptosis, granting immune evasion and promoting angiogenesis, proliferation and distant metastases [4].

One of the pathways used by tumor cells to proliferate is the PD-1/PD-L1, by overexpressing PD-L1 on the cancer cell surface or by inducing PD-L1 expression on the host's immune cells. Once activated, PD-L1 has the ability to exhaust and inhibit host T-cell response, allowing the tumor to escape immune surveillance. This is why the PD-1/PD-L1 complex is consider an ideal target for immunotherapeutic agents. There are different ways to quantify the expression of this complex; one is the combined positive score (CPS), which represents the percentage of PD-L1 expressing tumor and infiltrating immune cells within the total number of tumor cells. Another one is the tumor proportion score (TPS), which is the percentage of PD-L1 positive tumor cells. These scores can be used to identify possible responders to anti-PD-1 therapy.

Another pathway to escape and promote tumor growth is through CTLA-4. This homologue of the CD28 protein is a transmembrane protein expressed exclusively on activated T-cells. When CTLA-4 bounds to proteins, it prevents T cells from destroying other cells.

Immunotherapy includes all biologic/targeted agents that aim to obtain the balance back by modifying and/or blocking co-stimulatory signals, and therefore restoring the immune system's ability to detect and destroy cancer cells, known as immune-checkpoint inhibitors (ICIs) [4]. Different molecules that inhibit the link between PD-1 and PD-L1 are currently used for the treatment of gastrointestinal tumors and specifically for esophageal cancer: anti-PD-1 agents such as nivolumab, pembrolizumab, sintilimab and camrelizumab, or anti-PD-L1-agents such as atezolizumab and avelumab. The monoclonal antibodies used to inhibit upregulation of CTLA-4 are ipilimumab and tremelimumab.

Molecular Biomarkers for Immunotherapy

The selection of patients who will benefit from ICIs ("responders") is critical [9]. The role of predictive and prognostic molecular biomarkers has been investigated. PD-L1 expression is the most studied and used in previous trails and its overexpression can be found in up to 40–50% of ESCC [10]. Considering PD-L1 as a prognostic factor, various studies have focused on this matter, yet the results have been inconsistent. In the bulk of these studies, PD-L1 overexpression has been linked to unfavorable clinical outcomes. Nevertheless, it has been reported by others a better prognosis in PD-L1-positive patients over PD-L1-negtive [11, 12]. PD-L1 testing may be considered in patients with locally advanced, recurrent, or metastatic esophageal and gastroesophageal junction (GEJ) who are candidates for treatment with PD-1 inhibitors [13].

Research on others prognostic factors such as gene signatures have been done. However, the relationship between the expression of these genes and the response of patients receiving ICIs is not still clarified [14, 15]. Despite the promising prognostic value of gene-signatures for esophageal cancer, prospective studies are needed to validate and recommend their use. Regarding the predictive role of biomarkers, immunotherapy has shown to improve survival outcomes (HR: 0.71), mainly in patients with ESCC and PD-L1 CPS $\geq$ 10 [16].

Unfortunately, the prognostic significance of PD-L1 is unclear and diversity exists in the PD-L1 assessment, score and cut-off values. Figure 1 shows assessment and cut-off points of PD-L1 in different trials.

Non-metastatic Esophageal Cancer. Adjuvant and Neoadjuvant Scenario

Early stage ESCC and EAC are treated with upfront surgical resection. Patients with locally advanced disease are now managed with either preoperative chemoradiation or perioperative chemotherapy [2, 3]. Despite the improvement provided these systemic therapies, up to 30% of patients will present early recurrence within 12 months of surgery. As ICIs became a useful treatment strategy in the metastatic setting, research has recently moved to the non-metastatic scenario.

CheckMate 577 is the milestone trial that has changed the treatment paradigm, leading to the acceptance of adjuvant Nivolumab. This phase III trial enrolled patients with resected esophageal and GEJ tumors, who had received neoadjuvant chemoradiation and had evidence of residual pathological disease, and evaluated the safety and efficacy of adding of one year of adjuvant treatment with the anti-PD-1 nivolumab (N: 532) versus placebo (N: 262). The trial met its primary endpoint, by doubling the median disease-free survival (DFS) in the experimental arm compared to placebo (22.4 vs. 11 months, respectively; HR 0.69, $p < 0.001$) [17]. The study design did not used the tumor location as a stratification criterion. That being said, no significant benefit for

adjuvant nivolumab was shown for patients with GEJ tumors (HR 0.87). Another point to consider is that 71% of patients had EAC and only 29% ESCC. Although improvement was seen in both groups, the ESCC subgroup had a higher DFS benefit from nivolumab (HR, 0.61) than the EAC subgroup (HR, 0.75). In addition, the trial first studied and stratified patients with PD-L1 expression by TPS. When presenting the post hoc analysis, data regarding PD-L1 expression was shown with CPS, and 57% of patients in the nivolumab arm and 54% in the placebo arm had PD-L1 positive (CPS $\geq$ 5), and these patients presented a clear benefit over the negative ones (HR 0.62 and 0.89, respectively). Nivolumab was well tolerated, grade 3–4 adverse events occurred in 13% of patients in the nivolumab group and 6% in the placebo group. Overall, postoperative nivolumab is a new effective and recommended treatment option for patients at high risk for recurrence due to the presence of residual pathologic disease following preoperative chemoradiation and R0 resection [7, 13].

Data regarding neoadjuvant immunotherapy is scarce. In a recent systemic review and meta-analysis of 27 clinical trials with 815 patients the pooled rate of pathological complete response (pCR) was 31.4% (95% CI, 27.6–35.3%) with promising clinical and safety outcomes [18]. It is expected that in the near future many clinical trials will evaluate the role of neoadjuvant immunotherapy.

Advanced Esophageal Cancer

Platinum-based chemotherapy has been the standard treatment for advanced or unresectable esophageal cancer for more than 10 years [19]. The introduction of targeted therapy agents, mainly directed against human epidermal growth factor receptor 2 (HER2) [20] and PD-L1, represented a significant advance in esophageal cancer, as these agents improved survivals beyond one year for the first time.

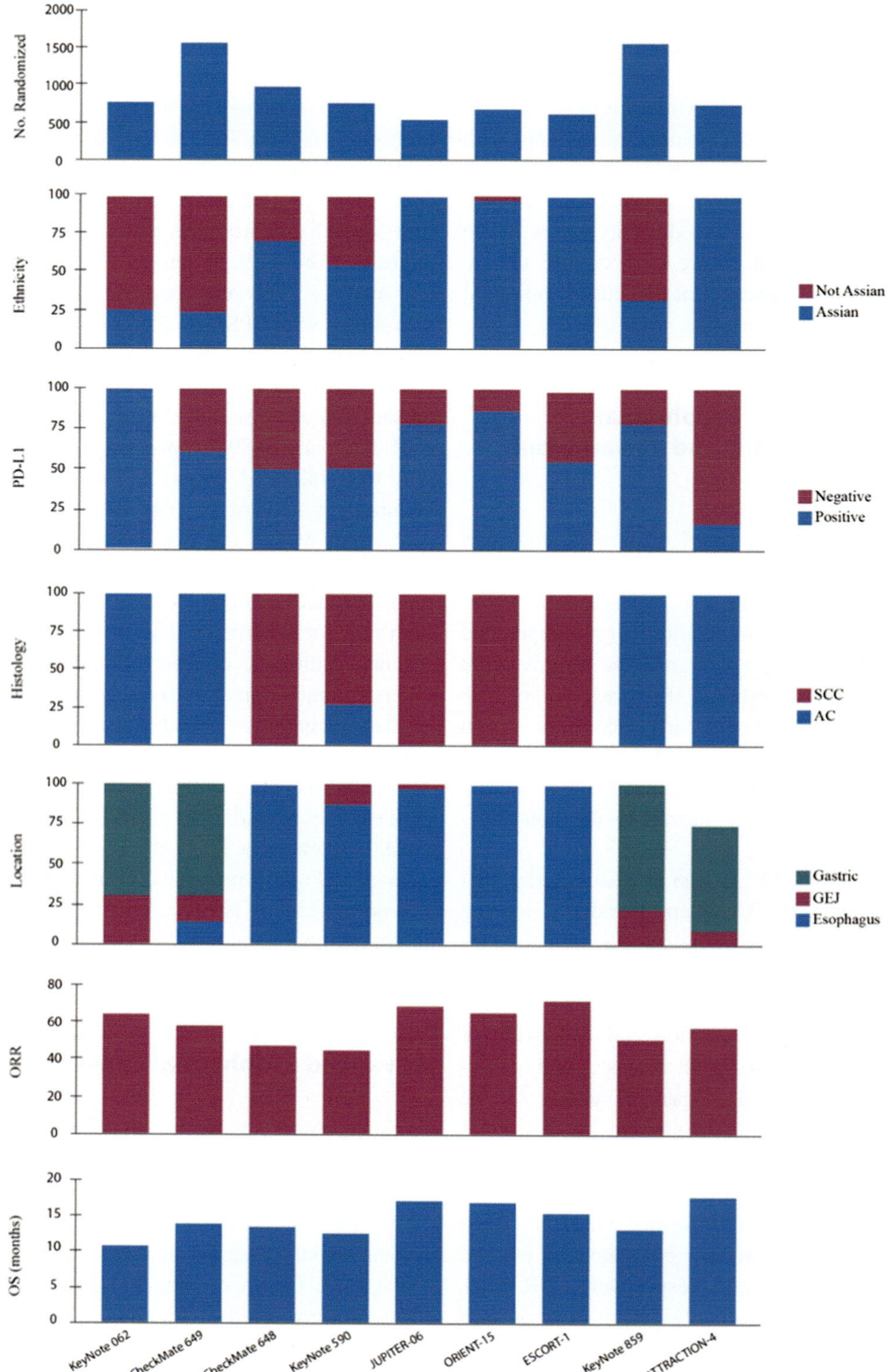

Fig. 1 First line trials of immunotherapy for advanced esophageal cancer (OS: Overall survival; ORR: Overall response rate; GEJ: Gastroesophageal Junction; AC: Adenocarcinoma; SCC: Squamous cell carcinoma)

First Line

The CheckMate-649 is a phase III study that restructured the first line treatment algorithm for GEJ tumors and EAC HER-2 negative [21]. It showed improvement in overall survival (OS) with the addition of nivolumab to standard chemotherapy (either capecitabine-oxaliplatin or 5-FU-leucovorin-oxaliplatin) in all randomly assigned patients (HR, 0.79; 95% CI 0.71–0.88) versus chemotherapy alone. The study also showed benefits in progression free survival (PFS) (HR, 0.79; 0.70–0.89). Even though the approval is regardless the PD-L1 expression, the greatest improvement in OS and PFS was shown in patients with a PD-L1 CPS $\geq$ 5 (HR 0.71; $p < 0.0001$ and HR 0.68; $p < 0.0001$, respectively).Therefore, this new therapeutic strategy was approved by the FDA, independent of PD-L1 expression and is currently recommended by NCCN as category 1 for patients with PD-L1 expression levels by CPS $\geq$ 5 or as category 2B when CPS < 5 [13]. It has also been approved by EMA and recommended by ESMO only when PD-L1 positive [22].

The phase III CheckMate 648 study randomized patients with treatment naive advanced ESCC to 3 arms: chemotherapy (cisplatine-5 FU), nivolumab plus chemotherapy or nivolumab plus ipilimumab, regardless the PD-L1 expression [23]. Patients treated with nivolumab plus chemotherapy had improved OS compared with patients treated with chemotherapy alone in the entire study population (13.2, 12.7 and 10.7 months in the nivolumab plus chemotherapy (HR: 0.74), nivolumab plus ipilimumab (HR: 0.78) and chemotherapy arm, respectively). This benefit was most pronounced in patients with PD-L1 $\geq$ 1%, with a 6-month improvement (HR 0.54; $p < 0.001$). PFS was also significantly improved by nivolumab plus chemotherapy in PD-L1 positive population (HR 0.65; p: 0.0023). But in all-randomized population, the benefit was a nonstatistical trend (HR = 0.81). Despite nivolumab plus ipilimumab improved OS compared with chemotherapy alone, this arm did not meet the PFS endpoint. While in the USA the recommendation for nivolumab plus chemotherapy or nivolumab plus ipilimumab in metastatic ESCC is regardless of the PD-L1 tumor expression, in Europe is restricted for PD-L1 $\geq$ 1 [7, 13].

KeyNote-062 randomized 763 patients with locally advanced/unresectable or metastatic gastric and GEJ adenocarcinoma with PD-L1 CPS $\geq$ 1 to pembrolizumab, pembrolizumab plus chemotherapy or chemotherapy alone [24]. Pembrolizumab showed no benefit compared to chemotherapy for OS (10.6 vs. 11.1 months; HR 0.91; 99.2% CI, 0.69–1.18). Although a benefit was seen in patients with CPS $\geq$ 10 (17.4 vs. 10.8 months; HR, 0.69; 95% CI, 0.49–0.97), this difference was not statistically tested.

The phase III KeyNote-590 trial evaluated addition of pembrolizumab to cisplatine plus 5FU in patients with untreated, advanced esophageal cancer or GEJ tumors (Siewert type I) [25]. The majority of patients in the study (73%) had ESCC. The greatest OS improvement was observed in patients with ESCC and elevated PD-L1 expression (CPS $\geq$ 10; HR 0.59; $p < 0.0001$), while in all randomized patients the median OS was 12.4 months (HR 0.73; $p < 0.0001$). A post hoc analysis suggested no benefit in patients with a PD-L1 CPS < 10. The FDA approved Pembrolizumab as a first-line option for patients with advanced and metastatic esophageal cancer independent of histological subtype and PD-L1 status. On the other hand, EMA approved it only for patients expressing PD-L1 CPS $\geq$ 10.

The KeyNote 859 phase III trial assessed the benefit of pembrolizumab plus chemotherapy versus chemotherapy alone in GEJ tumors and gastric cancer [26]. The combination of fluorouracil (5FU) and cisplatin or capecitabine plus oxalipaltin (CAPOX) were the chemotherapy choices (86% of patients received CAPOX). This trial showed a statistical benefit in OS for all the intention to treat, with a median benefit of 1.4 months (12.9 for pembrolizumab vs. 11.5 for chemotherapy, HR 0.78; $p < 0.0001$). When describing subgroups, the PD-L1 < 1 population only showed a HR 0.90 (0.701–1.148) and the CPS $\geq$ 10 a HR 0.62 (0.51–0.75).

In the advanced setting is also mandatory to investigate for other biomarkers. HER2 is a known marker for pathogenesis and poor outcomes. The ToGA trial showed that targeted treatment with trastuzumab improved survival when combined with chemotherapy in the first line setting in patients with gastric and GEJ adenocarcinoma [20]. Although this trial did not included patients with esophageal cancer, patients with HER2-positive EAC are usually treated based on the data of this trial.

The possibility of survival improvement in HER-2 positive patients not only with chemotherapy and trastuzumab but also with immunotherapy was firstly assessed with an investigator-initiated phase II trial. The study investigated the addition of pembrolizumab to the modified ToGA regimen with promising results. Thus, the phase III KEYNOTE-811 trial enrolled patients with metastatic HER2-positive gastric and GEJ adenocarcinoma (31% GEJ tumors) [27]. This trial demonstrated a significant benefit in objective response rate (ORR) with the combination of immunotherapy plus targeted therapy plus chemotherapy compared to targeted therapy plus chemotherapy (74.4% vs. 51.9%; p: 0.00006). These promising results led to the FDA to approve the addition of pembrolizumab to a backbone of FU/platinum with HER2-targeted therapy for HER2-positive gastric and GEJ adenocarcinoma, regardless of CPS score. This is also noted in the NCCN guidelines with the addition of pembrolizumab as a recommended first-line therapy.

Other phase III trials assessed the efficacy of immunotherapy in the first line setting in the Asian population. ESCORT-1 trial randomized 595 Chinese patients without previous treatment metastatic ESCC to receive chemotherapy (cisplatin plus paclitaxel) alone or in combination with camrelizumab [28]. The addition of camrelizumab to standard chemotherapy improved OS (HR: 0.70, p: 0.001) and PFS (HR: 0.56, p: 0.001) with a reasonable safety profile. Of note, the benefit in survival (OS, 3 months and PFS, 1.3 months improvement) is quite low considering this setting and there was no selection according to PD-L1 status. Another trial was the

phase III ORIENT-15 (97.1% of 659 patients randomized were Asian) [29] which investigated the benefit of adding sintilimab to chemotherapy versus chemotherapy alone as a first-line treatment for metastatic ESCC. Although patients were included regardless of PD-L1 status, the trial assessed PD-L1 positivity (by TPS and CPS scores). At the interim analysis, sintilimab with chemotherapy showed better OS and PFS compared with standard arm in all patients (median 16.7 vs. 12.5 months, HR 0.63, $P<0.001$; 7.2 vs. 5.7 months, 0.56, $P<0.001$, respectively). This improvement was higher in patients with $CPS \geq 10$.

The JUPITER-06 trial is a phase III trial that is evaluating the efficacy and safety of toripalimab as a first-line treatment for metastatic ESCC in Asian patients [30]. The trial randomized 514 patients to receive toripalimab plus chemotherapy (paclitaxel and cisplatin) or chemotherapy alone and continued with toripalimab as a maintenance treatment or placebo, regardless of PD-L1 expression. With the first results of PFS and OS, a significant improvement was observed by the addition of toripalimab to chemotherapy over the placebo arm (HR 0.58, $p<0.0001$ and HR 0.58, p: 0.0004, respectively). An East Asian phase II/III trial, ATTRACTION-4, enrolled 724 patients with previously untreated HER2-negative, unresectable, advanced or recurrent gastric or GEJ cancer (regardless of PD-L1 expression) and randomly assigned them to chemotherapy (oxaliplatin with either S-1 (SOX) or capecitabine (CAPOX) plus nivolumab or SOX/CAPOX with placebo [31]. They met their primary endpoint, with a median PFS of 10.4 versus 8.3 months (HR 0.68; p: 0.0007) favoring the IO arm. However, no benefit was observed in OS (17.45 months with nivolumab vs. 17.15 months with chemotherapy, HR 0.90; 95% CI 0·75–1·08; p: 0.26).

A new biomarker has emerged for the treatment of unresectable or metastatic GEJ and gastric adenocarcinomas as the SPOTLIGHT trial has recently presented [32]. It compared chemotherapy (FOLFOX) with chemotherapy plus zolbetuximab in HER2 negative population. Zolbetuximab is an antibody that targets claudin 18.2 (CLDN18.2), a tight junction protein present in approximately 30% of adenocarcinomas. The primary end point of PFS was met with a median of 10,6 vs. 8.76 months (HR 0.751, 0.58–0.94) with the addition of zolbetuximab. OS was also improved, median 18.23 vs. 15.54 months (HR 0.75, 0.61–0.93). Other potential biomarkers are currently been tested in clinical trials as FGFR with the drug bemarituzumab.

Overall, the addition of immunotherapy to a chemotherapy backbone should be considered for patients with advanced esophageal tumors. An increasing magnitude of benefit is noted in patients with higher levels of PDL1 (different cut off values regarding the drug and study) In ESCC patients who are unable to tolerate chemotherapy, nivolumab plus ipilimumab could be an option (Table 1 and Fig. 1).

Second and Subsequent Lines

As expected, the initial trials with immunotherapy agents evaluated its use in later lines of therapy. The trial KEYNOTE-059 was a global, phase II, single-arm, that studied pembrolizumab monotherapy in the third line setting for patients with advanced gastric or GEJ adenocarcinoma [33]. ORR was 11.6% with complete response in 2.3% of all patients. When stratified by PD-L1, ORR was 15.5% for PD-L1 positive versus 6.4% for PD-L1–negative tumors. Any-grade adverse events were reported in 95.8% of patients, with 61.4% experiencing one or more grade 3 to grade 5 adverse events, being the most common fatigue and anemia. This trial initiated the era on immunotherapy in esophageal cancer. Time then showed that benefits of immunotherapy are greater when using it in earlier lines.

The ATTRACTION-3 trial randomized 419 patients with ESCC to receive nivolumab or chemotherapy (paclitaxel or docetaxel) in the second line setting after failure of a fluoropyrimidine based treatment [34]. Even though this trial was global, only 18 patients (4%) were not Asian. It showed significantly superior OS for nivolumab when compared to chemotherapy (10.9 vs. 8.4 months, respectively; HR 0.77, p: 0.019). Despite the lack of improvement on PFS with nivolumab, when analyzing, the Kaplan-Meyer plot, the crossing of the curves exposed the need of selecting patients correctly in order to improve outcomes. And so, when looking at the responders' curves, they tend to have a plateau, interpreted as a maintenance of the response. While the objective response was higher in the chemotherapy arm rather than the nivolumab arm (22% vs. 19%, respectively), the duration of response was better in the nivolumab group. Based on these results, nivolumab received the approval from both USA and Europe as the new standard of care in the second-line treatment for metastatic ESCC after a fluoropyrimidine-based chemotherapy, regardless of PD-L1 status.

KEYNOTE-181 studied the benefit of pembrolizumab in the second line setting regardless of the histologic subtype [35]. Patients were randomly assigned to treatment with pembrolizumab or chemotherapy (paclitaxel, irinotecan or docetaxel). OS was higher with pembrolizumab in the Asian population, in those for patients with CPS $\geq$ 10, regardless of the histology (9.3 months vs. 6.7 months, HR: 0.69, $p = 0.0074$) and in ESCC tumors (8.2 vs. 7.1 months, HR: 0.78, p: 0.0095). In all randomly assigned patients, OS was equal for both arms, regardless of PD-L1 and histology. The results in the ESCC cohort did not reach the preplanned boundaries and thereby the trial did not meet the co-primary endpoint in median OS. Thus, pembrolizumab was only approved by the FDA in patients with ESCC whose tumors had PD-L1 CPS $\geq$ 10 expression as a second and further line therapy.

One novel immunotherapeutic agent was studied in the RATIONALE 302, a global phase III trial that investigated tislelizumab versus chemotherapy (paclitaxel, docetaxel, or irinotecan) in patients with ESCC [36]. This study found a significantly improved OS (8.6 vs. 6.3 months; HR 0.70; p: 0.0001) and ORR (20.3% vs. 9.8%), regardless PD-L1.

A phase III trial with only Asian population is the ESCORT [37]. This study randomized 457 patients with ESCC in the second line scenario

Table 1 First line trials of immunotherapy for advanced esophageal cancer

Study (date)	Regimens	N	PD-L1 assessment for end points	Tumor Histology	Location	Ethnicity	OS (months) outcomes	ORR	AE G ≥ 3
KeyNote062	a. Pembrolizumab	256	IHC 22C3	AC 100%	Gastric 69% GEJ 31%	Assian 24.5% Not Assian 75.5%	(a vs. c) 10.6 vs. 11.1 (HR 0.91)	57.1%	17.3%
	b. Pembrolizumab + Chemotherapy	257						64.7%	73.2%
	c. Chemotherapy	250						36.8%	69.3%
CheckMate 649 (2021)	a. Nivolumab + Chemoterapy	789	IHC 28.8	AC 100%	Gastric 70% GEJ 16.5% Esophagous 13.5%	Assian 24% Not Assian 76%	13.8 vs. 11.6 (HR 0.8)	58%	59% vs. 44%
	c. Placebo + Chemotherapy	792							
KeyNote 590 (2021)	a. Pembrolizumab + Chemotherapy	373	IHC 22C3	AC 27% SCC 73%	GEJ 12.2% Esophagous 87.8%	Assian 54% Not Assian 46%	12.4 vs. 9·8 (HR 0.73)	45%	72% vs. 68%
	b. Placebo + Chemotherapy	376							
Escort-1 (2021)	a. Camrelizumab + Chemotherapy	298	IHC 6E8	SCC 100%	Esophagous 100%	Assian 100%	15.3 vs. 12.0 (HR 0.70)	72.1%	63.4% vs. 67.7%
	b. Placebo + Chemotherapy	298							
Orient-15 (2022)	a. Sintilimab + Chemotherapy	327	IHC 22C3	SCC 100%	Esophagous 100%	Assian 97.3% Not Assian 2.7%	16.7 vs. 11 (HR 0.63)	66%	60% vs. 55%
	b. Chemotherapy + Placebo	332							
Jupiter-06 (2022)	a. Toripalimab + Chemotherapy	257	JS311	SCC 100%	GEJ 3% Esophagous 97%	Assian 100%	17 vs. 11 (HR 0.58)	69.3%	73.2% vs. 70%
	b. Chemotherapy + Placebo	257							
CheckMate 648 (2022)	a. Nivolumab + Chemoterapy	321	IHC 28.8	SCC 100%	Esophagous 100%	Assian 70.6% Not Assian 29.4%	(a vs. c) 13.2 vs. 10.7 (HR 0.74)	47%	(a vs. c) 47% vs. 36%
	b. Nivolumab + Ipilimumab	325							
	c. Placebo + Chemotherapy	324							
ATTRACTION-4 (2022)	a. Nivolumab + Chemotherapy	362	No selection	AC 100%	GEJ 18.56% Gastric 65.6%	Assian 100%	17.45 vs. 17.15 (HR 0.90)	57.5%	57.9% vs. 49.2%
	b. Chemotherapy + placebo	362							

(continued)

Table 1 (continued)

Study (date)	Regimens	N	PD-L1 assessment for end points	Tumor Histology	Location	Ethnicity	OS (months) outcomes	ORR	AE G≥3
KeyNote 589 (2023)	a. Pembrolizumab + Chemotherapy	790	IHC 22C3	AC 100%	GEJ 21.15% Gastric 78.85%	Assian 70.6%% Not Assian 29.4%	12.9 vs. 11.5 (HR 0.70)	51.3%	59.4% vs. 51.1%
	b. Chemotherapy + placebo	789							

OS overall survival, *ORR* overall response rate, *AE* adverse effect, *G* grade, *ICH* immunohistochemistry, *AC* adenocarcinoma, *SCC* squamous cell carcinoma, *GEJ* gastroesophageal junction, *HR* hazard ratio

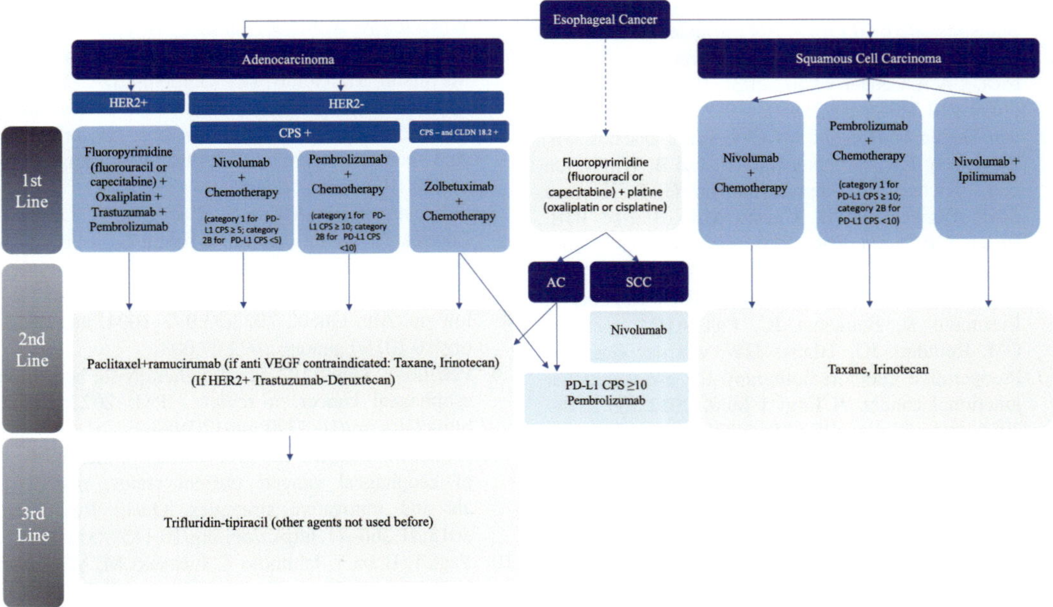

Fig. 2 Algorithm for the management of advanced esophageal cancer

to receive camrelizumab or chemotherapy (docetaxel), regardless of PD-L1 status. The immunotherapy arm showed improvement in the median OS in the study population (8.3 vs. 6.2 months, HR 0.71, *p*: 0.001) with an acceptable safety profile (grade 3–5 adverse events: 19% vs. 39%). Of note, patients with PD-L1 positive tumors (≥ 1% assessed by TPS) had the greatest benefit from camrelizumab. No benefit was reported for PFS, showing the same median PFS in both groups (1.9 vs. 1.9 months, respectively, HR 0.69, *p*: 0.00063). Camrelizumab appears to be a good therapeutic option in the second-line treatment for ESCC, regardless of the PDL1 expression. We should consider, however, that the trial included only Asian population.

A treatment algorithm for advanced esophageal cancer is presented in Fig. 2.

Conclusion

Immunotherapy, represented by immune checkpoint inhibitors, has become a research hotspot for the treatment of esophageal cancer. Significant improvements in survival have been obtained with the use immunotherapy, which have now changed the treatment algorithm in these patients.

References

1. Sung H, Ferlay J, Siegel RL, Laversanne M, Soerjomataram I, Jemal A, Bray F. Global Cancer Statistics 2020: GLOBOCAN estimates of incidence and mortality worldwide for 36 cancers in 185 countries. CA A Cancer J Clin. 2021;71:209–49. https://doi.org/10.3322/caac.21660.
2. van Hagen P, Hulshof MCCM, van Lanschot JJB, Steyerberg EW, Henegouwen MI, van B, Wijnhoven BPL, Richel DJ, Nieuwenhuijzen GAP, Hospers GAP, Bonenkamp JJ, Cuesta MA, Blaisse RJB, Busch ORC, ten Kate FJW, Creemers G-J, Punt CJA, Plukker JTM, Verheul HMW, Bilgen EJS, van Dekken H, van der Sangen MJC, Rozema T, Biermann K, Beukema JC, Piet AHM, van Rij CM, Reinders JG, Tilanus HW, van der Gaast A. Preoperative chemoradiotherapy for esophageal or junctional cancer. N Engl J Med. 2012;366:2074–2084. https://doi.org/10.1056/NEJMoa1112088.
3. Al-Batran S-E, Homann N, Pauligk C, Goetze TO, Meiler J, Kasper S, Kopp H-G, Mayer F, Haag GM, Luley K, Lindig U, Schmiegel W, Pohl M, Stoehlmacher J, Folprecht G, Probst S, Prasnikar N, Fischbach W, Mahlberg R, Trojan J, Koenigsmann M, Martens UM, Thuss-Patience P, Egger M, Block A, Heinemann V, Illerhaus G, Moehler M, Schenk M, Kullmann F, Behringer DM, Heike M, Pink D, Teschendorf C, Löhr C, Bernhard H, Schuch G, Rethwisch V, von Weikersthal LF, Hartmann JT, Kneba M, Daum S, Schulmann K, Weniger J, Belle S, Gaiser T, Oduncu FS, Güntner M, Hozaeel W, Reichart A, Jäger E, Kraus T, Mönig S, Bechstein WO, Schuler M, Schmalenberg H, Hofheinz RD. Perioperative chemotherapy with fluorouracil plus leucovorin, oxaliplatin, and docetaxel versus fluorouracil or capecitabine plus cisplatin and epirubicin for locally advanced, resectable gastric or gastro-oesophageal junction adenocarcinoma (FLOT4): a randomised, phase 2/3 trial. The Lancet. 2019;393:1948–57. https://doi.org/10.1016/S0140-6736(18)32557-1.
4. Teixeira Farinha H, Digklia A, Schizas D, Demartines N, Schäfer M, Mantziari S. Immunotherapy for esophageal cancer: state-of-the art in 2021. Cancers. 2022;14:554. https://doi.org/10.3390/cancers14030554.
5. Patruni S, Fayyaz F, Bien J, Phillip T, King DA. Immunotherapy in the management of esophago-gastric cancer: a practical review. JCO Oncol Pract. 2023;19:107–15. https://doi.org/10.1200/OP.22.00226.
6. Lawrence MS, Stojanov P, Polak P, Kryukov GV, Cibulskis K, Sivachenko A, Carter SL, Stewart C, Mermel CH, Roberts SA, Kiezun A, Hammerman PS, McKenna A, Drier Y, Zou L, Ramos AH, Pugh TJ, Stransky N, Helman E, Kim J, Sougnez C, Ambrogio L, Nickerson E, Shefler E, Cortés ML, Auclair D, Saksena G, Voet D, Noble M, DiCara D, Lin P, Lichtenstein L, Heiman DI, Fennell T, Imielinski M, Hernandez B, Hodis E, Baca S, Dulak AM, Lohr J, Landau D-A, Wu CJ, Melendez-Zajgla J, Hidalgo-Miranda A, Koren A, McCarroll SA, Mora J, Lee RS, Crompton B, Onofrio R, Parkin M, Winckler W, Ardlie K, Gabriel SB, Roberts CWM, Biegel JA, Stegmaier K, Bass AJ, Garraway LA, Meyerson M, Golub TR, Gordenin DA, Sunyaev S, Lander ES, Getz G. Mutational heterogeneity in cancer and the search for new cancer-associated genes. Nature. 2013;499:214–8. https://doi.org/10.1038/nature12213.
7. Obermannová R, Alsina M, Cervantes A, Leong T, Lordick F, Nilsson M, van Grieken NCT, Vogel A, Smyth EC. Oesophageal cancer: ESMO clinical practice guideline for diagnosis, treatment and follow-up. Ann Oncol. 2022;33:992–1004. https://doi.org/10.1016/j.annonc.2022.07.003.
8. Petrillo A, Smyth EC. Immunotherapy for squamous esophageal cancer: a review. JPM. 2022;12:862. https://doi.org/10.3390/jpm12060862.
9. Alsina M, Moehler M, Lorenzen S. Immunotherapy of esophageal cancer: current status, many trials and innovative strategies. Oncol Res Treat. 2018;41:266–71. https://doi.org/10.1159/000488120.
10. Yagi T, Baba Y, Ishimoto T, Iwatsuki M, Miyamoto Y, Yoshida N, Watanabe M, Baba H. PD-L1 expression, tumor-infiltrating lymphocytes, and clinical outcome in patients with surgically resected esophageal cancer. Ann Surg. 2019;269:471–8. https://doi.org/10.1097/SLA.0000000000002616.
11. Chen K, Cheng G, Zhang F, Zhang N, Li D, Jin J, Wu J, Ying L, Mao W, Su D. Prognostic significance of programmed death-1 and programmed death-ligand 1 expression in patients with esophageal squamous cell carcinoma. Oncotarget. 2016;7:30772–80. https://doi.org/10.18632/oncotarget.8956.
12. PD-L1 expression is a prognostic factor in patients with thoracic esophageal cancer treated without adjuvant chemotherapy. AR. 2017;37:1433–42. https://doi.org/10.21873/anticanres.11467.
13. Esophageal_blocks.pdf. https://www.nccn.org/professionals/physician_gls/pdf/esophageal_blocks.pdf.
14. Cao K, Ma T, Ling X, Liu M, Jiang X, Ma K, Zhu J, Ma J. Development of immune gene pair-based

signature predictive of prognosis and immunotherapy in esophageal cancer. Ann Transl Med. 2021;9:1591–1591. https://doi.org/10.21037/atm-21-5217.

15. Yao J, Duan L, Huang X, Liu J, Fan X, Xiao Z, Yan R, Liu H, An G, Hu B, Ge Y. Development and validation of a prognostic gene signature correlated with M2 macrophage infiltration in esophageal squamous cell carcinoma. Front Oncol. 2021;11:769727. https://doi.org/10.3389/fonc.2021.769727.

16. Leone AG, Petrelli F, Ghidini A, Raimondi A, Smyth EC, Pietrantonio F. Efficacy and activity of PD-1 blockade in patients with advanced esophageal squamous cell carcinoma: a systematic review and meta-analysis with focus on the value of PD-L1 combined positive score. ESMO Open. 2022;7:100380. https://doi.org/10.1016/j.esmoop.2021.100380.

17. Kelly RJ, Ajani JA, Kuzdzal J, Zander T, Van Cutsem E, Piessen G, Mendez G, Feliciano J, Motoyama S, Lièvre A, Uronis H, Elimova E, Grootscholten C, Geboes K, Zafar S, Snow S, Ko AH, Feeney K, Schenker M, Kocon P, Zhang J, Zhu L, Lei M, Singh P, Kondo K, Cleary JM, Moehler M. Adjuvant nivolumab in resected esophageal or gastroesophageal junction cancer. N Engl J Med. 2021;384:1191–203. https://doi.org/10.1056/NEJMoa2032125.

18. Ge F, Huo Z, Cai X, Hu Q, Chen W, Lin G, Zhong R, You Z, Wang R, Lu Y, Wang R, Huang Q, Zhang H, Song A, Li C, Wen Y, Jiang Y, Liang H, He J, Liang W, Liu J. Evaluation of clinical and safety outcomes of neoadjuvant immunotherapy combined with chemotherapy for patients with resectable esophageal cancer: a systematic review and meta-analysis. JAMA Netw Open. 2022;5:e2239778. https://doi.org/10.1001/jamanetworkopen.2022.39778.

19. Cunningham D, Starling N, Rao S, Iveson T, Nicolson M, Coxon F, Middleton G, Daniel F, Oates J, Norman AR. Capecitabine and oxaliplatin for advanced esophagogastric cancer. N Engl J Med. 2008;358:36–46. https://doi.org/10.1056/NEJMoa073149.

20. Bang Y-J, Van Cutsem E, Feyereislova A, Chung HC, Shen L, Sawaki A, Lordick F, Ohtsu A, Omuro Y, Satoh T, Aprile G, Kulikov E, Hill J, Lehle M, Rüschoff J, Kang Y-K. Trastuzumab in combination with chemotherapy versus chemotherapy alone for treatment of HER2-positive advanced gastric or gastro-oesophageal junction cancer (ToGA): a phase 3, open-label, randomised controlled trial. The Lancet. 2010;376:687–97. https://doi.org/10.1016/S0140-6736(10)61121-X.

21. Janjigian YY, Shitara K, Moehler M, Garrido M, Salman P, Shen L, Wyrwicz L, Yamaguchi K, Skoczylas T, Campos Bragagnoli A, Liu T, Schenker M, Yanez P, Tehfe M, Kowalyszyn R, Karamouzis MV, Bruges R, Zander T, Pazo-Cid R, Hitre E, Feeney K, Cleary JM, Poulart V, Cullen D, Lei M, Xiao H, Kondo K, Li M, Ajani JA. First-line nivolumab plus chemotherapy versus chemotherapy alone for advanced gastric, gastro-oesophageal junction, and oesophageal adenocarcinoma (CheckMate 649): a randomised, open-label, phase 3 trial. The Lancet. 2021;398:27–40. https://doi.org/10.1016/S0140-6736(21)00797-2.

22. Lordick F, Carneiro F, Cascinu S, Fleitas T, Haustermans K, Piessen G, Vogel A, Smyth EC. Gastric cancer: ESMO Clinical Practice Guideline for diagnosis, treatment and follow-up☆. Ann Oncol. 2022;33:1005–20. https://doi.org/10.1016/j.annonc.2022.07.004.

23. Doki Y, Ajani JA, Kato K, Xu J, Wyrwicz L, Motoyama S, Ogata T, Kawakami H, Hsu C-H, Adenis A, El Hajbi F, Di Bartolomeo M, Braghiroli MI, Holtved E, Ostoich SA, Kim HR, Ueno M, Mansoor W, Yang W-C, Liu T, Bridgewater J, Makino T, Xynos I, Liu X, Lei M, Kondo K, Patel A, Gricar J, Chau I, Kitagawa Y. Nivolumab combination therapy in advanced esophageal squamous-cell carcinoma. N Engl J Med. 2022;386:449–62. https://doi.org/10.1056/NEJMoa2111380.

24. Shitara K, Van Cutsem E, Bang Y-J, Fuchs C, Wyrwicz L, Lee K-W, Kudaba I, Garrido M, Chung HC, Lee J, Castro HR, Mansoor W, Braghiroli MI, Karaseva N, Caglevic C, Villanueva L, Goekkurt E, Satake H, Enzinger P, Alsina M, Benson A, Chao J, Ko AH, Wainberg ZA, Kher U, Shah S, Kang SP, Tabernero J. Efficacy and safety of pembrolizumab or pembrolizumab plus chemotherapy vs chemotherapy alone for patients with first-line, advanced gastric cancer: the KEYNOTE-062 Phase 3 randomized clinical trial. JAMA Oncol. 2020;6:1571. https://doi.org/10.1001/jamaoncol.2020.3370.

25. Sun J-M, Shen L, Shah MA, Enzinger P, Adenis A, Doi T, Kojima T, Metges J-P, Li Z, Kim S-B, Cho BC, Mansoor W, Li S-H, Sunpaweravong P, Maqueda MA, Goekkurt E, Hara H, Antunes L, Fountzilas C, Tsuji A, Oliden VC, Liu Q, Shah S, Bhagia P, Kato K. Pembrolizumab plus chemotherapy versus chemotherapy alone for first-line treatment of advanced oesophageal cancer (KEYNOTE-590): a randomised, placebo-controlled, phase 3 study. The Lancet. 2021;398:759–71. https://doi.org/10.1016/S0140-6736(21)01234-4.

26. Rha SY, Wyrwicz LS, Weber PEY, Bai Y, Ryu MH, Lee J, Rivera F, Alves GV, Garrido M, Shiu K-K, Fernández MG, Li J, Lowery M, Cil T, Cruz FJSM, Qin S, Yin L, Bordia S, Bhagia P, Oh D-Y. VP1-2023: pembrolizumab (pembro) plus chemotherapy (chemo) as first-line therapy for advanced HER2-negative gastric or gastroesophageal junction (G/GEJ) cancer: Phase III KEYNOTE-859 study. Ann Oncol. 2023;34:319–20. https://doi.org/10.1016/j.annonc.2023.01.006.

27. Janjigian YY, Kawazoe A, Yañez P, Li N, Lonardi S, Kolesnik O, Barajas O, Bai Y, Shen L, Tang Y, Wyrwicz LS, Xu J, Shitara K, Qin S, Van Cutsem E, Tabernero J, Li L, Shah S, Bhagia P, Chung HC. The KEYNOTE-811 trial of dual PD-1 and

HER2 blockade in HER2-positive gastric cancer. Nature. 2021;600:727–30. https://doi.org/10.1038/s41586-021-04161-3.

28. Luo H, Lu J, Bai Y, Mao T, Wang J, Fan Q, Zhang Y, Zhao K, Chen Z, Gao S, Li J, Fu Z, Gu K, Liu Z, Wu L, Zhang X, Feng J, Niu Z, Ba Y, Zhang H, Liu Y, Zhang L, Min X, Huang J, Cheng Y, Wang D, Shen Y, Yang Q, Zou J, Xu R-H, ESCORT-1st Investigators, Yuan X, Ma D, Liu L, Ye F, Liu T, Wang X, Liu L, Xia B, Ran F, Sun S, Miao Z, Bie J, Gao Y, Yu J, Chen L, He Y, Ren W, Luo S, Zhao G, Lin Y, Chen L, Guo Z, Hu C, Wang Y, Xu N, Chen B, Zhan X, Chen Y, Lu H, Qin S, Wang G, Chen L, Bai L, Zhang J. Effect of camrelizumab vs placebo added to chemotherapy on survival and progression-free survival in patients with advanced or metastatic esophageal squamous cell carcinoma: the ESCORT-1st randomized clinical trial. JAMA. 2021;326:916. https://doi.org/10.1001/jama.2021.12836.

29. Lu Z, Wang J, Shu Y, Liu L, Kong L, Yang L, Wang B, Sun G, Ji Y, Cao G, Liu H, Cui T, Li N, Qiu W, Li G, Hou X, Luo H, Xue L, Zhang Y, Yue W, Liu Z, Wang X, Gao S, Pan Y, Galais M-P, Zaanan A, Ma Z, Li H, Wang Y, Shen L. Sintilimab versus placebo in combination with chemotherapy as first line treatment for locally advanced or metastatic oesophageal squamous cell carcinoma (ORIENT-15): multicentre, randomised, double blind, phase 3 trial. BMJ. 2022;e068714. https://doi.org/10.1136/bmj-2021-068714.

30. Wang Z-X, Cui C, Yao J, Zhang Y, Li M, Feng J, Yang S, Fan Y, Shi J, Zhang X, Shen L, Shu Y, Wang C, Dai T, Mao T, Chen L, Guo Z, Liu B, Pan H, Cang S, Jiang Y, Wang J, Ye M, Chen Z, Jiang D, Lin Q, Ren W, Wang J, Wu L, Xu Y, Miao Z, Sun M, Xie C, Liu Y, Wang Q, Zhao L, Li Q, Huang C, Jiang K, Yang K, Li D, Liu Y, Zhu Z, Chen R, Jia L, Li W, Liao W, Liu H-X, Ma D, Ma J, Qin Y, Shi Z, Wei Q, Xiao K, Zhang Y, Zhang Y, Chen X, Dai G, He J, Li J, Li G, Liu Y, Liu Z, Yuan X, Zhang J, Fu Z, He Y, Ju F, Liu Z, Tang P, Wang T, Wang W, Zhang J, Luo X, Tang X, May R, Feng H, Yao S, Keegan P, Xu R-H, Wang F. Toripalimab plus chemotherapy in treatment-naïve, advanced esophageal squamous cell carcinoma (JUPITER-06): A multi-center phase 3 trial. Cancer Cell. 2022;40:277-288.e3. https://doi.org/10.1016/j.ccell.2022.02.007.

31. Kang Y-K, Chen L-T, Ryu M-H, Oh D-Y, Oh SC, Chung HC, Lee K-W, Omori T, Shitara K, Sakuramoto S, Chung I-J, Yamaguchi K, Kato K, Sym SJ, Kadowaki S, Tsuji K, Chen J-S, Bai L-Y, Oh S-Y, Choda Y, Yasui H, Takeuchi K, Hirashima Y, Hagihara S, Boku N. Nivolumab plus chemotherapy versus placebo plus chemotherapy in patients with HER2-negative, untreated, unresectable advanced or recurrent gastric or gastro-oesophageal junction cancer (ATTRACTION-4): a randomised, multicentre, double-blind, placebo-controlled, phase 3 trial. Lancet Oncol. 2022;23:234–47. https://doi.org/10.1016/S1470-2045(21)00692-6.

32. Shitara K, Lordick F, Bang Y.-J, Enzinger PC, Ilson DH, Shah MA, Van Cutsem E, Xu R, Aprile G, Xu J, Chao J, Pazo-Cid R, Kang Y-K, Yang J, Moran DM, Bhattacharya PP, Arozullah A, Wook Park J, Ajani JA. Zolbetuximab + mFOLFOX6 as first-line (1L) treatment for patients (pts) withclaudin-18.2+ (CLDN18.2+)/HER2—locally advanced (LA) unresectable or metastatic gastric or gastroesophageal junction (mG/GEJ) adenocarcinoma: primary results from phase 3 SPOTLIGHT study. JCO. 2023;41:LBA292–LBA292. https://doi.org/10.1200/JCO.2023.41.4_suppl.LBA292.

33. Fuchs CS, Doi T, Jang RW, Muro K, Satoh T, Machado M, Sun W, Jalal SI, Shah MA, Metges J-P, Garrido M, Golan T, Mandala M, Wainberg ZA, Catenacci DV, Ohtsu A, Shitara K, Geva R, Bleeker J, Ko AH, Ku G, Philip P, Enzinger PC, Bang Y-J, Levitan D, Wang J, Rosales M, Dalal RP, Yoon HH. Safety and efficacy of pembrolizumab monotherapy in patients with previously treated advanced gastric and gastroesophageal junction cancer: phase 2 clinical KEYNOTE-059 trial. JAMA Oncol. 2018;4:e180013. https://doi.org/10.1001/jamaoncol.2018.0013.

34. Kato K, Cho BC, Takahashi M, Okada M, Lin C-Y, Chin K, Kadowaki S, Ahn M-J, Hamamoto Y, Doki Y, Yen C-C, Kubota Y, Kim S-B, Hsu C-H, Holtved E, Xynos I, Kodani M, Kitagawa Y. Nivolumab versus chemotherapy in patients with advanced oesophageal squamous cell carcinoma refractory or intolerant to previous chemotherapy (ATTRACTION-3): a multicentre, randomised, open-label, phase 3 trial. Lancet Oncol. 2019;20:1506–17. https://doi.org/10.1016/S1470-2045(19)30626-6.

35. Kojima T, Shah MA, Muro K, Francois E, Adenis A, Hsu C-H, Doi T, Moriwaki T, Kim S-B, Lee S-H, Bennouna J, Kato K, Shen L, Enzinger P, Qin S-K, Ferreira P, Chen J, Girotto G, de la Fouchardiere C, Senellart H, Al-Rajabi R, Lordick F, Wang R, Suryawanshi S, Bhagia P, Kang SP, Metges J-P. on behalf of the KEYNOTE-181 Investigators: randomized phase III KEYNOTE-181 study of pembrolizumab versus chemotherapy in advanced esophageal cancer. JCO. 2020;38:4138–48. https://doi.org/10.1200/JCO.20.01888.

36. Shen L, Kato K, Kim S-B, Ajani JA, Zhao K, He Z, Yu X, Shu Y, Luo Q, Wang J, Chen Z, Niu Z, Zhang L, Yi T, Sun J-M, Chen J, Yu G, Lin C-Y, Hara H, Bi Q, Satoh T, Pazo-Cid R, Arkenau H-T, Borg C, Lordick F, Li L, Ding N, Tao A, Shi J, Van Cutsem E. For the RATIONALE-302 investigators: tislelizumab versus chemotherapy as second-line

treatment for advanced or metastatic esophageal squamous cell carcinoma (RATIONALE-302): a randomized phase III study. JCO. 2022;40:3065–76. https://doi.org/10.1200/JCO.21.01926.

37. Huang J, Xu J, Chen Y, Zhuang W, Zhang Y, Chen Z, Chen J, Zhang H, Niu Z, Fan Q, Lin L, Gu K, Liu Y, Ba Y, Miao Z, Jiang X, Zeng M, Chen J, Fu Z, Gan L, Wang J, Zhan X, Liu T, Li Z, Shen L, Shu Y, Zhang T, Yang Q, Zou J, Luo S, Peng F, Wu G, Xu N, Zhao L, Ma D, Qin S, Ren W, Li E, Lu H, Pan Y, Xiong J, Yuan Y, Bai Y, Chen L, Hu Y, Zhang L, Gao Y. Camrelizumab versus investigator's choice of chemotherapy as second-line therapy for advanced or metastatic oesophageal squamous cell carcinoma (ESCORT): a multicentre, randomised, open-label, phase 3 study. Lancet Oncol. 2020;21:832–42. https://doi.org/10.1016/S1470-2045(20)30110-8.

Anesthesia for Esophageal Surgery

Jacob Jackson and Alessia Pedoto

Abstract

Esophageal surgery for cancer can be curative but is associated with significant morbidity and mortality. Scrutinizing the perioperative anesthetic management for the procedure seeks to understand its impact on outcomes and discover opportunities for improvement. Moreover, surgical approaches to esophagectomy continue to evolve with the advent of minimally invasive techniques and robotic surgery, and anesthetic methods and concerns must evolve in parallel.

Keywords

Esophageal cancer · Anesthesia · One-lung ventilation · Goal directed fluid therapy · Regional anesthesia · Thoracic epidural analgesia · Enhanced recovery after surgery

Introduction

Esophageal surgery for cancer can be curative but is associated with significant morbidity and mortality. Scrutinizing the perioperative anesthetic management seeks to understand its impact on outcomes and discover opportunities for improvement. Moreover, surgical approaches to esophagectomy continue to evolve with the increased adoption of minimally invasive techniques and robotic surgery, and anesthetic methods and concerns must evolve in parallel.

The anesthesiologist plays a crucial role throughout the perioperative period, ensuring an appropriate preoperative evaluation and optimization of modifiable conditions, intraoperative management, and recovery. As esophagectomy care further develops through research and innovation, the role of the anesthesia provider during the perioperative period will likely become even more pronounced.

Preoperative Evaluation

Initial Assessment and Testing

Patients presenting for esophagectomy may have several comorbidities pertinent to their anesthetic management in addition to their esophageal pathology. Appropriate patient selection and evaluation is necessary to mitigate potential

J. Jackson (✉) · A. Pedoto
Department of Anesthesiology and Critical Care Medicine, Memorial Hospital, Memorial Sloan Kettering Cancer Center, 1275 York Avenue, New York, NY 10065, USA
e-mail: jacksoj1@mskcc.org

A. Pedoto
e-mail: pedotoa@mskcc.org

complications of what is already a highly morbid procedure.

Gastroesophageal reflux disease (GERD) and dysphagia are commonly associated with esophageal lesions and predispose to pulmonary aspiration. Severe GERD can cause pharyngolaryngitis, chronic cough, or asthma-like symptoms; chronic aspiration can lead to pulmonary fibrosis.

Smoking and alcohol use should be assessed with consideration for presence of chronic obstructive pulmonary disease (COPD) and hepatic dysfunction, respectively. Active smoking at the time of surgery, especially if combined with excessive alcohol use, is associated with an increase in postoperative complications after esophagectomy, such as decreased wound healing and increased cardiovascular and respiratory adverse events [1]. Tobacco smokers should quit at least 30 days prior to surgery. Electronic cigarette (e-cigarette) or vaping use has been associated with lung injury, which, if present, can place patients at increased morbidity risk. However, there are currently no evidence-based guidelines for perioperative management or cessation [2]. Perioperative medical or recreational cannabis use may have implications for airway reactivity, altered drug metabolism, unpredictable effects of anesthetics, and postoperative withdrawal symptoms—intoxication may prompt a delay in the procedure. *Cannabis withdrawal syndrome* has been described 24–72 h post cessation in heavy marijuana users (> 1.5 g/day inhales or > 20 mg/day PO) as irritability or anger, anxiety, insomnia, decreased appetite, restlessness, altered mood, and discomfort. Symptoms peak at one week and can last for two weeks [3]. *Heavy alcohol* users (more than 24 gm/day in women, 35 gm/day in men) are at increased risk for general morbidity, infections, pulmonary complications, increased hospital length of stay, intensive care unit admission and 30-day mortality. *Acute alcohol withdrawal* can occur within 6–8 h of abstinence, manifesting as hallucinations, seizures, and status epilepticus. *Delirium tremens* is observed after 48–96 h and can last up to two weeks. Cognitive dysfunction is common in this phase [4]. Risks from

smoking and alcohol use may be reversible, depending on the duration of smoking and the interval of abstinence [5].

Poor nutritional status, resulting from the disease state, poor oral intake, or chemoradiation toxicity, decreases physiologic tolerance to the procedure and impairs healing and recovery [6]. Electrolyte impairment and coagulopathy can develop, as well as hypoalbuminemia with an effect on drug binding. A poor preoperative nutritional status has been associated with a worse postoperative outcome. Parameters used to assess nutrition include albumin, cholesterol, and total lymphocyte count [7].

Neoadjuvant chemoradiation is often used in the preoperative period to decrease tumor size, increase the curative success of surgery, and decrease distant micrometastases [8, 9]. *Chemotherapeutic agents* can cause bone marrow suppression with anemia and thrombocytopenia. Anemia increases the chances of red blood cell transfusion with its associated complications. Thrombocytopenia may exacerbate intraoperative bleeding or preclude neuraxial blockade. Platinum derivatives can cause renal dysfunction or impaired hearing [10], while fluorouracil is associated in rare cases with cardiomyopathy, hyperammonemia and encephalopathy [11]. *Immunotherapy*, a successful treatment for melanoma and lung cancer, is being investigated in patients with esophageal tumors, showing some promising results [12]. These drugs specifically target T-cells and their receptors, re-activating the immune system against cancer cells. Their potency seems to be increased after exposure to radiation treatment and because of their mechanism of action, they can activate several immune-related side effects within 3–6 months of exposure. The severity is variable and, in most cases, transient. Skin rashes and diarrhea are the most common side effects. Hypophysitis, hypothyroidism, diabetes mellitus, and adrenal insufficiency with secondary hyponatremia have been reported. Hypoparathyroidism with hypocalcemia has also been observed but is extremely rare. Mild cases are usually monitored and managed conservatively, while for severe cases, steroid treatment with thyroid replacement is recommended [13, 14]. Immunotherapy is usually continued unless severe symptoms are present.

After completing a thorough history and physical exam, appropriate *laboratory studies* should include a comprehensive metabolic panel to analyze electrolytes, renal function, and hepatic function, and a complete blood count to quantify anemia and thrombocytopenia, if present. *Coagulation studies* are relevant for patients with a bleeding diathesis or who are taking anticoagulants but also serve to evaluate hepatic function and safety of neuraxial blockade. Severe malnutrition may be associated with abnormal coagulation studies.

Comorbid *cardiovascular disease* can significantly increase patient mortality risk and should be evaluated in accordance with American College of Cardiology/American Heart Association guidelines (ACC/AHA) [15]. *Twelve-lead electrocardiogram* is performed as indicated for patients with known coronary heart disease, significant arrhythmia, peripheral arterial disease, cerebrovascular disease, or other significant structural heart disease, or may be performed as screening for myocardial ischemia or arrhythmia. More invasive cardiac testing (e.g., *stress test, angiogram*) is indicated in patients at high risk, such as those with unstable angina, decompensated chronic heart failure, arrhythmias, and severe valvular disease [15]. *Preoperative angina* in patients with previous myocardial infarction (MI) is associated with a higher incidence of postoperative adverse cardiac events, such as MI and/or cardiac arrest [16]. If patients require revascularization, elective surgery needs to be postponed. The dilemma of how long to wait needs to be discussed with the surgeon and oncologist due to the concern for potential disease progression [17]. *Cardiac stents*, especially drug-eluting ones, represent a significant problem due to the prolonged need for anticoagulation. Stopping dual antiplatelet therapy (DAPT) (aspirin plus a $P2Y_{12}$ inhibitor) is associated with increased risk of stent thrombosis, while continuing DAPT leads to increased risk of intra- and postoperative bleeding and precludes neuraxial anesthetic

techniques [18]. The duration of DAPT prior to undergoing elective noncardiac surgery is based upon the type of stent: bare metal stents require 30 days after implantation, while drug-eluting stents require 6 months for purely elective procedures and 3 months for cases in which the risk of further delay in surgery is greater than the expected risks of stent thrombosis. If the $P2Y_{12}$ inhibitor therapy is stopped prior to surgery, it is recommended that aspirin be continued if possible and the $P2Y_{12}$ platelet receptor inhibitor (clopidogrel, prasugrel, or ticagrelor) be restarted as soon as possible after surgery [19].

Patients with a history of COPD, prior lung resection, chronic lung disease or morbid obesity should undergo *pulmonary function testing (PFTs)* in anticipation of one-lung ventilation (OLV). A computed tomography (CT) scan or positron emission tomography (PET) scan of the chest done for cancer staging or to assess chemotherapeutic treatment response may also be used by the anesthesiologist to evaluate airway abnormalities or lung disease. Poor PFTs are associated with an increased incidence of respiratory complications, with potential benefits from preoperative pulmonary rehabilitation or training (i.e., incentive spirometry, deep diaphragmatic breathing, coughing). Respiratory rehabilitation has been proposed as part of a multidisciplinary approach to improve respiratory mechanics and decrease complications [20].

Preoperative staging involves cross-sectional imaging and *endoscopic ultrasound (EUS) evaluation*, the latter of which is done as an outpatient procedure and requires an anesthetic [21]. The decision between sedation versus general anesthesia is based on the severity of symptoms and the experience of the provider.

Patient Selection

Predicting which patients are going to have a complicated recovery or increased mortality following esophagectomy is valuable information for all involved. In general, poor overall health and preexisting organ system dysfunction negatively impact esophagectomy outcomes [22].

The use of *scoring algorithms* can add objectivity to the selection criteria.

- The *Glasgow Prognostic Score* (GPS) and modified GPS (mGPS) combine elevated C-Reactive protein and hypoalbuminemia as markers of systemic inflammation. Seven studies of the GPS and mGPS in esophageal cancer have shown prognostic value independent of tumor stage and pathological features [23]. While GPS for squamous cell carcinoma correlates strongly with mortality after esophagectomy [24], mGPS for adenocarcinoma correlates with disease severity but not mortality [25].
- The Physiological and Operative Severity Score for the enumeration of Mortality and Morbidity (*POSSUM*), Portsmouth *(P) POSSUM* and upper gastrointestinal *(O) POSSUM* models were developed for calculating risk-adjusted mortality using a two-part scoring system: a 12-factor physiological score and a six-factor operative severity score. A comparison of the three models showed that P-POSSUM provided the most accurate prediction of in-hospital mortality after esophagectomy [26]. A comparison of POSSUM models with mGPS showed that the POSSUM physiology score was useful in predicting postoperative morbidity, while mGPS was the best predictor of cancer-specific survival [27].

Cardiopulmonary exercise testing (CPET) is a method for determining a patient's physiological capacity to tolerate the stress of surgery. The test involves exercising against increasing levels of known resistance in the form of a cycle ergometer, treadmill, or a hand crank for approximately ten minutes while recording ventilatory parameters, inspiratory and expiratory gases, blood pressure, and electrocardiogram. From this data, the body's maximum oxygen uptake and the anaerobic threshold (the point at which anaerobic metabolism exceeds aerobic metabolism) are determined [28]. In elderly patients undergoing major abdominal or thoracic surgery, results of CPET have shown that an anaerobic threshold (AT) of < 11 ml/kg/min predicted postoperative cardiopulmonary deaths [28]. The utility of CPET for assessment of preoperative exercise capacity and as a tool for risk stratification for esophagectomy patients was previously studied and shown to correlate well with postoperative cardiopulmonary morbidity; however, CPET did not previously demonstrate adequate discriminatory ability [29, 30]. The topic was revisited by Patel et al. in 2019, who found that patients with $VO_{2peak} < 17$ mL/kg/min (VO_{2peak} is the highest volume of oxygen use achieved during the final 30 s of the test) and AT < 10.5 ml/kg/min were over twice as likely to develop major morbidity after esophagectomy [32]. The results have renewed interest in CPET, though in the setting of cost and resource limitations, simpler ergometric testing (e.g., shuttle walk test or stair climb test) or assessment of functional status by metabolic equivalents may be favored.

In sum, patient assessment for surgery based on scoring systems and assessment of functional status can help with patient selection and risk stratification, but should not be used in isolation for clinical decision-making. Experienced judgment of the surgeon and anesthesiologist, who consider multiple factors, still takes precedent.

Optimization

Reduction of modifiable risk factors is the main focus in preparation for surgery, with an emphasis on smoking cessation, correction of anemia, and improved nutritional state.

1. In a retrospective analysis, the incidence of pneumonia decreased with a longer duration of *smoking cessation* prior to esophagectomy. It is unclear how long is needed to decrease postoperative complications, with some providers suggesting at least 4–8 weeks [33]. Another study showed smoking cessation ≤ 30 days was an independent risk factor for pneumonia and smoking cessation ≤ 90 days was an independent risk factor for other severe morbidities [34]. It is strongly recommended that the perioperative

provider counsel patients at the preoperative visit and may suggest behavioral and pharmacological interventions [5]. Respiratory physiotherapy has been studied (i.e., inspiratory muscle training) and shown to improve respiratory function but not incidence of postoperative pneumonia after esophagectomy [35].

2. *Anemia* is commonly found with esophageal cancer and increases the likelihood of red blood cell transfusion, which is significantly associated with higher overall complications and increased risk of surgical site infections [36]. Iron deficiency anemia may be corrected preoperatively with oral or intravenous iron supplementation; oral iron takes two weeks to increase the serum hemoglobin level and two months to normalize it [37]. Intravenous iron infusions can correct anemia faster—a dose of 1000–1500 mg has 50% effect in five days and full effect in three weeks. It is unclear if the use of iron supplements with or without erythropoietin decrease the need for transfusion [38] or have beneficial effect with respect to outcomes after major upper gastrointestinal surgery [39].

3. *Malnutrition* is likely to predispose to postoperative complications and is exacerbated by surgical stress and metabolic demands of recovery. While nutrition is not easily improved in patients with dysphagia, a nutritional assessment should be performed and attempts to improve nutrient intake should be made. *Carbohydrate loading* prior to appropriate preoperative fasting may attenuate the surgical stress response, insulin resistance and subsequent hyperglycemia, as well as muscle breakdown of the patient [40, 41]. In severe cases of malnutrition, feeding tubes can be placed prior to surgery. However, elective enteral nutrition has not been shown to improve outcome prior to neoadjuvant treatment and therefore should not be recommended unless deemed necessary [42].

Prehabilitation has been suggested to improve outcome. Supervised exercise programs, in addition to smoke cessation programs and dietary assessment especially in malnourished patients, have the theoretical advantage to improve fitness and provide a faster return to baseline preoperative functional status [43]. The literature has yet to demonstrate a convincing relationship between prehabilitation and oncological outcomes [44]. In addition, many programs require 2–4 weeks for success, potentially delaying a curative operation.

Intraoperative Management

Surgical Approach

The anesthetic preparation must consider the planned surgical approach, as each has its own considerations. Independent of the technique (open versus minimally invasive) and the type of operation (Ivor Lewis, McKeown, transhiatal, etc.), patients undergoing esophagectomy are at risk of aspiration on induction and emergence and require optimal analgesia. Invasive m onitoring is commonly used independently of the technique, due to the potential arrhythmias during the thoracic dissection or in the postoperative period. Proper positioning to avoid neuropathy is essential for cases of long duration [45]. *Extubation* at the end of the case is recommended to avoid ventilation associated respiratory injury and hemodynamic instability as a consequence of the sedation required to tolerate the ventilator.

Open approaches involve large incisions and violate both the peritoneal and pleural cavities, making it a painful procedure for the patient. Inadequate pain control can complicate extubation and impair effective pulmonary toilet and ambulation during recovery without a multimodal analgesic plan in place. Proper analgesia is important, usually in the form of epidural or paravertebral catheters, removed within 2–3 days if the patient is enrolled in an enhanced recovery after surgery (ERAS) pathway.

Minimally invasive esophagectomy (MIE) has become more popular since the early 2000s, particularly at high-volume academic centers, with the goal of decreasing risk and improving outcomes by decreasing surgical stress, inducing less postoperative pain, and easing recovery overall. All forms of dissections can be performed minimally invasively [45], with similar morbidity and mortality to the open approach [46–48]. The main concerns for these cases are related to the positioning, the creation of pneumoperitoneum and pneumothorax, and arrhythmias during the thoracic phase. In most cases, patients are first in reverse Trendelenburg followed by the lateral decubitus. However, the prone position is used in some centers for the thoracoscopic dissection [49]. Steep reverse Trendelenburg requires a secured patient to prevent falls and padding of the feet to avoid pressure sores. Hypotension can occur soon after positioning, it is exacerbated by decreased venous return from abdominal insufflation, and may require intravascular volume loading, vasopressors, or inotropes. At the time of the crural dissection, a left pneumothorax may develop and require desufflation of the peritoneal cavity, fluid and vasopressor/inotrope administration, leveling of the operating room table, and decompression of the pleural cavity with chest tube placement in severe cases [50].

Intraoperative Monitoring

The duration and complexity of esophagectomy require the ability to monitor patient hemodynamics and metabolic state comprehensively and expeditiously. Standard monitoring should include pulse oximetry, noninvasive blood pressure monitoring, electrocardiography, and temperature monitoring. Placement of an arterial line for continuous blood pressure monitoring is commonly used to guide hemodynamic support and ventilator settings, especially for OLV. Furthermore, surgical dissection in the thorax and manipulation of the mediastinum has the potential for large vessel compression or injury and stimulation of cardiac dysrhythmias that need to be detected and intervened upon quickly. Arterial blood samples from the arterial line may be used for point-of-care analysis of hemoglobin level, electrolyte balance, acid–base status, arterial oxygenation and lactic acid concentration. Central venous access is usually unnecessary except in cases of difficult intravenous access or if desired for vasopressor infusion. If a cervical surgical incision is being employed, left internal or external jugular venous cannulation should be avoided and implanted ports in the left chest wall should not be used. A temperature probe can be placed in the oropharynx, nasopharynx, external auditory canal, bladder, or rectum. However, care should be taken to avoid placement of temperature probes or other devices in the esophagus except in conjunction with the surgical team.

Induction and Airway Management

Induction of anesthesia for esophagectomy should be done with comorbid conditions in mind—particularly that of aspiration risk. While some patients may be able to swallow normally with minimal or no GERD, or have complete resolution of dysphagia after neoadjuvant chemotherapy, anesthesiologists must be vigilant for this risk and take precautions when appropriate. The head-of-bed should be kept elevated at 30 degrees until the airway is secured. A rapid sequence induction is advocated using an intravenous induction agent, such as propofol, and succinylcholine or rocuronium for rapid-onset neuromuscular blockade. A double lumen tube (DLT) or single lumen tube (SLT) with bronchial blocker may be used to provide OLV during transthoracic procedures, especially for minimally invasive techniques [51]. Fiberoptic bronchoscopy confirms the correct placement of either device after intubation and after the change in patient position. If the surgical team is planning an initial flexible bronchoscopy for evaluation of airway involvement or if the patient has disadvantageous anatomy, a SLT may be placed and subsequently exchanged for a DLT or kept in place for use with a bronchial blocker. Attempting a rapid sequence induction for placement of a DLT can be challenging even for experienced providers and should be approached thoughtfully and with a plan in case of difficult intubation. Videolaryngoscopy or fiberoptic bronchoscopy can greatly improve glottic view for easier DLT placement and can be part of the primary or backup plan [52]. A supraglottic airway device may be placed for rescue of failed intubation, though it is not ideal for patients at risk for aspiration. Once in place, it may be exchanged for an endotracheal tube. Finally, awake intubation may be necessary for patients who have an anticipated difficult airway.

Ventilator Management

Protective lung strategies have been advocated intraoperatively due to the potential for lung injury that can be more pronounced after OLV. Postoperative pulmonary complications remain the most common type of complication after esophagectomy, with a prevalence of 20–40% according to National Surgical Quality Improvement Program (NSQIP) data [53]. Perioperative acute lung injury is multifactorial, resulting from surgical trauma, alveolar inflammation, and ventilator-induced lung injury (VILI). Protective strategies include maintaining low tidal volumes based on predicted body weight, optimizing end expiratory positive pressure (PEEP), performing routine recruitment maneuvers, reducing inspired oxygen concentration, avoiding high peak inspiratory and plateau airway pressures, and limiting the duration of OLV [54, 55]. Precise guidelines for ventilation parameters are yet to be elucidated. For patients with difficulty oxygenating during OLV, continuous positive airway pressure (CPAP) can be a useful technique to apply to the lung on the operative side of transthoracic surgery when performed in agreement with the surgical team. However, due to the potential of lung expansion, CPAP is usually only adopted after changes in the ventilator parameters and confirmation that the lung isolation device is still in good position.

Analgesia

Effective pain control for esophagectomy can have widespread benefits for the patient, and it is an important component of many enhanced recovery pathways. *Thoracic epidural analgesia* (TEA) remains the gold standard for open esophagectomy, reducing the systemic inflammatory response and providing better pain relief than parenteral opioids [56, 57]. Epidural catheters are usually placed preoperatively at a thoracic level that allow coverage from T4 to L1. Commonly used medications include a diluted local anesthetic with or without opioid—typically bupivacaine or ropivacaine with fentanyl or hydromorphone. There is some evidence that preemptive analgesia with TEA reduces acute postoperative pain for thoracotomy when compared to TEA initiated at completion of surgery [58], but there are no studies dedicated to esophagectomy. In addition to effective pain control, demonstrated benefits of TEA include facilitation of early extubation, better analgesia for postoperative mobility, and reduced incidence of pneumonia and anastomotic leak [57, 59]. TEA can have complications, such as urinary retention, hypotension, and failed or incomplete block [59].

Paravertebral block (PVB) or catheters are an alternative to TEA, providing equivalent analgesia with fewer pulmonary complications and more favorable overall side effect profile when used for thoracotomy [60]. PVB is a more challenging procedure than epidural placement, as it requires injection or catheter placement in a deep space. With the advent of ultrasound guidance the success rate has improved. Paravertebral catheters can be placed intraoperatively under direct vision by the surgeon before chest closure. The main advantage for PVB is its unilaterality; the main disadvantage is the lack of coverage for the abdominal incision. To date, there are no prospective studies that have compared PVB versus TEA for thoracolaparotomy or esophagectomy, though a Cochrane review of PVB versus TEA for thoracotomy supported PVB use to reduce the risks of developing minor complications and supported its efficacy as noninferior to TEA in controlling acute pain [61].

Peripheral nerve blocks may be used when neuraxial techniques are contraindicated. Intercostal nerve blocks and transversus abdominis plane blocks are viable opioid-sparing regional techniques. Early reports show the serratus plane block and erector spinae plane block may also be effective for thoracotomy pain with low-risk profiles [62, 63]. Even so, peripheral nerve blocks provide suboptimal analgesia alone; opioids and adjuvants are still needed. Various intravenous and oral medications may be added to the analgesic regimen, such as acetaminophen, nonsteroidal anti-inflammatory drugs (NSAIDs), alpha-2 agonists (e.g., dexmedetomidine), NMDA antagonists (e.g., ketamine), and gabapentinoids (e.g., gabapentin and pregabalin). Studies specific to the efficacy of these analgesic adjuvants for esophagectomy are lacking. Of note, concern has risen with the use of NSAIDs for colorectal surgery because of an association with impaired anastomotic healing and increased rate of leakage, and their use in esophagectomy patients may be unfavorable [64, 65]. Gabapentin has been associated with sedation and respiratory depression after laparoscopic surgery especially in the elderly patients and when combined with long-acting opioids and benzodiazepines [66]. Gabapentinoids as a class have fallen out of favor for widespread analgesic use in the perioperative setting [67].

Currently, there is no gold standard analgesic for MIE. Unlike for open esophagectomy, use of TEA for minimally invasive procedures is variable and mostly dependent on patient respiratory comorbidities. Multiple port sites and fields of operation still cause enough pain that multimodal analgesia is required for patient comfort and recovery. If not contraindicated for the patient, a thoracic epidural should be placed preoperatively for MIE if there is a high likelihood of conversion to an open procedure. Patients with chronic opioid use and tolerance, history of side effects or allergy to opioids, poor respiratory function, propensity for delirium, or other conditions that make opioid use less effective or desirable will also likely benefit from TEA for MIE. Truncal fascial plane blocks with or without catheter techniques may be implemented as part of a multimodal, opioid-sparing analgesic approach.

Fluid Management

There is still a lack of evidence on the appropriate amount of intravenous fluid needed during esophagectomy. As for any other surgery, fluid management should target euvolemia, homeostasis and normal physiology. The volume and the type of fluid used should be customized to the patient and the type of surgery [68]. Fluid restriction to the point of hypovolemia could decrease cardiac output and tissue oxygen delivery, compromising renal function and perfusion of the esophagogastric anastomosis. Conversely, liberal fluid administration to the point of excess could cause shifts into the interstitial space, impairing anastomotic healing and bowel function and contributing to pulmonary complications [69]. Balanced crystalloids are recommended. Colloids may be added given a lack of evidence that they increase morbidity or mortality in various types of shock. Moreover, unfavorable outcome data from prolonged use of colloids may not be applicable to the surgical population, which is exposed for limited time intervals. Based on data extrapolated from existing studies on fluid administration and complication rates after thoracic surgery and esophagectomy, one review has suggested total intraoperative fluid volume should be between 3 ml/kg/hr and 10 ml/kg/hr [70]. However, emphasis should be made that individual fluid requirements vary widely, and there is no strong evidence for fixed fluid replacement recommendations by total volume or by rate on outcomes.

A more tailored approach to fluid replacement is based on *goal directed fluid therapy* (GDFT), which focuses on objective measures or estimates of volume status and responsiveness. The challenge for using GDFT in esophagectomy is that flow-related hemodynamic endpoints (e.g., stroke volume variation and pulse pressure variation) may be inaccurate with an open hemithorax or in the presence of pneumoperitoneum. They are also affected by the presence of arrhythmias, mechanical ventilation with low tidal volumes (< 8 cc/kg IBW), and decreased chest wall compliance. Unfortunately, neither esophageal Doppler nor transesophageal echocardiography can be used for GDFT during surgery on the esophagus. Some advanced hemodynamic parameters (and trends in more conventional hemodynamic parameters) provide valid information related to preload, afterload, and contractility during the procedure and can help dynamically guide fluid and vasopressor administration. A decrease in the incidence of pneumonia has been observed in the GDFT arm of an observational quality improvement project where GDFT with a noninvasive cardiac output monitor was compared to standard treatment in patients undergoing either MIE or open esophagectomy [71].

NPO status guidelines have changed, especially with the advent of ERAS pathways, allowing patients to have clears until 2 h preoperatively. Thus, preoperative intravascular volume depletion is minimal (200–400 cc) with no need for replacement. Bowel preparation is also not used routinely, contributing to less preoperative volume deficit [68]. Intraoperative blood loss for open and minimally invasive procedures is also usually minimal; insensible losses during open esophagectomy may be consequential but are negligible during MIE.

Perfusion of the Esophagogastric Anastomosis

Anastomotic leak due to ischemia of the esophagogastric anastomosis is a devastating complication after esophagectomy. Preservation of perfusion of the gastric conduit for adequate tissue oxygenation of the anastomotic site is key. Blood supply to the gastric fundus, which is used to construct the conduit, is reduced in the process of ligating arteries for gastric mobilization. Thus, blood flow to the anastomosis is heavily reliant on the local microvascular network within the fundus ventriculi. For the anesthesiologist, avoidance of hypotension is important for perfusion, though supranormal mean arterial pressures do not improve gastric conduit perfusion in experimental models [72]. Hypotension due to anesthesia or TEA can be readily corrected with vasopressor or inotrope administration [73]. The belief that vasopressors should be completely avoided during esophagectomy is not supported by the literature. A study using laser speckle contrast imaging to intraoperatively assess microcirculation 1 mm below the tissue surface showed that changes in perfusion were related more to the operative procedure than to TEA-use or phenylephrine support [74]. Moreover, a 2021 retrospective study of vasopressor use in open and minimally invasive esophagectomies did not find an association between vasopressor administration and anastomotic leak rates [75]. New modalities are needed to ensure healing of the esophagogastric anastomosis, and some promise has been shown with intraoperative use of indocyanine green fluorescein imaging to forewarn of areas of poor perfusion [76].

Postoperative Recovery

Complications

Adverse outcomes can occur postoperatively in up to 60% of esophagectomy patients [77].

Pulmonary complications are the most common, and primarily include pneumonia, aspiration pneumonitis, acute lung injury (ALI), acute respiratory distress syndrome (ARDS), bronchopleural fistula, atelectasis, and pulmonary embolism. ARDS is the most critical pulmonary complication with mortality rates up to 50% [78]. There are a multitude of factors that contribute to these adverse pulmonary outcomes [79]. Intraoperative mechanical ventilation may be a significant component especially when combined with surgical manipulation and lung isolation. Poor analgesia or excessive sedation can lead to poor respiratory efforts, contributing to hypoventilation. Opioid-related sedation can also contribute to aspiration.

Cardiovascular complications also account for significant morbidity and mortality after esophagectomy, predominantly in the form of arrhythmias. Supraventricular tachyarrhythmias, mostly atrial fibrillation, occur in about 18% of cases [80] and lead to a higher rate of ICU admission, longer hospital stay and higher 30-day mortality rate [81]. Several protocols are in place for the treatment, mainly relying on pharmacological cardioversion (amiodarone, sotalol) or rate control with beta blockers, calcium channel blockers, or amiodarone. Age, gender, type of procedure and elevated brain natriuretic peptide (BNP > 30 pg/ml) have been associated with an increased postoperative risk of developing atrial fibrillation [82]. Amiodarone or calcium channel blockers are the drugs of choice for prophylaxis. Beta-blockers should be continued in patients already taking them. Magnesium, statins, and ACE inhibitors have also been proposed as weak prophylactic agents.

Esophageal anastomotic leakage adds to the morbidity of recovery and significantly increases the mortality in the postoperative period.

Other less common but notable complications include chylothorax, recurrent laryngeal nerve injury, ileus, abscess formation and wound infection. These are complications that may require surgical treatment and therefore the need of an anesthetic.

Enhanced Recovery Pathway

Formalizing results from well-conducted, peer-reviewed studies into a streamlined protocol of perioperative care known as an enhanced recovery after surgery (ERAS) pathway has been successful in minimizing complications and speeding recovery for a variety of surgical populations [38]. This approach is now being evaluated for its effectiveness in esophagectomy care, given that a comprehensive set of interventions is likely needed to see an overall improvement in outcomes. The general focus of an ERAS pathway is on five categories of care: (1) preoperative assessment, planning, and preparation before admission; (2) reducing the physiologic stress of the operation; (3) a structured approach to immediate postoperative and perioperative management, including pain relief; (4) early mobilization; and (5) early enteral feeding [83]. In 2019, ERAS guideline recommendations were published specific to esophagectomy [84].

Currently, there is minimal evidence for individual interventions for esophagectomy, with many recommendations derived from non-esophageal thoracoabdominal surgery. Yet, adapting existing ERAS protocols to esophagectomy is a logical approach and has promise to make surgical treatment of esophageal cancer safer for the patient thanks in part to better teamwork and education.

Conclusions

Anesthetic perspectives on esophagectomy care continue to evolve with increasing focus on multidisciplinary teams, multimodal monitoring and analgesia, and minimally invasive techniques. As enhanced recovery pathways further develop, the role of the anesthesiologist will become more active in the coordination of care from the time of prehabilitation through the continuum of surgery, recovery, and follow-up. Optimizing the functional status in the preoperative period, planning each aspect of the anesthetic, and preventing medical complications in the postoperative period are all goals for a successful patient experience. Achieving these goals will require continued efforts to research and implement best practices specific to esophageal cancer patients.

References

1. Mantziari S, Hübner M, Demartines N, Schäfer M. Impact of preoperative risk factors on morbidity after esophagectomy: is there room for improvement? World J Surg. 2014;38(11):2882–90.
2. Rusy DA, Honkanen A, Landrigan-Ossar MF, et al. Vaping and e-cigarette use in children and

adolescents: implications on perioperative care from the American Society of Anesthesiologists Committee on Pediatric Anesthesia, Society for Pediatric Anesthesia, and American Academy of Pediatrics Section on Anesthesiology and Pain Medicine. Anesth Analg. 2021;133:562–8.

3. Shah S, Schwenk ES, Sondekoppam RV, et al. ASRA Pain Medicine consensus guidelines on the management of the perioperative patient on cannabis and cannabinoids. Reg Anesth Pain Med. 2023;48:97–117.

4. Eliasen M, Grønkjær M, Skov-Ettrup LS, et al. Preoperative alcohol consumption and postoperative complications: a systematic review and meta-analysis. Ann Surg. 2013;258(6):930–42.

5. Yousefzadeh A, Chung F, Wong DT, et al. Smoking cessation: the role of the anesthesiologist. Anesth Analg. 2016;122(5):1311–20.

6. Nozoe T, Kimura Y, Ishida M, et al. Correlation of pre-operative nutritional condition with postoperative complications in surgical treatment for oesophageal carcinoma. Eur J Surg Oncol. 2002;28(4):396–400.

7. Yoshida N, Baba Y, Shigaki H, et al. Preoperative nutritional assessment by controlling nutritional status (CONUT) is useful to estimate postoperative morbidity after esophagectomy for esophageal cancer. World J Surg. 2016;40(8):1910–7.

8. Burt BM, Groth SS, Sada YH, et al. Utility of adjuvant chemotherapy after neoadjuvant chemoradiation and esophagectomy for esophageal cancer. Ann Surg. 2017;266(2):297–304.

9. Klevebro F, Johnsen G, Johnson E, et al. Morbidity and mortality after surgery for cancer of the oesophagus and gastro-oesophageal junction: a randomized clinical trial neoadjuvant chemotherapy vs. neoadjuvant chemoradiation. Eur J Surg Onc. 2015;41(7):920–6.

10. Dilruba S, Kalayda GV. Platinum-based drugs: past, present and future. Cancer Chemother Pharmacol. 2016;77(6):1103–24.

11. Thomas SA, Grami Z, Mehta S, Patel K. Adverse effects of 5-fluorouracil: Focus on rare side effects. Cancer Cell Microenviron. 2016;3:e1266.

12. Farinha HT, Digklia A, Schizas D, et al. Immunotherapy for esophageal cancer: state-of-the art in 2021. Cancers. 2022;14(3):554.

13. Cukier P, Santini FC, Scaranti M, Hoff AO. Endocrine side effects of cancer immunotherapy. Endocr Relat Cancer. 2017;24(12):T331–47.

14. Lewis AL, Chaft J, Girotra M, Fischer GW. Immune checkpoint inhibitors: a narrative review of considerations for the anaesthesiologist. Br J Anaesth. 2020;124(3):251–60.

15. Fleisher L, Fleischmann K, Auerbach A, et al. 2014 ACC/AHA guideline on perioperative cardiovascular evaluation and management of patients undergoing noncardiac surgery. J Am Coll Cardiol. 2014;64(22):e77–137.

16. Pandey A, Sood A, Sammon JD, et al. Effect of Preoperative angina pectoris on cardiac outcomes in patients with previous myocardial infarction undergoing major noncardiac surgery (data from ACS-NSQIP). Am J Cardiol. 2015;115(8):1080–4.

17. McFalls EO, Ward HB, Moritz TE, et al. Coronary-artery revascularization before elective major vascular surgery. N Engl J Med. 2004;351(27):2795–804.

18. Spahn DR, Howell SJ, Delabays A, Chassot PG. Coronary stents and perioperative anti-platelet regimen: dilemma of bleeding and stent thrombosis. Br J Anaesth. 2006;96(6):675–7.

19. Levine GN, Bates ER, Bittl JA, et al. 2016 ACC/AHA guideline focused update on duration of dual antiplatelet therapy in patients with coronary artery disease: a report of the American College of Cardiology/American Heart Association Task Force on Clinical Practice Guidelines: an update of the 2011 ACCF/AHA/SCAI guideline for percutaneous coronary intervention, 2011 ACCF/AHA guideline for coronary artery bypass graft surgery, 2012 ACC/AHA/ACP/AATS/PCNA/SCAI/STS guideline for the diagnosis and management of patients with stable ischemic heart disease, 2013 ACCF/AHA guideline for the management of ST-elevation myocardial infarction, 2014 AHA/ACC guideline for the management of patients with non–ST-elevation acute coronary syndromes, and 2014 ACC/AHA guideline on perioperative cardiovascular evaluation and management of patients undergoing noncardiac surgery. Circulation. 2016;134(10):e123–55.

20. Yamana I, Takeno S, Hashimoto T, et al. Randomized controlled study to evaluate the efficacy of a preoperative respiratory rehabilitation program to prevent postoperative pulmonary complications after esophagectomy. Dig Surg. 2015;32(5):331–7.

21. Schreurs LMA, Janssens ACJW, Groen H, et al. Value of EUS in determining curative resectability in reference to CT and FDG-PET: the optimal sequence in preoperative staging of esophageal cancer?. Ann Surg Oncol. 2016;23(suppl 5):1021–8.

22. Bartels H, Stein HJ, Siewert JR. Preoperative risk analysis and postoperative mortality of oesophagectomy for resectable oesophageal cancer. Br J Surg. 1998;85(6):840–4.

23. Mcmillan DC. The systemic inflammation-based Glasgow prognostic score: a decade of experience in patients with cancer. Cancer Treat Rev. 2013;39(5):534–40.

24. Kobayashi T, Teruya M, Kishiki T, et al. Inflammation-based prognostic score, prior to neoadjuvant chemoradiotherapy, predicts postoperative outcome in patients with esophageal squamous cell carcinoma. Surgery. 2008;144(5):729–35.

25. Walsh SM, Casey S, Kennedy R, et al. Does the modified Glasgow Prognostic Score (mGPS) have a prognostic role in esophageal cancer? J Surg Oncol. 2016;113:732–7.

26. Bosch DJ, Pultrum BB, Bock GHD, et al. Comparison of different risk-adjustment models in assessing short-term surgical outcome after transthoracic esophagectomy in patients with esophageal cancer. Am J Surg. 2011;202(3):303–9.

27. Dutta S, Al-Mrabt NM, Fullarton GM, et al. A comparison of POSSUM and GPS models in the prediction of post-operative outcome in patients undergoing oesophago-gastric cancer resection. Ann Surg Oncol. 2011;18(10):2808–17.

28. Smith TB, Stonell C, Purkayastha S, et al. Cardiopulmonary exercise testing as a risk assessment method in non cardio-pulmonary surgery: a systematic review. Anaesthesia. 2009;64(8):883–93.

29. Older P, Smith R, Courtney P, et al. Preoperative evaluation of cardiac failure and ischemia in elderly patients by cardiopulmonary exercise testing. Chest. 1993;104(3):701–4.

30. Forshaw MJ, Strauss DC, Davies AR, et al. Is cardiopulmonary exercise testing a useful test before esophagectomy? Ann Thorac Surg. 2008;85(1):294–9.

31. Moyes L, Mccaffer C, Carter R, et al. Cardiopulmonary exercise testing as a predictor of complications in oesophagogastric cancer surgery. Ann R Coll Surg Engl. 2013;95(2):125–30.

32. Patel N, Powell AG, Wheat JR, et al. Cardiopulmonary fitness predicts postoperative major morbidity after esophagectomy for patients with cancer. Physiol Rep. 2019;7(14): e14174.

33. Turan A, Koyuncu O, Egan C, et al. Effect of various durations of smoking cessation on postoperative outcomes: a retrospective cohort analysis. Eur J Anaesthesiol. 2017;34:1–10.

34. Yoshida N, Baba Y, Hiyoshi Y, et al. Duration of smoking cessation and postoperative morbidity after esophagectomy for esophageal cancer: how long should patients stop smoking before surgery? World J Surg. 2016;40(1):142–7.

35. Dettling DS, Schaaf MVD, Blom RL, et al. Feasibility and effectiveness of pre-operative inspiratory muscle training in patients undergoing oesophagectomy: a pilot study. Physiother Res Int. 2013;18(1):16–26.

36. Melis M, Mcloughlin JM, Dean EM, et al. Correlations between neoadjuvant treatment, anemia and perioperative complications in patients undergoing esophagectomy for cancer. J Surg Res. 2009;153(1):114–20.

37. Muñoz M, García-Erce JA, Cuenca J, et al. On the role of iron therapy for reducing allogeneic blood transfusion in orthopaedic surgery. Blood Transfus. 2012;10(1):8–22.

38. Findlay JM, Gillies RS, Millo J, et al. Enhanced recovery for esophagectomy: a systematic review and evidence-based guidelines. Ann Surg. 2014;259(3):413–31.

39. Richards T, Baikady RR, Clevenger B, et al. Preoperative intravenous iron to treat anemia before major abdominal surgery (PREVENTT): a randomized, double-blind, controlled trial. The Lancet. 2020;396:1353–61.

40. Li L, Wang Z, Ying X, et al. Preoperative carbohydrate loading for elective surgery: a systematic review and meta-analysis. Surg Today. 2012;42(7):613–24.

41. Yuill KA, Richardson RA, Davidson HI, et al. The administration of an oral carbohydrate-containing fluid prior to major elective upper-gastrointestinal surgery preserves skeletal muscle mass postoperatively—a randomised clinical trial. Clin Nutr. 2005;24(1):32–7.

42. Jenkins TK, Lopez AN, Sarosi GA, et al. Preoperative enteral access is not necessary prior to multimodality treatment of esophageal cancer. Surgery. 2017;S0039–6060(17):30694–703.

43. Molenaar CJL, Papen-Botterhuis NE, Herrle F, et al. Prehabilitation, making patients fit for surgery—a new frontier in perioperative care. Innov Surg Sci. 2019;4:132–8.

44. Tukanova KH, Chidambaram S, Guidozzi N, et al. Physiotherapy regimens in esophagectomy and gastrectomy: a systematic review and meta-analysis. Ann Surg Oncol. 2022;29:3148–67.

45. Sihag S, Kosinski AS, Gaissert HA, et al. Minimally invasive versus open esophagectomy for esophageal cancer: a comparison of early surgical outcomes from the Society of Thoracic Surgeons National Database. Annals Thorac Surg. 2016;101(4):1281–8.

46. Luketich JD, Pennathur A, Awais O, et al. Outcomes after minimally invasive esophagectomy: review of over 1000 patients. Ann Surg. 2012;256(1):95–103.

47. Luketich JD, Pennathur A, Franchetti Y, et al. Minimally invasive esophagectomy: results of a prospective phase II multicenter trial-the eastern cooperative oncology group (E2202) study. Ann Surg. 2015;261(4):702–7.

48. Biere SS, Cuesta MA, van der Peet DL. Minimally invasive versus open esophagectomy for cancer: a systematic review and meta-analysis. Minerva Chir. 2009;64(2):121–33.

49. Palanivelu C, Prakash A, Senthilkumar R, et al. Minimally invasive esophagectomy: thoracoscopic mobilization of the esophagus and mediastinal lymphadenectomy in prone position—experience of 130 patients. J Am Coll Surg. 2006;203(1):7–16.

50. Rucklidge M, Sanders D, Martin A. Anaesthesia for minimally invasive oesophagectomy. Continuing Educ Anaesthesia Crit Care Pain. 2010;10(2):43–7.

51. Narayanaswamy M, McRae K, Slinger P, et al. Choosing a lung isolation device for thoracic surgery: a randomized trial of three bronchial blockers versus double-lumen tubes. Anesth Analg. 2009;108(4):1097–101.

52. Yamakazi T, Ohsumi H. The airway scope is a practical intubation device for a double-lumen tube during rapid-sequence induction. J Cardiothorac Vasc Anesth. 2009;23(6):926.

53. Molena D, Mungo B, Stern M, et al. Incidence and risk factors for respiratory complications in patients undergoing esophagectomy for malignancy: a NSQIP analysis. Semin Thorac Cardiovasc Surg. 2014;26(4):287–94.

54. Shen Y, Zhong M, Wu W, et al. The impact of tidal volume on pulmonary complications following minimally invasive esophagectomy: a randomized and controlled study. J Thorac Cardiovasc Surg. 2013;146(5):1267–73.

55. Lohser J, Slinger P. Lung injury after one-lung ventilation: a review of the pathophysiologic mechanisms affecting the ventilated and the collapsed lung. Anesth Analg. 2015;121(2):302–18.

56. Rudin A, Flisberg P, Johansson J, et al. Thoracic epidural analgesia or intravenous morphine analgesia after thoracoabdominal esophagectomy: a prospective follow-up of 201 patients. J Cardiothorac Vasc Anesth. 2005;19(3):350–7.

57. Flisberg P, Törnebrandt K, Walther B, et al. Pain relief after esophagectomy: thoracic epidural analgesia is better than parenteral opioids. J Cardiothorac Vasc Anesth. 2001;15(3):282–7.

58. Bong CL, Samuel M, Ng JM, et al. Effects of preemptive epidural analgesia on post-thoracotomy pain. J Cardiothorac Vasc Anesth. 2005;19(6):786–93.

59. Wei L, Yongchun L, Qingyuan H, et al. Short and long-term outcomes of epidural or intravenous analgesia after esophagectomy: a propensity-matched cohort study. PLoS ONE. 2016;11(4):e0154380.

60. Davies RG, Myles PS, Graham JM. A comparison of the analgesic efficacy and side-effects of paravertebral vs epidural blockade for thoracotomy—a systematic review and meta-analysis of randomized trials. Br J Anaesth. 2006;96(4):418–26.

61. Yeung JHY, Gates S, Naidu BV, et al. Paravertebral block versus thoracic epidural for patients undergoing thoracotomy. Cochrane Database Syst Rev. 2016;2:CD009121.

62. Blanco R, Parras T, McDonnell JG, Prats-Galino A. Serratus plane block: a novel ultrasound-guided thoracic wall nerve block. Anesthesia. 2013;68(11):1107–13.

63. Forero M, Adhikary SD, Lopez H, et al. The erector spinae plane block: a novel analgesic technique in thoracic neuropathic pain. Reg Anesth Pain Med. 2016;41(5):621–7.

64. Gorissen KJ, Benning D, Berghmans T, et al. Risk of anastomotic leakage with non-steroidal anti-inflammatory drugs in colorectal surgery. Br J Surg. 2012;99(5):721–7.

65. Rushfeldt CF, Sveinbjørnsson B, Søreide K, Vonen B. Risk of anastomotic leakage with use of NSAIDs after gastrointestinal surgery. Int J Colorectal Dis. 2011;26(12):1501–9.

66. Cavalcante AN, Sprung J, Schroeder DR, Weingarten TN. Multimodal analgesic therapy with gabapentin and its association with postoperative respiratory depression. Anesth Analg. 2017;125(1):141–6.

67. Verret M, Lauzier F, Zarychanski R, et al. Perioperative use of gabapentinoids for the management of postoperative acute pain: a systematic review and meta-analysis. Anesthesiology. 2020;133:265–79.

68. Navarro LH, Bloomstone JA, Auler JO Jr, et al. Perioperative fluid therapy: a statement from the international Fluid Optimization Group. Periop Med. 2015;4:3.

69. Holte K, Sharrock NE, Kehlet H. Pathophysiology and clinical implications of perioperative fluid excess. Br J Anaesth. 2002;89(4):622–32.

70. Durkin C, Schisler T, Lohser J. Current trends in anesthesia for esophagectomy. Curr Opin Anaesthesiol. 2017;30(1):30–5.

71. Veelo DP, van Berge Henegouwen MI, Ouwehand KS, et al. Effect of goal-directed therapy on outcome after esophageal surgery: a quality improvement study. PLoS ONE. 2017;12(3):e0172806.

72. Klijn E, Niehof S, de Jonge J, et al. The effect of perfusion pressure on gastric tissue blood flow in an experimental gastric tube model. Anesth Analg. 2010;110(2):541–6.

73. Pathak D, Pennefather SH, Russell GN, et al. Phenylephrine infusion improves blood flow to the stomach during oesophagectomy in the presence of a thoracic epidural analgesia. Eur J Cardiothorac Surg. 2013;44(1):130–3.

74. Walsh KJ, Zhang H, Tan KS, et al. Use of vasopressors during esophagectomy is not associated with increased risk of anastomotic leak. Dis Esophagus. 2021;34(4):1–7.

75. Ambrus R, Achiam MP, Secher NH, et al. Evaluation of gastric microcirculation by laser speckle contrast imaging during esophagectomy. J Am Coll Surg. 2017;225(3):395–402.

76. Ohi M, Toiyama Y, Mohri Y, et al. Prevalence of anastomotic leak and the impact of indocyanine green fluorescein imaging for evaluating blood flow in the gastric conduit following esophageal cancer surgery. Esophagus. 2017;14(4):351–9.

77. McCulloch P, Ward J, Tekkis PP, et al. Mortality and morbidity in gastro-oesophageal cancer surgery: initial results of ASCOT multicentre prospective cohort study. BMJ. 2003;327(7425):1192–7.

78. Tandon S, Batchelor A, Bullock R, et al. Perioperative risk factors for acute lung injury after elective oesophagectomy. Br J Anaesth. 2001;86(5):633–8.

79. McKevith JM, Pennefather SH. Respiratory complications after oesophageal surgery. Curr Opin Anaesthesiol. 2010;23(1):34–40.

80. Chebbout R, Heywood EG, Drake TM, et al. A systematic review of the incidence of and risk factors for postoperative atrial fibrillation following general surgery. Anaesthesia. 2018;73(4):490–498.

81. Amar D, Burt ME, Bains MS, Leung DH. Symptomatic tachydysrhythmias after esophagectomy: incidence and outcome measures. Ann Thorac Surg. 1996;61(5):1506–9.
82. Amar D. Postoperative atrial fibrillation: Is there a need for prevention? J Thorac Cardiovasc Surg. 2016;151(4):913–5.
83. Carney A, Dickinson M. Anesthesia for esophagectomy. Anesthesiol Clin. 2015;33(1):143–63.
84. Low DE, Allum W, Manzoni GD, et al. Guidelines for perioperative care in esophagectomy: enhanced recovery after surgery (ERAS®) society recommendations. World J Surg. 2019;43:299–330.

Transhiatal Esophagectomy

Francisco Schlottmann, Manuela Monrabal Lezama,
Fernando A. M. Herbella and Marco G. Patti

Abstract

Transhiatal esophagectomy with cervical anastomosis is an established procedure for the treatment of esophageal cancer. It is important to select the proper patients for this procedure. For instance, this approach is not ideal for patients with severe mediastinal adhesions secondary to prior operations or radiotherapy or those with T4 tumors. Cancer of the distal esophagus and esophago-gastric junction are well suited for this procedure, as most of the dissection of the area involved by the cancer can be done under direct vision.

F. Schlottmann (✉) · M. Monrabal Lezama
Department of Surgery, Hospital Alemán of
Buenos Aires, 1640 Pueyrredon Ave, Buenos Aires,
Argentina
e-mail: fschlottmann@hotmail.com

F. Schlottmann
Department of Surgery, University of Illinois at
Chicago, Chicago, IL, USA

F. A. M. Herbella
Department of Surgery, Federal University of Sao
Paulo, Sao Paulo, Brazil
e-mail: herbella.dcir@epm.br

M. G. Patti
Department of Surgery, University of Virginia,
Charlottesville, VA, USA

Keywords

Esophageal cancer · Transhiatal
esophagectomy · Mediastinal dissection ·
Cervical anastomosis · Laparotomy

Introduction

Transhiatal esophagectomy (THE) with cervical anastomosis is an established procedure for the treatment of esophageal cancer. It is important to select the proper patients for this procedure, mostly avoiding patients with severe mediastinal adhesions secondary to prior operations or radiotherapy, or those with a T4 tumor. Cancers of the distal esophagus are well suited for this procedure, as most of the dissection of the area involved by the cancer can be done under direct vision. The advantages of THE include reduction of respiratory morbidity as a thoracotomy is not performed, and avoidance of mediastinitis in case an anastomotic leak occurs (i.e. a leak at the cervical level is often less complex to treat). The oncologic properties of THE have been questioned because, contrary to a transthoracic esophagectomy (TTE), it does not allow dissection of lymph nodes in the posterior mediastinum. However, previous studies have shown no significant differences in survival between THE and TTE. This suggests that the key determinant of survival is mostly related to the stage of the disease at diagnosis and the biological behavior of the cancer [1–8].

In this chapter, we will focus on the technique of THE and the prevention and treatment of the most common complications related to the procedure.

Surgical Technique

Patients are admitted the morning of the operation. A thoracic epidural catheter is inserted in the pre-operative area. Heparin, 5000 units subcutaneously, and intravenous antibiotics are given before induction, and pneumatic compression devices are applied to the lower extremities. A single lumen endotracheal tube and a nasogastric tube are inserted. A radial artery catheter is essential for monitoring of the blood pressure, particularly during the blunt mediastinal dissection. The patient is placed supine on the operating room table with a blanket between the shoulders. The arms are secured at the side of the table, and the patient's head is turned towards the right. The operating field extends from the left ear to the pubis, and laterally all the way to the posterior axillary line so that chest tubes can be inserted if the pleural cavities are entered during the mediastinal dissection.

The THE has three components: abdominal, mediastinal and cervical.

Abdominal Phase

The abdominal cavity is entered through a midline incision extending from the xiphoid process to the umbilicus. A self-retained retractor is used, particularly to lift the right and left costal margins and provide exposure to the subdiaphragmatic area. The abdomen is inspected carefully to rule out metastases in the liver, carcinomatosis or ascites.

The left triangular ligament is incised in order to retract the left lateral segment of the liver towards the right and expose the gastro-hepatic ligament and the esophageal hiatus. The gastro-hepatic ligament is incised all the way to the right pillar of the crus. The right gastric artery is usually preserved. The phreno-esophageal membrane overlying the esophagus is divided. A window is opened between the right pillar of the crus and the esophagus, and the posterior mediastinum is entered. Gentle dissection will determine if the tumor can be freed from the surrounding structures.

After identification of the right gastroepiploic artery, the gastro-colic omentum is opened initially towards the pylorus and then along the greater curvature. The short gastric vessels are then divided all the way to the left pillar of the crus. During this phase of the dissection it is of paramount importance to avoid injury to the spleen. This problem is usually caused by traction exerted in order to provide exposure, particularly to the upper short gastric vessels. It can be minimized by using a long 5 mm laparoscopic bipolar instrument to coagulate and divide these vessels, avoiding the use of ligatures. If a small splenic capsule tear occurs, use of the cautery and gentle packing will frequently stop the bleeding. Dissection is then continued between the esophagus and the left pillar of the crus, and a Penrose drain is passed around the esophagus. Particularly when dealing with distal or esophago-gastric junction tumors, it is possible to determine under direct vision if the tumor is mobile and can be separated from the surrounding structures. After this determination is made, the coronary vein, the left gastric artery and the surrounding nodal tissue are dissected. The vessels are transected at their base with an Endo-GIA stapler with a vascular cartridge. Posterior gastric adhesions are divided.

The duodenum is often mobilized in order to obtain a tension-free gastric conduit (sometimes a Kocher maneuver is needed). Adhesions with the gallbladder and the porta hepatis are divided. A loop of jejunum 30–40 cm distal to the ligament of Treitz is chosen for the placement of a feeding jejunostomy. A Weitzel tunnel is created with interrupted 3–0 silk sutures, and the jejunal loop is then fixed to the abdominal wall.

Cervical Phase

A 6 cm incision is made along the anterior border of the left sternocleidomastoid muscle (Fig. 1). The platysma is divided, the omohyoid muscle is exposed and divided. The carotid sheath is retracted laterally, and the prevertebral fascia is exposed by blunt dissection. The inferior thyroid artery is ligated: the recurrent laryngeal nerve is usually visible just deep and medial to this vessel. The trachea and the larynx are gently retracted medially with a finger; metal retractors are not recommended to retract the trachea in order to avoid injuring the recurrent laryngeal nerve. The esophagus is then encircled with a right-angle clamp and a narrow Penrose drain is passed around the esophagus. The esophagus is then dissected bluntly until the upper mediastinum is reached (Figs. 2 and 3).

Mediastinal Phase

The initial part of the mediastinal dissection can be performed under direct vision. This is facilitated by the division of 1 or 2 cm of the rim of the esophageal hiatus anterior to the esophagus, in between sutures. The anterior and posterior vagus nerves are divided. Most of the dissection can be performed with the same instrument used for the division of the gastro-colic omentum and the short gastric vessels (e.g. Ligasure), usually reaching all the way to the carina. The remaining mediastinal dissection is done blindly, and some rules must be followed to avoid damage to mediastinal structures. It is very useful to have a large nasogastric tube inside the esophagus and feel it with your hand all the way up during the dissection. Initially, the posterior plane is developed along the prevertebral fascia, separating

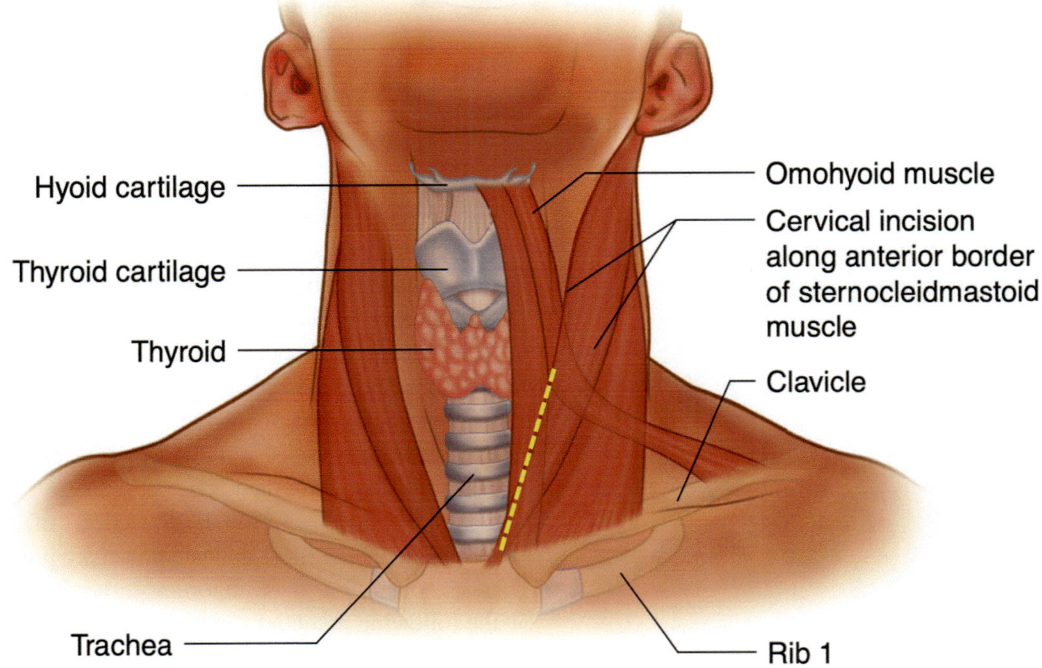

Fig. 1 Cervical incision (yellow dotted line)

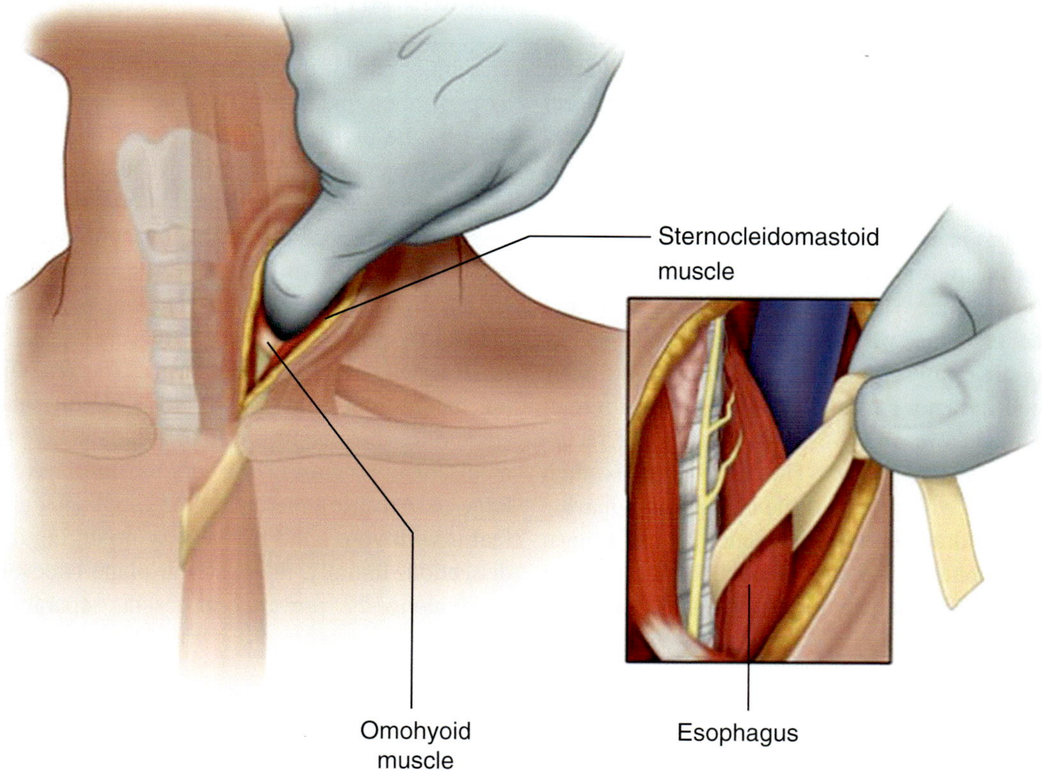

Fig. 2 The tracheoesophageal groove and recurrent nerve are constantly protected with the surgeon's finger, and a Penrose drain is used to encircle the esophagus

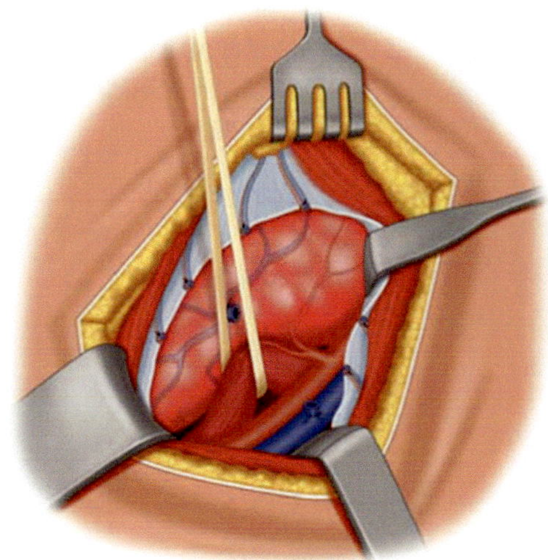

Fig. 3 The middle thyroid vein and inferior thyroid artery divided

the esophagus from the spine. Then the anterior plane is developed with the surgeon's hand turned down so that the palm is in contact with the anterior aspect of the esophagus (Fig. 4). This maneuver displaces the airway anteriorly. At this point, the esophagus is quite mobile, and the lateral attachments of the middle and upper esophagus can be easily divided, reaching the dissection started in the neck.

The blind mediastinal dissection of the esophagus is the most delicate and risky portion of the operation. It is important to be aware of the following potential complications:

- Hypotension. This is caused by mechanical compression of the surgeon's hand. It can be prevented by having good filling pressures

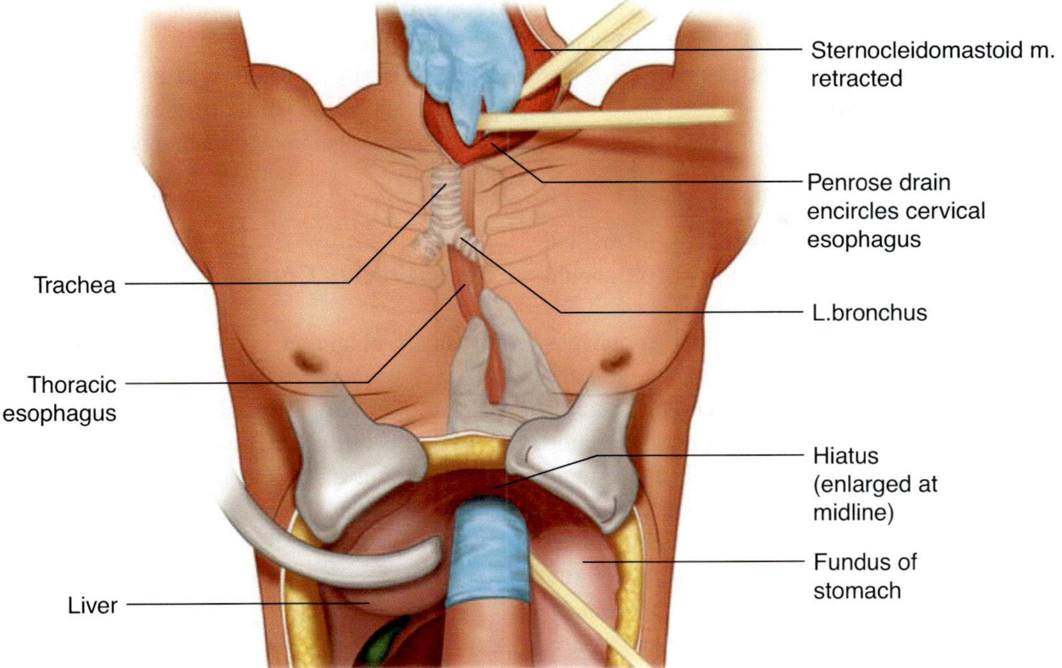

Fig. 4 Transhiatal dissection of the esophagus

before the dissection is started, and is usually treated by simply withdrawing the hand, allowing the blood pressure to normalize.

- Cardiac arrhythmias. Usually self-limited, and caused by the irritation of the pericardium.
- Violation of one or both pleural spaces. If it occurs, it requires placement of chest tubes.
- Bleeding. It is key to keep the dissecting hand in continuous contact with the esophagus so that the feeding blood vessels are transected when they enter the esophageal wall and then contract. Massive bleeding is usually secondary to a torn azygos vein. If this occurs, the mediastinum should be immediately packed tightly and a thoracotomy is performed to control the bleeding.
- Tracheal laceration. Lacerations of the membranous portion of the trachea are quite rare. They manifest with loss of large volumes of the insufflated gas and inadequate patient's ventilation. In these cases, the single lumen endotracheal tube should be advanced into the left mainstem bronchus to prevent significant loss of insufflated tidal volume. Tears just above the carina are best repaired through a right thoracotomy. Higher tears can be approached through the cervical incision or require a partial sternal split.

The conduit is then prepared using multiple fires of a stapler, in order to create a gastric tube whose blood supply is based on the right gastroepiploic artery and the right gastric artery. The nasogastric tube is pulled back all the way to the oro-pharynx and the esophagus is transected in the neck. A wide Penrose drain is attached to the distal esophagus. When the esophagus is delivered through the abdominal incision, the Penrose drain is attached to the tip of the gastric fundus with interrupted sutures and using a combination of pushing and gentle pulling, the gastric conduit is delivered into the neck incision. The stomach must be oriented so that the greater curvature is toward the patient's left. The esophageal hiatus is then narrowed with interrupted sutures in order to avoid herniation of viscera such as the colon. However, compression of the gastric vessels must be avoided.

Cervical Anastomosis

We usually perform a side-to-side, semi-stapled anastomosis (4–5 cm of gastric conduit should lay above the left clavicle without tension for this anastomosis). The transected esophagus is placed over the anterior wall of the stomach and stay sutures are placed between the anterior wall of the stomach and the right and left side of the esophagus. Additional 4–0 silk sutures are placed anteriorly and laterally including all the esophageal layers in order to avoiding proximal sliding of the mucosa. A 2 cm gastrotomy is then made next to the cut edge of the esophagus, and a 30 mm Endo-GIA stapler with a vascular cartridge is inserted, with one arm in the stomach and one in the esophagus. By firing the stapling device, an anastomosis is made between the posterior wall of the esophagus and the anterior wall of the stomach. The staple line is inspected for bleeding, and minor oozing can be stopped using cautery. The nasogastric tube is then advanced down the esophagus into the stomach. The anterior opening is closed in two layers, an inner layer of running 3–0 absorbable suture and an outer layer of interrupted 3–0 silk sero-muscular Lembert sutures.

If a side-to-side anastomosis would be under tension, it is preferable to perform a hand sutured end-to-end anastomosis, using an inner layer of running absorbable 3–0 sutures, and an outer layer of interrupted 3–0 silk Lembert sutures.

Before closing the cervical incision in layers, a Jackson-Pratt drain (exteriorized lateral to the upper portion of the incision) is placed next to the anastomosis and in the upper mediastinum. Because of its suction action, this type of drain is more effective than a Penrose drain in case of a leak (the Penrose does not prevent the leakage

to reach the mediastinum when the patient is in the upright position).

The abdominal incision is then closed and the operation is completed. Extubation is done if all the respiratory and hemodynamic parameters are satisfactory.

Postoperative Course

We usually obtain an imaging study (i.e. upper GI) on postoperative day three. If no leak is detected, the nasogastric tube is removed and a liquid diet is initiated. The diet is then advanced as per tolerance. If a complication occurs or the patient is unable to take enough calories by mouth, tube feedings are started. Patients are often discharged on postoperative day 7–10.

References

1. Orringer MB, Sloan H. Esophagectomy without thoracotomy. J Thorac Cardiovasc Surg. 1978;76:643–54.
2. Hulscher JB, Tijssen JG, Obertop H, van Lanschot JJ. Transthoracic versus transhiatal resection for carcinoma of the esophagus: a meta-analysis. Ann Thorac Surg. 2001;72:306–13.
3. Orringer MB, Marshall B, Chang AC, Lee J, Pickens A, Lau CL. Two thousand transhiatal esophagectomies: changing trends, lessons learned. Ann Surg. 2007;246:363–72.
4. Chang AC, Ji H, Birkmeyer NJ, Orringer MB, Birkmeyer JD. Outcomes after transhiatal and transthoracic esophagectomy for cancer. Ann Thorac Surg. 2008;85:424–9.
5. Connors RC, Reuben BC, Neumayer LA, Bull DA. Comparing outcomes after transthoracic and transhiatal esophagectomy: a 5-year prospective cohort of 17,395 patients. J Am Coll Surg. 2007;205:735–40.
6. Orringer MB. Transhiatal esophagectomy: how I teach it. Ann Thorac Surg. 2016;102(5):1432–7.
7. Akhtar NM, Chen D, Zhao Y, et al. Postoperative short-term outcomes of minimally invasive versus open esophagectomy for patients with esophageal cancer: an updated systematic review and meta-analysis. Thoracic Cancer. 2020;11(6):1465–75.
8. Gottlieb-Vedi E, Kauppila JH, Mattsson F, et al. Long-term survival in esophageal cancer after minimally invasive esophagectomy compared to open esophagectomy. Ann Surg. 2022;276(6):e744–8.

McKeown Esophagectomy

Ian Wong and Simon Law

Abstract

The classical three-phase esophagectomy was described by McKeown in 1976. It is widely adopted in centers worldwide for the treatment of esophageal carcinoma. Since its inception, surgeons have modified the procedure based on new technologies and experiences. Morbidity and mortality rates have also improved. Nonetheless, the procedure itself is technically demanding. In this chapter, the technical steps of the procedure are detailed.

Keywords

Esophagectomy · Esophageal cancer · Lymphadenectomy · Thoracotomy · Laparotomy · Recurrent laryngeal nerve injury

Introduction

For squamous cell carcinoma, the majority of intrathoracic esophageal carcinomas are located at the middle and lower esophagus. For adenocarcinoma, 75% are located at distal esophagus or around the gastroesophageal junction. Two-phase esophagectomy with laparotomy and right thoracotomy was first described independently by Lewis and Tanner in 1946 and 1947 respectively. McKeown, in 1976, described a three-phase esophagectomy which began with the abdominal approach, followed by right thoracotomy and cervical phase. Three-phase esophagectomy has its advocates. It provides maximal proximal margin from the primary tumor. When superior mediastinal lymph node dissection is performed (especially indicated for squamous cell cancers), it makes sense to perform the anastomosis in the neck since the upper esophagus has been mobilized. Although leak rates are generally reported to be higher for a cervical anastomosis as compared to an intrathoracic anastomosis, it is easier to manage as drainage via the neck wound is generally effective. When a neck anastomosis is chosen, the conduit for esophageal replacement can be brought up via the posterior mediastinal, retrosternal as well as subcutaneous route. The ability to choose different routes are important, e.g. when colonic interposition is required, or in cases of palliative resection or when postoperative radiotherapy to the mediastinum is planned, the retrosternal route is often preferred. Other advantages of the retrosternal route include the avoidance of conduit infiltration by recurrent tumors in the posterior mediastinum, and in

I. Wong · S. Law (✉)
Division of Esophageal and Upper Gastrointestinal Surgery, Department of Surgery, Queen Mary Hospital, School of Clinical Medicine, The University of Hong Kong, Hong Kong, China
e-mail: slaw@hku.hk

the authors' experience, delayed gastric emptying occurs less frequently compared to the posterior mediastinal route, provided that there is no conduit mal-rotation. In this chapter, the important points in open surgical technique, available adjuncts, and tips on intraoperative trouble-shooting are described. Video assisted thoracoscopy and laparoscopic techniques are not described here, although the dissection should be the same, only carried out in a minimally invasive manner.

Surgical Technique

The McKeown operation (three-phase esophagectomy) involves thoracic esophageal mobilization and lymphadenectomy; abdominal exploration, gastric mobilization and lymphadenectomy; and cervical incision for anastomosis. Modifications of the initial publication in 1976 are many, depending on: (1) The approach: open, video-assisted thoracoscopic (VATS), laparoscopic, hybrid or robotics; (2) The sequence: the initial Mc Keown operation started with abdominal phase, followed by thoracic and right cervical incision. Most centers now start with thoracic phase followed by abdominal and cervical phase in a supine position and the patient would only need to change position once. (3) The construction of gastric conduit: The original approach used the whole stomach. A narrower gastric tube of around 3–4 cm in diameter is more commonly utilized; the conduit is lengthened and there is also less chance of delayed gastric emptying. (4) The technique of anastomosis: different centers favor different methods in terms of suture material, number of layers of sutures, and use of linear or circular stapler. Regardless of the modification, the fundamental steps of the operation include the abdominal, thoracic and the cervical phase which are described in detail below.

Thoracic Phase

The authors perform the procedure through a right thoracotomy in the left lateral decubitus position. A single-lumen endotracheal tube with right bronchial blocker is preferred over a double lumen tube for one-lung ventilation. A single lumen tube is less traumatic and stiff, and allows easier retraction of the trachea and left main bronchus during superior mediastinal lymphadenectomy. However, the blocker is often displaced by retraction and needs close cooperation and communication with the anaesthetist. If superior mediastinal dissection is not planned, a double-lumen tube ensures more certain lung collapse.

An anterolateral thoracotomy is usually made at the fifth intercostal space. Depending on the site of tumour, extent of (superior mediastinal) lymphadenectomy and the anatomy of the patient, the fourth space can be chosen for the thoracotomy. A controlled fracture of the posterior fifth or sixth rib is made, after careful dissection to avoid injury of the intercostal pedicle. Bleeding at the bony cut end is controlled with bone wax. The intercostal space can be further enlarged by gradual retraction using two rib spreaders, placed diagonally to each other. Sometimes extensive adhesions are encountered, and may be time-consuming to free.

Starting at the lower esophagus, the inferior pulmonary ligament is divided. The dissection plane proceeds along the posterior surface of the pericardium, superiorly towards the root of inferior pulmonary vein and posteriorly towards the left side of the pleura. In case of locally advanced tumour, the left side pleura and part of the pericardium can be resected en-bloc. A separate incision is made at the mediastinal pleura posterior to the esophagus, joining the dissection plane anteriorly behind the pericardium, to encircle the lower esophagus. The lower esophagus can now be slung with a suture for retraction. The mediastinal pleural incision is continued inferiorly to circumscribe the hiatus, exposing both crura and removing the supradiaphragmatic lymph nodes en-bloc. The thoracic duct is identified close to the hiatus by isolating the tissue between the azygos vein and the surface of the aorta. The duct is ligated to prevent chylothorax and is marked with metal clip as a radiological guide in case of leakage. The incision at the posterior mediastinal pleura is continued proximally along the azygos vein until the arch of azygos is reached. The arch of azygos vein is isolated and divided between ligature, or a linear stapler can be used. The right bronchial artery beneath the azygos vein can be sacrificed. Lymphadenectomy is performed by removing the tissue on the surface of the aorta together with the thoracic duct. Anteriorly, along the plane of the posterior pericardium, the dissection should reach the right main bronchus and the tracheal bifurcation. Careful lymphadenectomy is performed at the subcarina and bilateral bronchi. Bleeding may be encountered but is usually self-limiting and can be controlled by gauze packing with or without hemostatic material. Sharp or thermal injury to the airway should be prevented. This concludes the dissection of the middle and lower esophagus. In case of bulky tumour with difficult retraction, the lower end of the thoracic esophagus can be divided with a stapler and the stump can be retracted cranially to aid exposure.

In the superior mediastinum, the plane between the trachea and esophagus is entered posterior to the right vagus nerve. Posteriorly, the pleura opening is extended from inferiorly at the arch of the azygos vein up to the apex superiorly. The aortic arch is exposed and the esophagus is dissected away from the spine and left side pleura. Another suture can be used to sling the esophagus. The superior mediastinal and recurrent laryngeal nerve lymphadenectomy is essential for squamous cell cancers. The pleura on the tracheoesophageal groove is incised along the right vagus nerve and traced upwards to the lower surface of the right subclavian artery. With gentle blunt dissection, the right recurrent laryngeal nerve should be found

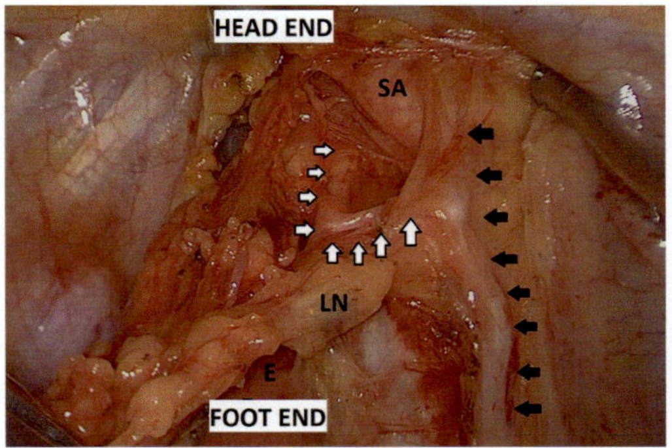

Fig. 1 Right recurrent laryngeal nerve lymphadenectomy. *SA* Subclavian artery, *E* esophagus, *LN* lymph node. Black arrow: right vagus nerve. White arrow: right recurrent laryngeal nerve

as a thin glistering white structure branching off from the right vagus nerve, travelling postero-inferior to the right subclavian artery within the fatty tissue. The location and integrity of the nerve can be checked by nerve stimulator. Sizable lymph nodes are often found next to the right recurrent nerve (Fig. 1). These lymph nodes are contiguous with the cervical chain of paratracheal and para-esophageal lymph nodes. Dissection around the nerve has to be carefully performed, avoiding excessive heat energy from instruments such as diathermy and ultrasonic energy sources.

The esophagus is dissected away from the membranous part of the trachea until the left side of the cartilaginous trachea C-ring is reached. The trachea is rotated in a clockwise direction and retracted anteriorly and the esophagus is pulled posteriorly by the sling to expose the left tracheoesophageal groove. With blunt dissection, the left recurrent laryngeal nerve should be identified along the left side of the trachea. The sympathetic nerve runs in parallel to and sometimes mimics the left recurrent laryngeal nerve. The integrity and location of the nerve can be checked by nerve stimulator (Fig. 2). Extra care should be taken in the subaortic lymph node dissection to prevent injury to the pulmonary artery, which is potentially lethal. The whole thoracic esophageal dissection is now completed. A Fr 24 chest drain is inserted towards the apex. The authors prefer a Fr 19 round fluted

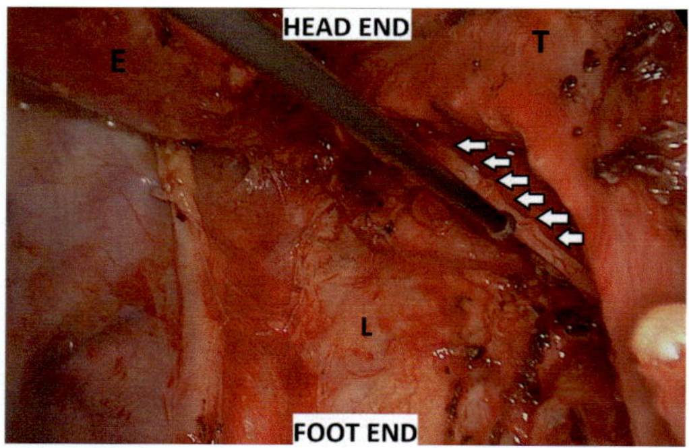

Fig. 2 Left recurrent laryngeal nerve lymphadenectomy. *E* Esophagus (retracted posteriorly), *T* Trachea (retracted anteriorly), *L* Left lung. White arrow: left recurrent laryngeal nerve (after lymphadenectomy). The integrity of the left recurrent laryngeal nerve is checked by the ball-tip intermittent nerve stimulator

drain connected to vacuum drainage. This tube is much softer and smaller, and without the need of an underwater seal device is much more comfortable and allows easy ambulation. A formal chest tube is only inserted when extensive adhesiolysis has been performed since air leak is more efficiently drained by a conventional chest tube with underwater seal. After confirming lungs expansion, ribs are approximated with suture. Muscle and skin are closed in layers.

Abdominal Phase

Patient is placed in a supine and reversed Trendelenburg position. Upper midline or a bilateral subcostal incision is usually used. The authors prefer the bilateral subcostal incision as it gives excellent exposure to the upper abdomen, hiatus and the left subphrenic region, which may be difficult especially in obese patients. The spleen is brought forward by placing a piece of gauze posteriorly to prevent traction injury. The mobilization of stomach begins by dividing the gastrocolic ligament away from the right gastroepiploic arcade. Care is taken during manipulation and retraction of the stomach to prevent injury to the arcade. Once the lesser sac is reached, dissection can be continued towards the direction of the spleen. Complete omentectomy is not needed. Large pieces of omentum will make the conduit

bulky and make delivery of the stomach to the neck difficult. The anastomosis between left and right gastroepiploic vessels is often incomplete. The pancreatic tail acts as a landmark for the origin of the left gastroepiploic vessels, where they should be divided. Short gastric vessels should be ligated or divided with energy device. One should be cautious to prevent injury to the spleen. Small lacerations of the spleen can be controlled by simple packing or haemostatic agents. An easier way to prevent splenic injury is to dissect close to the gastric wall. The gastric fundus is rotated medially, after dividing the attachment to the diaphragm to expose the left crus. The dissection of the right side of the gastrocolic ligament continued until the right gastroepiploic origin is reached. Posterior adhesions between the stomach and the pancreatic capsule is divided until the gastroduodenal artery is visualized.

The gastrohepatic ligament is incised to expose the right crus, celiac trifurcation and supra-pancreatic region. Aberrant left hepatic artery, which originates from left gastric artery, is not uncommon. A sizable vessel, if sacrificed, can result in deranged liver function or even liver necrosis. It can be preserved by dissecting from the origin of the left gastric artery to remove any surrounding lymph nodes, and divide distally on the stomach side after branching off the aberrant left hepatic artery. For dissection of the celiac axis, the lesser curve of the stomach should be retracted anteriorly, and the pancreas should be retracted downwards. The dissection should begin at the superior border of the pancreas, to the right, along the anterior surface of the hepatic artery proper, limit by the hepatoduodenal ligament. Attention should be made to prevent injury to the right gastric artery which is branching off from the common hepatic artery. To the left, dissection is performed along the splenic artery which is often tortuous. The left gastric (coronary) vein is found draining either anteriorly to the splenic vein or posteriorly to the portal vein. It should be isolated and divided. A lot of lymphatic channels are running through this area, large lymphatics should be ligated, clipped or cauterized by energy source to prevent chyle leakage. With the upward retraction of the stomach, the left gastric artery should be clearly running vertically, and it should be divided at its origin. The lymphadenectomy is continued along the surface of the aorta towards the hiatus. With careful dissection, the whole procedure can be a bloodless exercise. The phreno-esophageal ligament between the right crus and abdominal esophagus is divided, meeting the dissection plane on the left. The whole hiatus and abdominal esophagus should now be mobilized. For advanced lower esophageal tumour that have transmural involvement at this level, part of the crural muscle can be resected en-bloc. A sling, such as a cotton tape, Pen-rose drain or latex tube can be looped around the abdominal esophagus for better retraction. The mobilization of stomach is complete and is ready for gastric conduit creation after retrieval of the specimen.

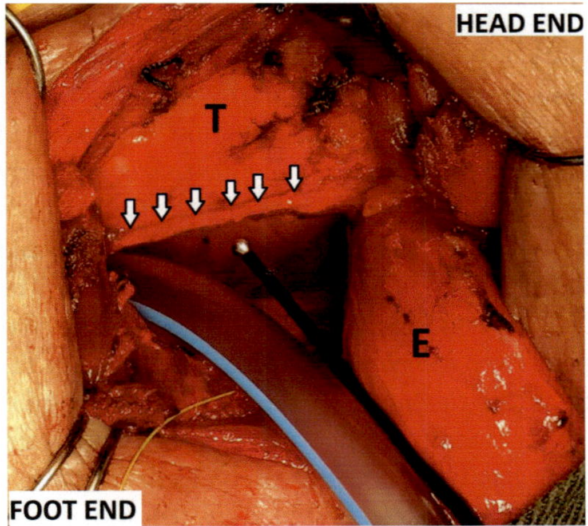

Fig. 3 Left recurrent laryngeal nerve after dissection at cervical phase. *T* Trachea, *E* proximal esophageal stump (transected and retracted cranially). White arrow: left recurrent laryngeal nerve tested by a ball-tip intermittent nerve stimulator. Chest drain is attached to the distal esophageal stump and delivered to the abdomen via the posterior mediastinal route

Cervical Phase

The author opts for a left supraclavicular incision because the esophagus is more inclined to the left side at this level. The incision is extended medially from midline to just beyond the sternocleidomastoid muscle laterally. The strap muscles are divided with electrocautery, exposing the thyroid gland underneath. The thyroid and trachea are retracted to the right side, exposing the carotid sheath. The middle thyroid vein is now visible and should be divided to gain exposure. Along the dissection plane medial to the carotid sheath and prevertebral fascia posteriorly, signs of apical dissection from the thoracic phase should be evident. The esophagus can easily be slung by a finger or a cotton tape, where it is identified anterior to the spine and posterior to the trachea. One should be extra cautious with the recurrent laryngeal nerves as they are unprotected after extensive dissection at the thoracic phase (Fig. 3). The detail of cervical lymphadenectomy will not be discussed here. The cervical esophagus can now be divided at a desirable location with an adequate margin from the tumour. The proximal esophageal stump is opened and anchored at four directions with stay sutures. The distal stump is closed and tagged to a chest tube. The esophageal specimen together with the distal end of the chest tube is retrieved through the abdomen. An alternative method is to divide the abdominal esophagus and retrieved the specimen via the neck. This is the authors' preferred technique. The reason for this is to maximise the preservation of esophageal length in preparation for the esophago-gastric anastomosis. In case the gastric conduit's blood supply is suboptimal and resection of part of the stomach is required, this allows an adequate length of the esophagus. In some cases, the chest could be re-opened and an intrathoracic anastomosis performed. This is only possible if esophageal length is preserved.

Creation of Gastric Conduit and Anastomosis

After delivering the esophageal specimen and the mobilized stomach outside the abdomen, the gastric conduit is created. On the lesser curvature, the right and left gastric arcade anastomosis is divided at a point distal to the third branch of the left gastric artery. This point is chosen for oncological reasons. It has been documented that the majority of lymph node metastases are found in proximity to the origin of the left gastric artery and the risk is relatively negligible distal to its third branch. The stomach is then straightened and gently stretched, and the highest point is marked at the fundus. The lesser curvature is transected with linear staplers from the arcade division point towards the tip of the fundus to create a narrow gastric tube (Figs. 4 and 5). A narrow gastric tube theoretically has better gastric emptying than a whole stomach. A Heineke-Mikulicz pyloroplasty is performed in two layers with continuous absorbable monofilament sutures to further enhance the drainage. Pyloromyotomy, as advocated by Mc Keown, is equally effective. The perfusion of the gastric conduit is checked, and the tip of the fundus is tagged to the distal end of the chest tube. Indocyanine green fluorescence angiography is a very useful adjunct to ensure adequate perfusion of the conduit, and is available with laparoscopic or open instruments. If the retrosternal route is chosen, dissection begins just below the xiphoid. The substernal plane is entered, blunt dissection with a wide metal blade is usually sufficient. Dissection stays in the midline to avoid too big a tunnel in order not to breach the mediastinal pleurae on either side. Dissection of the tunnel in the neck begins by opening the plane just posterior to the insertion of the strap muscles. By insertion 3 fingers into the substernal space, the metal blade inserted via the abdomen is guided to the neck. This dissection should be a relatively bloodless exercise as the retrosternal tunnel is avascular. Two long gauzes can be introduced into the tunnel for transient packing for hemostasis. The conduit is then delivered to the neck via the posterior mediastinal or retrosternal route inside a transparent plastic bag. One should pay extra attention to the axis of the lesser curve and the staple line to ensure that there is no rotation.

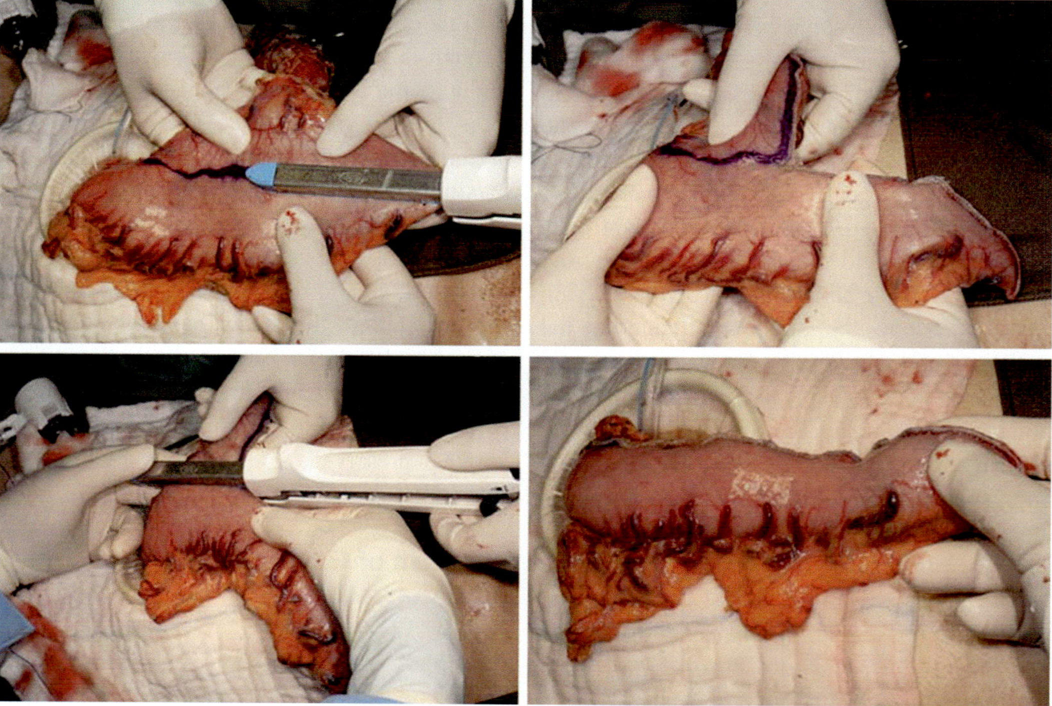

Fig. 4 Gastric conduit construction. Serial linear staplers are applied from the tip of the fundus along the predesigned path towards lesser curvature (the third branch distal to the origin of the left gastric artery). It would result in a narrow gastric tube of around 3–4 cm in width

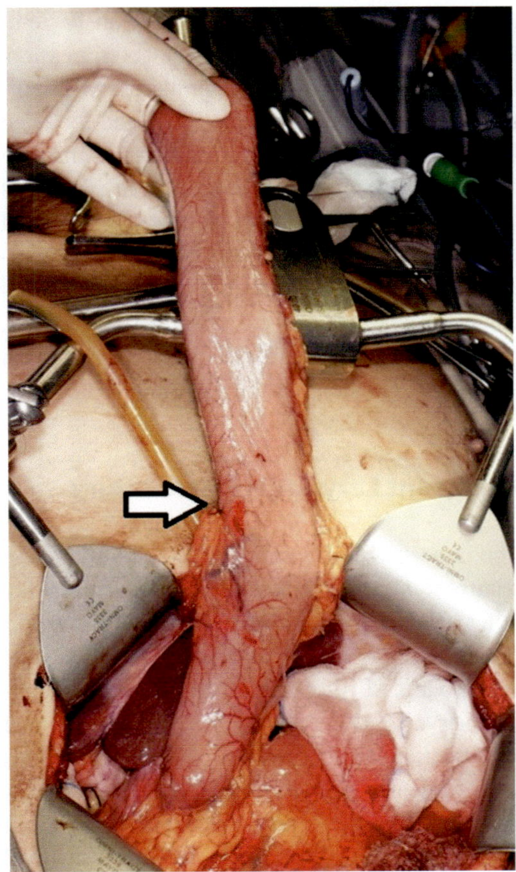

Fig. 5 Gastric conduit construction. White arrow: Division of the lesser curvature arcade at the third branch distal to the origin of the left gastric artery. Linear staplers can also be applied from this point towards the tip of the fundus. Adequate length of the conduit is checked by bringing up the tip of the conduit extracorporeally, which should be able to reach the neck without tension

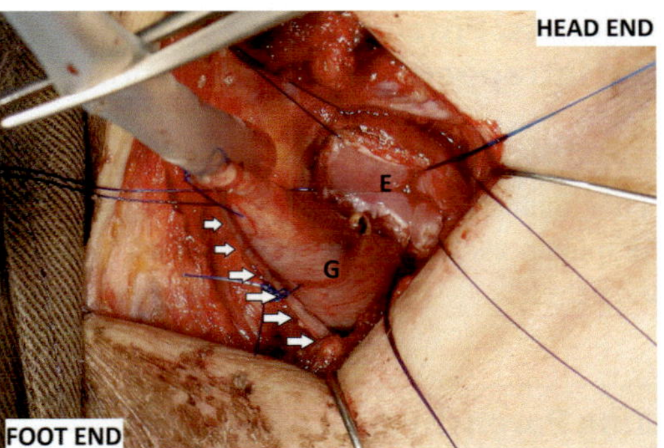

Fig. 6 Esophagogastric anastomosis. *E* Proximal esophageal stump opened up with stay sutures, anchoring at 4 corners at 3, 6, 9, 12 o'clock position. Extra suture in blue is the temporary anchoring stitch for the nasogastric tube. *G* Tip of gastric conduit connected to a chest tube that has been pulled up via the posterior mediastinal route. White arrows: the staple line along the lesser curvature which is now facing anteriorly

After haemostasis, the abdomen is closed in layers without drainage.

Esophago-gastric anastomosis can be performed with handsewn technique, circular or linear staplers. Stricture rate tends to be higher when a small-sized circular stapler is used. There is no difference in leakage rate across different methods of anastomosis. The authors prefer handsewn anastomosis as it is more economical, less dependent on length and position of the conduit, and more controllable. The tip of the gastric fundus is opened up for anastomosis (Fig. 6). The anastomosis is performed in a single-layer continuous manner with a double needle monofilament absorbable sutures. It starts with the distal angle of the esophagus and stomach. The posterior layer is first completed in a continuous manner, across the proximal angle to the anterior wall at the proximal end. The other end of the needle is then used to complete the anterior layer from distally, incorporating and inverting the staple line (T-Junction) into the anastomosis until it reaches the suture at the proximal end. Before completion of the anastomosis, a Fr 16 nasogastric tube is inserted into the gastric lumen under direct vision. The two ends of the needle are tied, and the anastomosis is complete. A metal clip is applied near the knot for a radiological guide in case of postoperative leakage. A Fr 15 round fluted drain is inserted close to the anastomosis. The platysmas and skin are closed in layers. The method of anastomosis is probably less important than its proper application. The surgeon's experience and preference are important, as long as it adheres to the principle of avoiding tension, adequate perfusion of the conduit, and its meticulous construction.

Adjuncts, Pitfalls and Intraoperative Complications

For every surgical complication, prevention is better than cure. However, when intraoperative complications occur, one should react promptly and calmly.

Lung Parenchyma and Airway Injury

In patients with previous pulmonary insults, e.g. tuberculosis or other inflammatory conditions, extensive adhesiolysis is expected. Lung parenchymal injury may result in significant air leak, subsequent pneumothorax, and surgical emphysema postoperatively. One should actively check for such injury by communicating with the anaesthetist in terms of ventilator readings and search for any active air leak under positive ventilation. Small injuries can be managed conservatively or by commercially available tissue glue or fibrin sealant patch. Larger air leak may require wedge resection of the diseased lung. A formal chest drain should be inserted and put on low suction postoperatively.

Aortic or Major Vascular Injury

During lymphadenectomy along the surface of the aorta, we usually work on an avascular plane. However, in advanced tumour or a tumour with previous neoadjuvant therapy, desmoplastic or fibrotic changes may occur and make the dissection plane less well-defined. Thinning of the aortic adventitia or tearing of small intercostal or bronchial branches from the aorta may cause torrential bleeding. One should remain calm as the defect is usually small and can be temporarily controlled with digital compression. Communication with the anaesthetist is important for potential heavy blood loss and the need for blood product replacement. After confirming the anatomy and site of injury, smaller defects can be repaired by pledged sutures. Tight control of blood pressure intraoperative and postoperatively is important. For larger defect, cardiovascular surgeons should be consulted for repair. Staged procedure with delayed reconstruction should be considered if the patient is unstable.

Recurrent Laryngeal Nerve Injury

The importance of lymphadenectomy around the recurrent nerves cannot be overstated. On the other hand, the risk of vocal cord paralysis after esophagectomy can be as high as 60–70%. Due to the variability of the anatomy of the recurrent nerves and their high sensitivity to thermal and traction injury, technology has helped us to confidently identify the nerves and potentially prevent the injury. Intermittent recurrent nerve monitoring has been well documented in thyroid surgery. The same can be applied to esophagectomy with a longer probe and a ball tip to accustom to the deep thoracic cavity. The newer continuous nerve monitoring system works through autonomic periodic stimulation of the vagus nerve to ensure the completeness of the circuit. Any drop in the amplitude of the electromyography of the vocalis muscle or the latency of nerve conduction beyond the threshold will trigger an alarm to notify the surgeon of potential nerve injury. The authors have demonstrated that nerve monitoring can help improve the quality of lymph node dissection and prevent potential complications (Fig. 7).

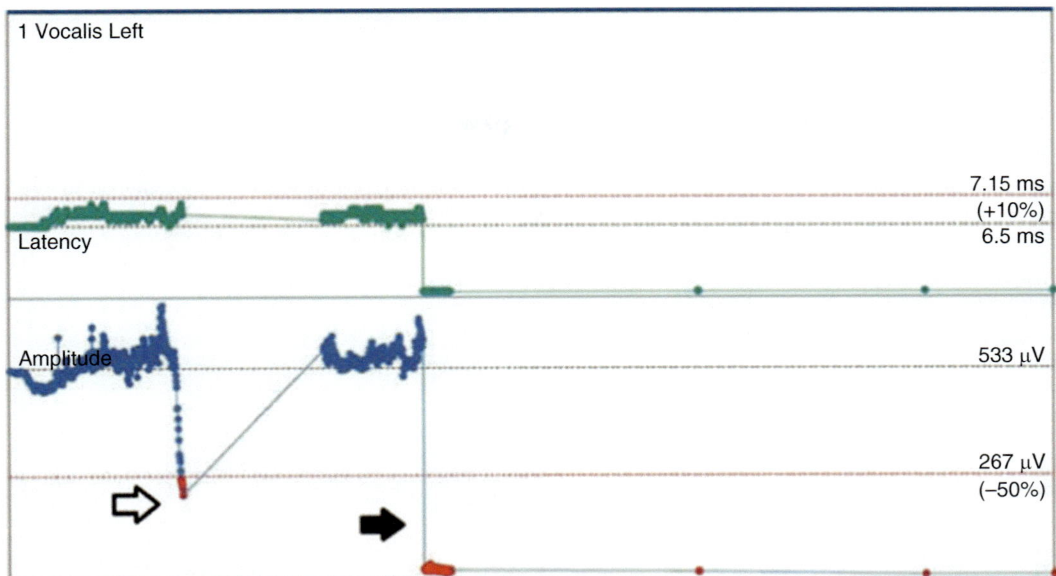

Fig. 7 Continuous intraoperative left recurrent laryngeal nerve monitoring—autonomic periodic stimulation reading. White arrow: a transient drop in amplitude for more than 50% of baseline in left vocalis electromyography. It can be due to minor traction. Black arrow: permanent drop in both latency and amplitude to minimal reading. It can be due to transection of the nerve or dislodgement of vagus nerve probe

Gastric Conduit Ischaemia

Conduit ischaemia although rare, is a potentially lethal complication. Patients surviving the initial sepsis would have prolonged hospitalization, repeated operations, delayed adjuvant treatment, and significant residual morbidity. Traditionally, determination of conduit vascularity relies mostly on naked eyes assessment on its colour, turgor and back bleeding at cut edges. Various methods have been utilized to enhance the detection rate (e.g. laser doppler flowmetry, transmural oxygen saturation, spectrophotometry, etc.) but none has shown to be reliable. Indocyanine green fluorescence angiography has gained its popularity in recent years to provide a real-time quantitative assessment of conduit vascularity. Depending on the different hardware and software available, some may give fluorescence or superimposed coloured images for surgeons to determine the cut-off for satisfactory blood supply. Data analysis can show detailed inflow and outflow velocity of Indocyanine green at a particular site of the conduit. The intraoperative decision can be altered and the site for anastomosis with satisfactory perfusion can be determined with confidence (Fig. 8).

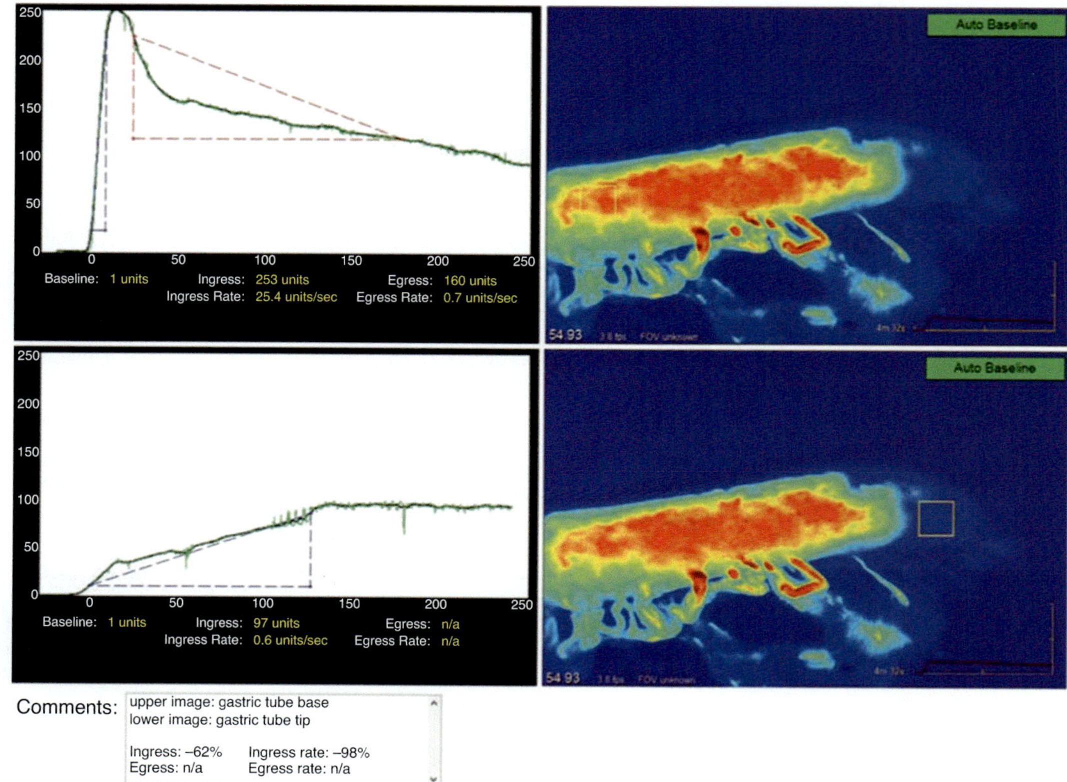

Fig. 8 Software for ICG perfusion data analysis. Upper images with "square" placed at distal (antral) end of the gastric conduit, showing good ingress and egress of ICG as demonstrated by the steep slopes in the graphs. Lower images with "square" placed at proximal (fundal) end of the gastric conduit, showing slow ingress and no egress of ICG. The poorly perfused segment is resected and anastomosis should be placed at site balancing the optimal perfusion adequate length of the conduit

Conclusions

The surgical technique on three-phase esophagectomy has evolved throughout the years but the basic concept persists. A good surgical outcome depends on patient selection, surgical skills, prevention of complication, and vigilance in the management of potential complications. New technology on energy device, stapling device, and other adjuncts has helped the surgeon to perform a safer and better surgery.

Hybrid (Laparoscopy—Thoracotomy) Esophagectomy

Francisco Schlottmann, Manuela Monrabal Lezama,
Fernando A. M. Herbella and Marco G. Patti

Abstract

The hybrid esophagectomy combines a laparoscopic approach for preparation of the gastric conduit and lymphadenectomy, followed by a right muscle sparing thoracotomy for resection of the esophagus, gastric pull-up, and esophago-gastric anastomosis. In this chapter, we will review the critical surgical steps for the operation.

Keywords

Esophageal cancer · Esophagectomy · Laparoscopy · Thoracotomy · Hybrid esophagectomy

F. Schlottmann (✉) · M. Monrabal Lezama
Department of Surgery, Hospital Alemán of Buenos Aires, Buenos Aires, Argentina
e-mail: fschlottmann@hotmail.com

F. Schlottmann
Department of Surgery, University of Illinois at Chicago, Chicago, IL, USA

F. A. M. Herbella
Department of Surgery, Federal University of Sao Paulo, Sao Paulo, Brazil
e-mail: herbella.dcir@epm.br

M. G. Patti
Department of Surgery, University of Virginia, Charlottesville, VA, USA

Introduction

The hybrid esophagectomy combines a laparoscopic approach for preparation of the gastric conduit and lymphadenectomy, followed by a right muscle sparing thoracotomy for resection of the esophagus, gastric pull-up, and esophago-gastric anastomosis. This technique offers a safe and effective approach for the surgical treatment of esophageal cancer [1–8].

Surgical Technique

The hybrid esophagectomy combines a laparoscopic approach for preparation of the gastric conduit and lymphadenectomy, followed by a right muscle sparing thoracotomy for resection of the esophagus, gastric pull-up, and esophago-gastric anastomosis. Before starting the operation, the anesthesiologist places an epidural catheter, a double lumen endotracheal tube, and an arterial catheter.

Laparoscopic Phase

The patient is placed over an inflated beanbag and the legs are extended on stirrups with the knee flexed 20 to 30°. Pneumatic compressions stockings are used as prophylaxis against deep vein thrombosis. The surgeon stands between the patient's legs, with one assistant on the patient's right side and another on the patient's left side. If the surgeon is right-handed, the scrub nurse will stand over the patient's left foot (Fig. 1).

Five trocars are used for the operation. Port A is placed in the midline, about 18 cm below the xiphoid process, and it is used for the insertion of a 30° scope. Ports B and C are placed about 1 inch below the right and left costal margins (forming an angle of about 120°) and are used for dissection. Port D is placed at the level of port A in the right mid-clavicular line, and it is used for the liver retractor. Port E is placed at the level of port A in the left mid-clavicular line, and it is used for a Babcock clamp, for insertion of a bipolar instrument to take down the short gastric vessels, and for insertion of a stapling device to transect the coronary vein and the left gastric artery. If a pyloroplasty is performed, an additional port is placed in between ports A and D, usually about 2 inches below them (Fig. 2).

The dissection is started by identifying the right gastroepiploic artery and opening the gastro-colic omentum (Fig. 3). The dissection is then continued taking down all the short gastric vessels all the way to the left pillar of the crus, which is then separated from the esophagus. The gastro-hepatic ligament is then divided respecting the right gastric artery. The esophagus is separated from the right pillar of the crus. The phreno-esophageal membrane is then divided, and dissection of the esophagus is performed in the posterior mediastinum for about 2 inches. A window is created between the esophagus, the left pillar of the crus and the stomach, and a Penrose drain is passed around the esophagus and pushed as high as possible. The drain will help with the thoracic dissection, and it will be retrieved from the chest.

The coronary vein and the left gastric artery are dissected all the way to their base in order to retrieve as many lymph nodes as possible (Fig. 4), and then are transected using a laparoscopic stapler with a vascular cartridge (Fig. 5). Upon completion of this step, the blood supply of the stomach is based on the right gastric and right gastroepiploic arteries. Posterior adhesions between the posterior wall of the stomach and the pancreas are then taken down using the cautery. We do not perform a Kocher maneuver.

After a final inspection, the trocars are removed, the trocars sites are closed, local anesthesia is injected, and sterile dressings are applied.

Thoracic Phase

After the laparoscopic component of the operation is completed, the patient is positioned in a left lateral decubitus. The chest is entered through a muscle sparing thoracotomy in the fifth intercostal space (Fig. 6). Resection of a 1.5-cm long segment of the posterior portion of the 6th rib facilitates the positioning of a retractor to achieve the optimal exposure of the surgical field. Initially, the inferior pulmonary ligament is divided, and the pleura is opened above and below the azygous vein. An Endo-GIA linear stapler with a vascular cartridge is used to divide the azygous vein (Fig. 7). Then, the dissection of the esophagus and surrounding lymph nodes is performed beginning about 3 cm above the azygous vein all the way down to the gastroesophageal junction, thus joining the mediastinal dissection previously performed by laparoscopy. The stomach is pulled up into the chest, a window is opened along the lesser curvature about 8 cm below the gastroesophageal junction, and transection of the upper portion of the stomach along the lesser curvature is performed with multiple fires of an Endo-GIA stapler. After the gastric conduit is created, 5 mg of indocyanine green (ICG) are injected intravenously as a bolus in order to assess the adequate perfusion of the conduit with fluorescence imaging (Fig. 8).

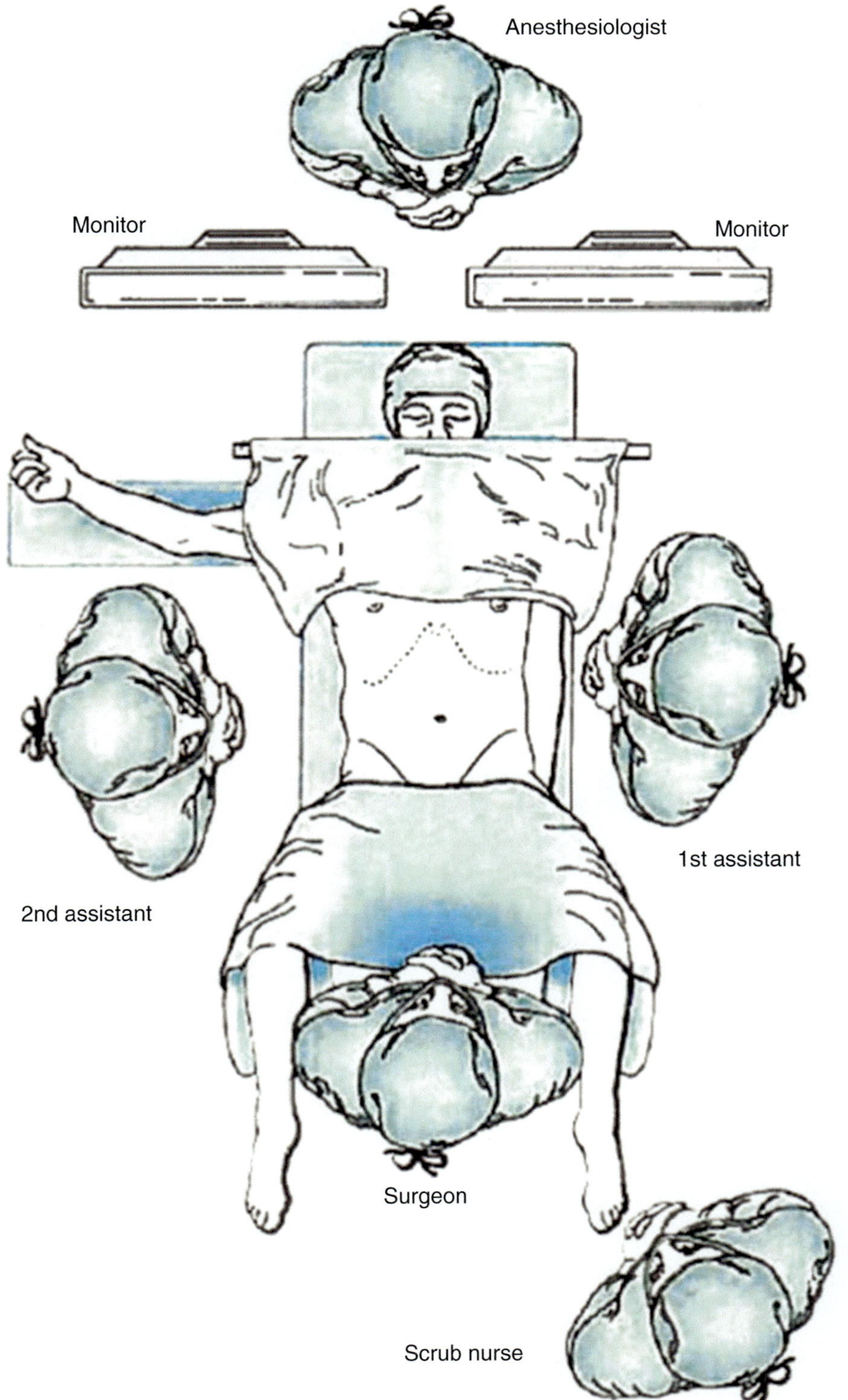

Fig. 1 Position of the operating team. Reproduced with permission from Atlas of Esophageal Surgery, P. Marco Fisichella, Marco G. Patti editors, Springer

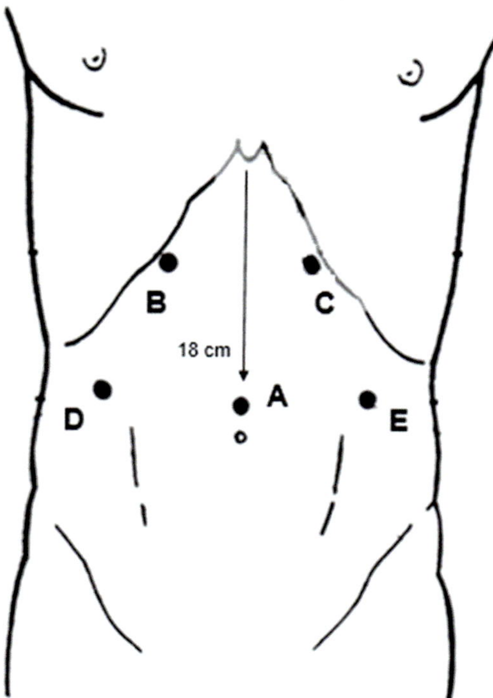

Fig. 2 Placement of abdominal ports

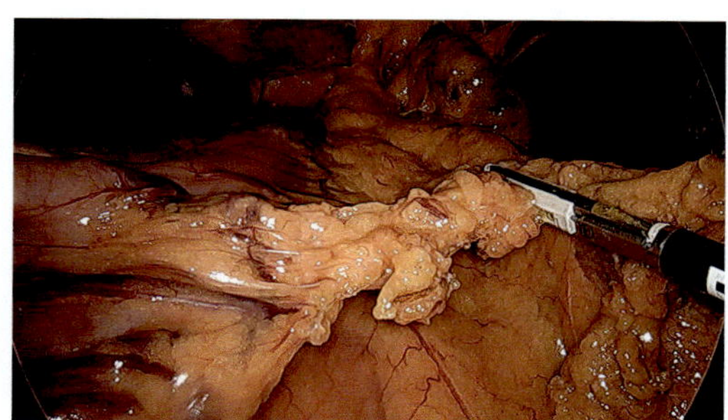

Fig. 3 Dissection along the greater curvature of the stomach

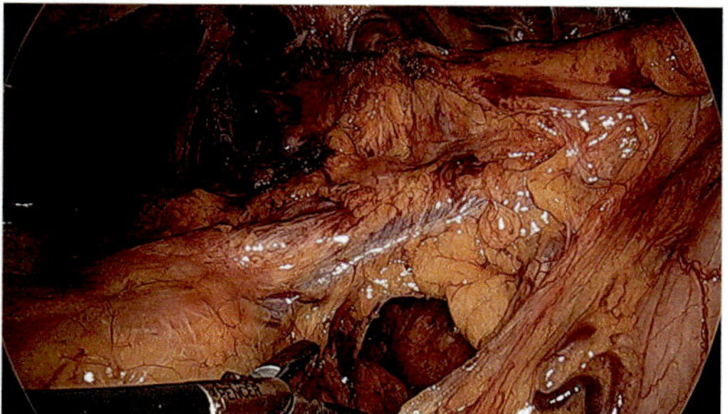

Fig. 4 The coronary vein and left gastric artery are dissected all the way to their base

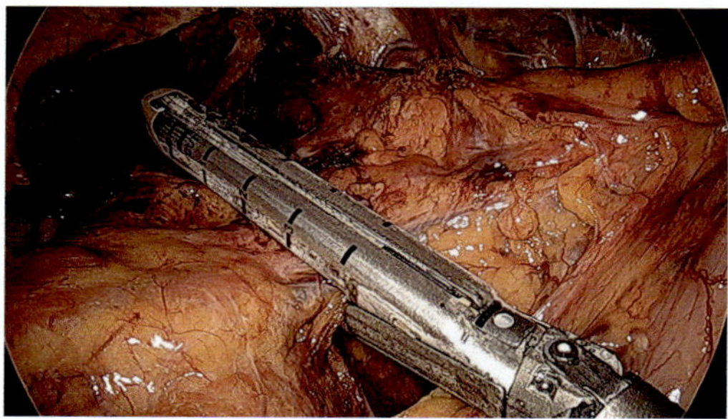

Fig. 5 An Endo GIA™ stapler (Covidien, Minneapolis MN) with a 45-mm vascular cartridge is used for the transection of the coronary vein and left gastric artery

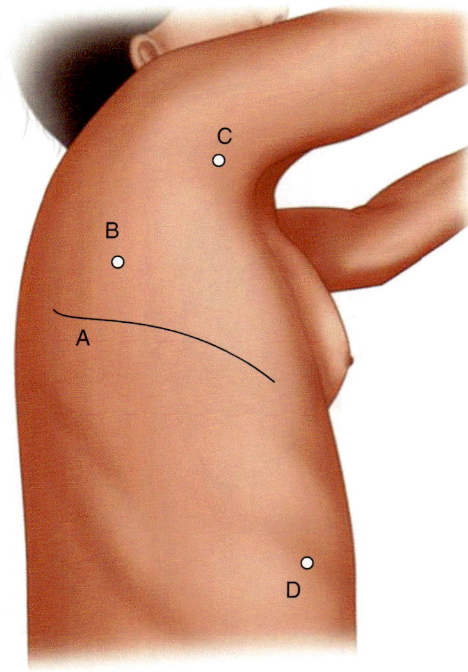

Fig. 6 Position of patient for right thoracotomy. **a** Thoracotomy in 5th intercostal space. **b** Inferior angle of scapula. **c** Posterior axillary line. **d** Port for *Ligasure* dissection and chest tube in 8th or 9th intercostal space, anterior to anterior iliac spine

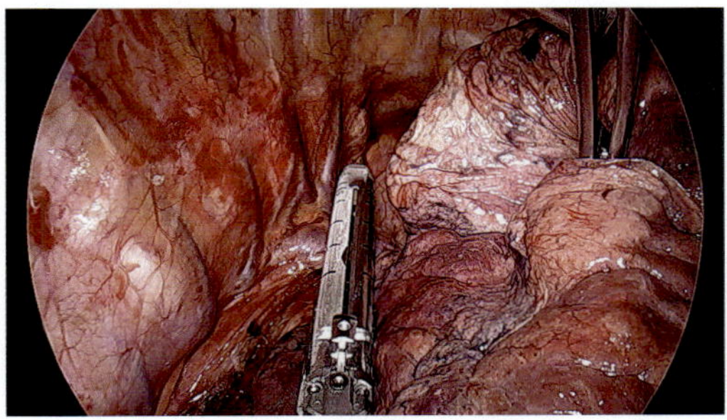

Fig. 7 Division of azygous vein with an Endo GIA™ stapler (Covidien, Minneapolis MN) with a 45-mm vascular cartridge

Intrathoracic Anastomosis

The esophagus is placed over the anterior wall of the stomach, clamped with a Satinsky clamp to avoid separation of the mucosa from the muscular layers, and transected about 3 cm above the azygous vein (Fig. 9). Full-thickness 3-0 silk stay sutures are placed to keep the posterior wall of the esophagus aligned with the anterior wall of the gastric fundus. Sliding of the esophageal mucosa when the stapler is inserted is avoided by placing 3-0 silk stay sutures at the four edges of the esophageal opening that keep together the mucosa with the other layers of the esophageal wall (Fig. 10). The anterior wall of the stomach is opened just distal to the esophageal transection line and interrupted 3-0 silk stiches are used to fix the gastrotomy to the posterior wall of the esophagus. After inserting the thinner branch of a 45 mm Endo-GIA stapler into the stomach and the thicker branch into the esophagus, the stapler is fired, thus constructing a 4 cm long side-to-side anastomosis between the posterior wall of the esophagus and the anterior wall of the stomach (Fig. 11). A nasogastric tube is passed under direct vision into the stomach so that the tip is above the diaphragm. The closure of the anterior aspect of the anastomosis is obtained in two layers: an inner layer of running 3-0 absorbable suture, followed by an outer layer of interrupted 3-0 silk sutures (Fig. 12).

One chest tube is placed, and after direct visual evaluation of the expansion of the lung, the thoracotomy is closed in layers.

Postoperative Course

The patient is extubated in the operating room and transferred to the intensive care unit. Liquid diet is often started on postoperative day 4 and advanced as per tolerance. Patients are usually discharged on postoperative day 7–10.

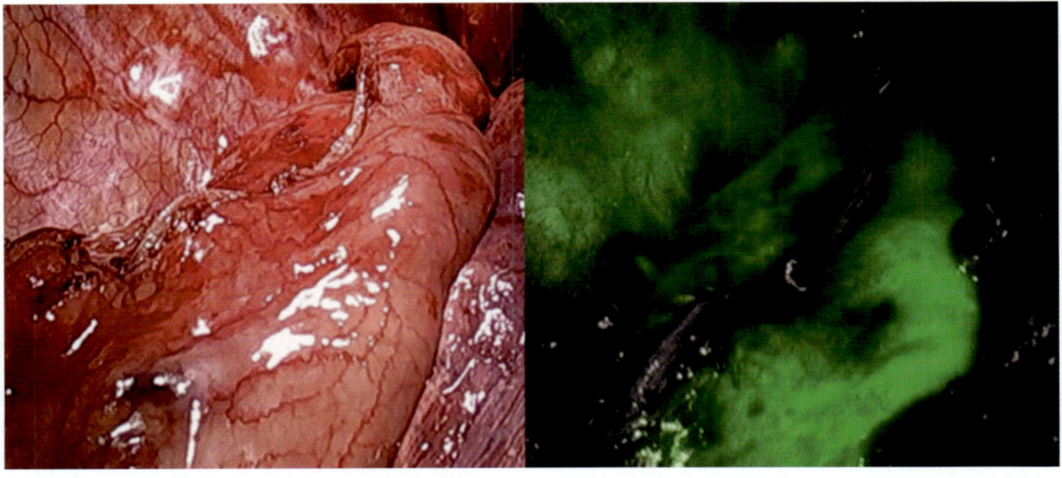

Fig. 8 Perfusion assessment of the gastric conduit with ICG fluorescence imaging

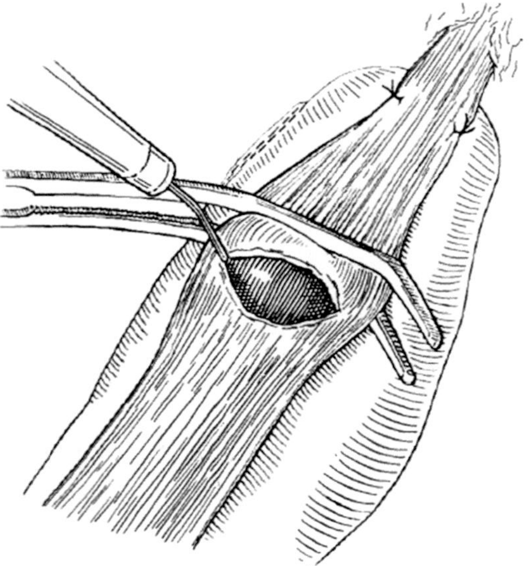

Fig. 9 Transection of the esophagus with electrocautery. The Satinsky clamp is key to avoid separating the mucosa from the muscle layers. Reproduced with permission from Atlas of Esophageal Surgery, P. Marco Fisichella, Marco G. Patti editors, Springer

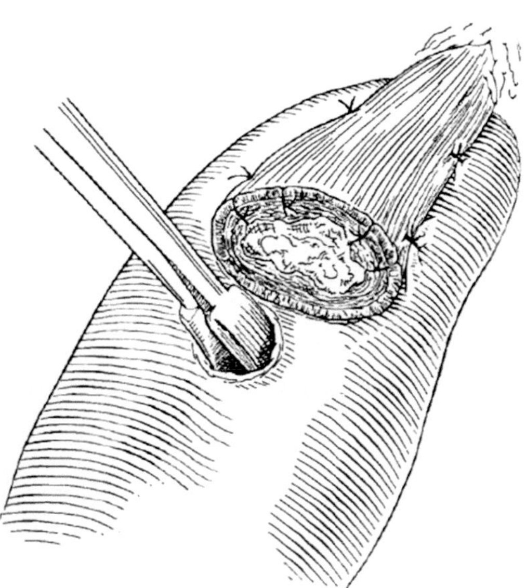

Fig. 10 Placement of stay sutures laterally and anteriorly in the esophagus to avoid sliding of the mucosa when the stapler is inserted. Reproduced with permission from Atlas of Esophageal Surgery, P. Marco Fisichella, Marco G. Patti editors, Springer

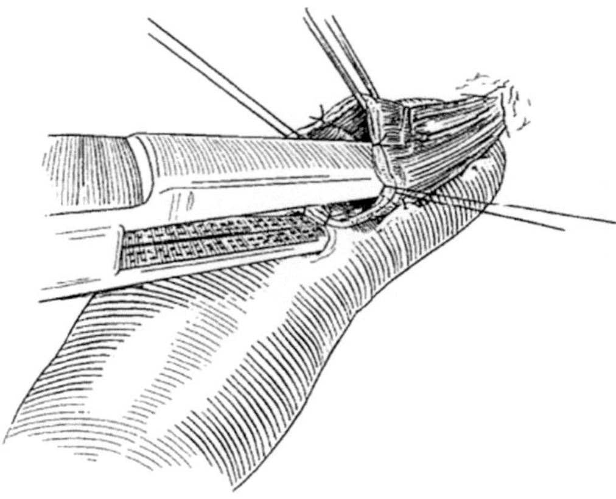

Fig. 11 Insertion of the stapler, with the thinner arm into the stomach and the thicker arm into the esophagus. Reproduced with permission from Atlas of Esophageal Surgery, P. Marco Fisichella, Marco G. Patti editors, Springer

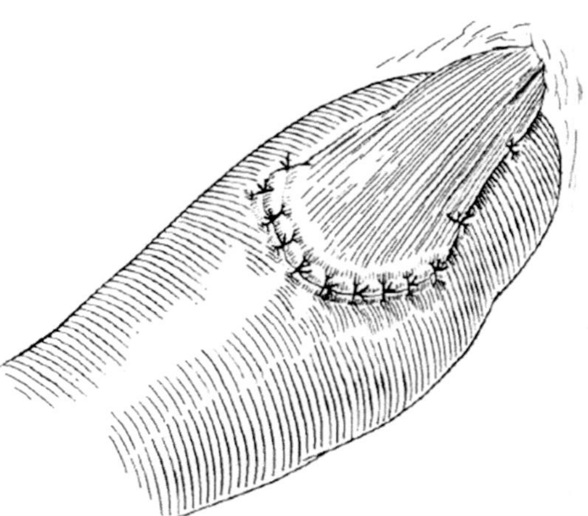

Fig. 12 Closure of the anterior aspect of the anastomosis. Reproduced with permission from Atlas of Esophageal Surgery, P. Marco Fisichella, Marco G. Patti editors, Springer

References

1. Allaix ME, Herbella FA, Patti MG. Hybrid trans-thoracic esophagectomy with side-to-side stapled intrathoracic esophagogastric anastomosis for esophageal cancer. J Gastrointest Surg. 2013;17:1972–9.
2. Nagpal K, Ahmed K, Vats A, et al. Is minimally invasive surgery beneficial in the management of esophageal cancer? A meta-analysis. Surg Endosc. 2010;24:1621–9.
3. Bierre SS, van Berge Henegouwen MI, Maas KW, et al. Minimally invasive versus open

oesophagectomy for patients with esophageal cancer: a multi centre, open-label, randomized controlled trial. Lancet. 2012;379:1887–92.

4. Mariette C, Meunier B, Pezet D, et al. Hybrid mini-invasive versus open oesophagectomy for patients with oesophageal cancer: a multicenter open-label, randomized phase III controlled trial. The MIRO trial. J Clin Oncol. 2015;33(suppl 3; abstr 5).

5. Messager M, Pasquer A, Duhamel A, et al. Laparoscopic gastric mobilization reduces post-operative mortality after esophageal cancer surgery. A French nationwide study. Ann Surg. 2015;262:817–23.

6. Mariette C, Markar SR, Dabakuyo-Yonli TS, et al. Hybrid minimally invasive esophagectomy for esophageal cancer. N Engl J Med. 2019;380(2):152–62.

7. Nuytens F, Dabakuyo-Yonli TS, Meunier B, et al. Five-year survival outcomes of hybrid minimally invasive esophagectomy in esophageal cancer: results of the MIRO randomized clinical trial. JAMA Surg. 2021;156(4):323–32.

8. van Workum F, Klarenbeek BR, Baranov N, Rovers MM, Rosman C. Totally minimally invasive esophagectomy versus hybrid minimally invasive esophagectomy: systematic review and meta-analysis. Dis Esophagus. 2020;33(8):doaa021.

Laparoscopic and Thoracoscopic Ivor Lewis Esophagectomy

Simon R. Turner and Daniela Molena

Abstract

Esophagectomy is one of the most potentially morbid procedures in thoracic surgery, and patients with esophageal cancer frequently have multiple comorbidities related to obesity, smoking and/or alcohol use. Minimally invasive Ivor Lewis esophagectomy minimizes surgical morbidity to the patient, while providing oncologic benefit that is equal or superior to open approaches. This allows for better patient outcomes, especially in patients with multiple medical problems. In this chapter we provide our approach to minimally invasive Ivor Lewis esophagectomy, including surgical tips to avoid complications and intraoperative trouble shooting.

Keywords

Esophageal cancer · Esophagectomy · Minimally invasive · Laparoscopy · Thoracoscopy · Ivor Lewis

S. R. Turner
Division of Thoracic Surgery, Department of Surgery, University of Alberta, Edmonton, AB, Canada

D. Molena (✉)
Thoracic Surgery Service, Department of Surgery, Memorial Sloan Kettering Cancer Center, New York, NY, USA
e-mail: molenad@mskcc.org

Introduction

Minimally invasive Ivor Lewis esophagectomy (MIE) is a technically challenging procedure, requiring advanced skills in both thoracoscopy and laparoscopy. With experience, the procedure can be performed with excellent patient outcomes, both in terms of perioperative morbidity and oncologic efficacy, with only a modest increase in operative time compared to open approaches [1–7]. By avoiding open incisions, especially regarding thoracotomy, the minimally invasive approach results in less pain and blood loss and fewer pulmonary complications [4, 5, 8–13]. Accordingly, length of stay is also reduced [5, 7, 9, 14–16]. While several studies have demonstrated no difference in anastomotic leak rate [5, 6, 8–10], at least two recent studies did find a higher rate of leak with the minimally invasive approach [15, 16] and some studies have demonstrated a small but significant increased need for reintervention compared to open esophagectomy [4, 6, 15]. In several of these studies overall morbidity and length of stay were lower in the MIE group despite the higher incidence of leak. Importantly, oncologic outcomes, including completeness of resection, number of nodes removed, recurrence, and 3- and 5-year survival appear equivalent, if not improved with minimally invasive esophagectomy [7–9, 14]. Potential oncologic benefits of the minimally invasive approach include improved visualization for more complete lymphadenectomy, especially in obese patients, and less immune dysfunction related to surgical stress and blood transfusion. Quality of life at 1 year is also improved compared to open esophagectomy [5, 11–13, 17].

Operative Technique

The patient is intubated with a left-sided double lumen endotracheal tube, and two large bore IVs, a radial arterial line and urinary catheter are inserted. An epidural catheter is not required, an added benefit of avoiding laparotomy and thoracotomy incisions and allowing for faster removal of urinary catheters and less post-operative hypotension. If the patient has not had a recent upper endoscopy prior to surgery, this is performed prior to making incisions to determine the extent of the tumor and any associated Barrett's esophagus, to confirm the suitability of the stomach as a conduit and assess the patency of the pylorus. A pyloric drainage procedure is unnecessary in most patients and may increase long term morbidity and need for reintervention, so we do not routinely perform it [18]. If Botox pyloromyotomy is being performed (see below), there is an option to perform it endoscopically at this point, with or without pyloric dilation, but always care must be taken to minimize the amount of air insufflated into the stomach, which will hinder laparoscopy. The stomach is suctioned out with the scope and an orogastric tube is placed to completely decompress the stomach.

The patient is positioned supine on a bean bag. The feet are secured to a padded footboard with tape. The arms are comfortably abducted to allow access to the abdomen. The abdomen is widely prepped and draped. Reverse Trendelenburg position, used during laparoscopy to aid in visualization of the upper abdomen, is introduced gradually to avoid sudden hypotension.

Abdominal Port Placement

A 5 mm port is placed under direct visualization just under the left costal margin in the midclavicular line; after abdominal insufflation with CO_2 at 15 mmHg the other ports are placed as followed: a 5 mm camera port in the midline just below the falciform ligament, a 10 mm port in the right flank and a 5 mm port in the right upper quadrant such that instruments will have an easy trajectory under the liver and falciform ligament and towards the hiatus. An optional additional 5 mm port may be placed in the left upper quadrant for the assistant. A Nathanson liver retractor is placed just below the xiphoid to elevate the left lobe of the liver and expose the hiatus (Fig. 1). Most of the work is done by the primary surgeon standing on the patient's right, with an atraumatic grasper in the left hand and Harmonic scalpel (Ethicon, Somerville, NJ) in the right. The first assistant stands at the

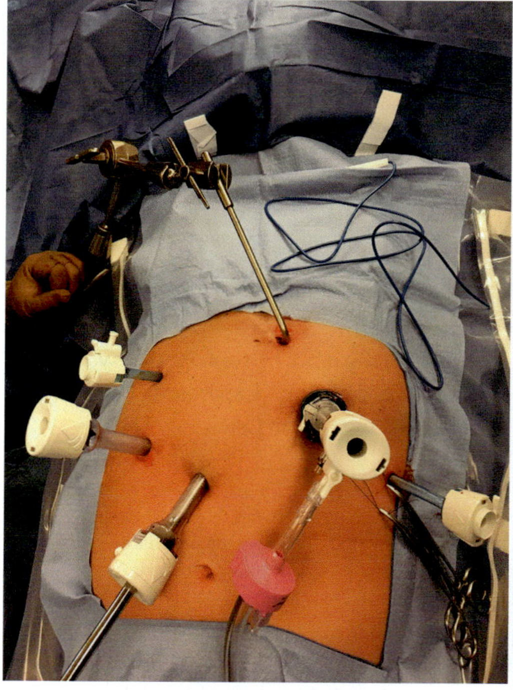

Fig. 1 Abdominal port placement

patient's left and uses a grasper in each hand to assist with retraction. The camera operator stands to the patient's right below the primary surgeon. Mobilization of the most cranial and caudal extents of greater curvature of the stomach is done by the surgeon standing on the patient's left, especially the division of the highest short gastric vessels and mobilization of the pylorus.

Abdominal Lymphadenectomy and Gastric Mobilization

The dissection begins with division of the gastrohepatic ligament, proceeding superiorly until reaching the right crus. The left gastric, splenic and common hepatic arteries are identified in order to perform a complete dissection of their associated nodes. Exposure is facilitated by the assistant lifting the stomach with a closed grasper along the lesser curve, behind the stomach and to the left of the left gatric pedicle. This puts the left gastric vessels in a vertical orientation toward the ceiling and allows optimal visualization of the lesser sac. Dissection is started at the superior aspect of the pancreas and the hepatic artery is identified. This artery is skeletonized superiorly to the takeoff of the left gastric and splenic arteries. Once the left gastric

artery is identified, the lymph nodes are swept upwards into the specimen so that the artery and vein can be divided at their origin using a vascular stapler (Fig. 2). By retracting the stomach anteriorly, access is gained to the celiac artery nodes found between the left gastric artery stump and the base of the diaphragmatic crus. Using this exposure, posterior gastric attachments can start to be divided and the tip of the fundus can be partially mobilized from behind, which can facilitate the later dissection along the greater curve.

Attention then returns to the hiatus. The dissection is carried to the base of the hiatus and into the posterior mediastinum. The left crus is dissected from phrenoesophageal attachments toward the angle of His. Fibers of the crura should be preserved if possible while staying wide enough to ensure an adequate radial margin from the tumor. Muscle of the crura may be resected en bloc if there is concern for invasion by bulky disease at the gastroesophageal junction. The hiatus should be repaired in case of partial resection or when a large paraesophageal hernia is encountered. Leaving a large diaphragmatic crural opening will likely lead to paraconduit herniation of abdominal content into the mediastinum, a complication more commonly seen with minimally invasive esophagectomy, possibly due to lack of intraabdominal adhesions

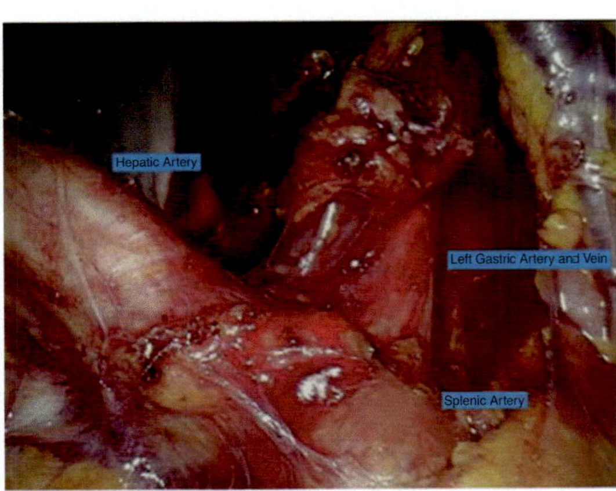

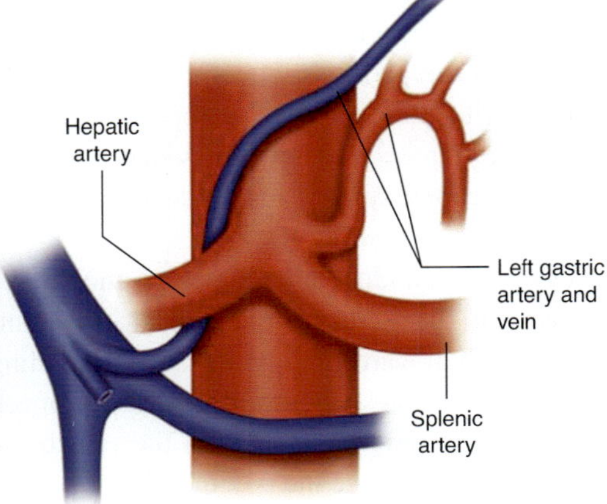

Fig. 2 The hepatic and splenic arteries are skeletonized superiorly and the left gastric vessels are completely dissected at their base before division with vascular stapler

[19]. The esophagus should not be completely encircled at this time, nor should extensive transhiatal dissection yet be performed, to avoid pneumothorax and hemodynamic instability early in the procedure.

Careful handling of the stomach throughout the procedure will help preserve the submucosal collateral vessels that are the only vascular supply of the conduit in the area of the anastomosis. Where possible the stomach should be retracted bluntly with closed instruments, avoiding grasping the stomach as much as possible in the area which will constitute the conduit. Attention is turned to dissecting the greater curvature of the stomach. The stomach is gently retracted anteriorly and to the right, exposing the gastrocolic ligament. The right gastroepiploic artery is visualized and must be preserved to perfuse the gastric conduit. Staying well away from this artery, the gastrocolic ligament is divided along the greater curve toward the fundus. While preserving this arterial pedicle it is still important not to stray to far from the greater curve, which risks injury to the transverse colon. Eventually the artery terminates, though there are sometimes horizontal collaterals with one or two short gastric arteries which should be preserved. Above this level, it is safest to stay close to the stomach. Doing so allows the short gastric arteries to be divided with a long stump on the splenic side. Care is taken not to injure the spleen as mobilization continues towards the previous dissection along the left crus. It is generally easier to divide the last attachments holding the fundus while standing at the patient's left. If posterior attachments of the stomach to the retroperitoneum are encountered these can now be divided. Posterior gastric arterial branches may also be identified and divided.

Once the fundus is completely mobilized, division of the gastrocolic ligament is continued caudally towards the pylorus. Fully dividing these attachments between the distal stomach and the colon reduces tension on the anastomosis and helps decrease the risk of colonic herniation via the hiatus. The pylorus should be freely mobile and the colon completely separated from the stomach and proximal duodenum. The pylorus will nearly reach the hiatus and a Kocher maneuver is neither required nor encouraged, as excessive duodenal mobility may result in herniation of the duodenum into the chest with kinking of the gastric conduit.

Pyloric Drainage and Feeding Jejunostomy

A pyloric drainage procedure is not necessary and we do not typicaly perform one. If a pyloric drainage procedure is being performed, 100 units of Botox in 5 cc of sterile saline are injected into the muscle of the pylorus using a transabdominal needle.

The decision to perform feeding jejunostomy should also be individualized to each patient. If a feeding tube is required, the bed is leveled for the jejunostomy placement. The colon is lifted superiorly to identify the ligament of Treitz at the base of the transverse mesocolon. A proximal loop of jejunum that reaches easily to the abdominal wall of the left mid abdomen is selected for jejunostomy placement. Four absorbable sutures are placed in a diamond pattern on the anti-mesenteric aspect of the bowel, surrounding the planned jejunostomy site. Each suture is brought through the abdominal wall with a Carter-Thompson fascial closure device and secured loosely with hemostats. A Seldinger technique is then used to perform a percutaneous jejunostomy (Fig. 3). Care is taken to ensure the tube is intraluminal and not dissecting within the wall of the bowel and is directed antegrade. Once the tube has been inserted, the four anchoring sutures are tied externally within the subcutaneous layer, securing the jejunum to the anterior abdominal wall. Next an anti-torsion stitch is placed about 2 cm distal to the jejunostomy itself. The tube is secured to the skin with non-absorbable sutures. The tube should be flushed after securing it to ensure patency. After the jejunostomy is completed, the transverse colon and the omentum are returned to their standard position.

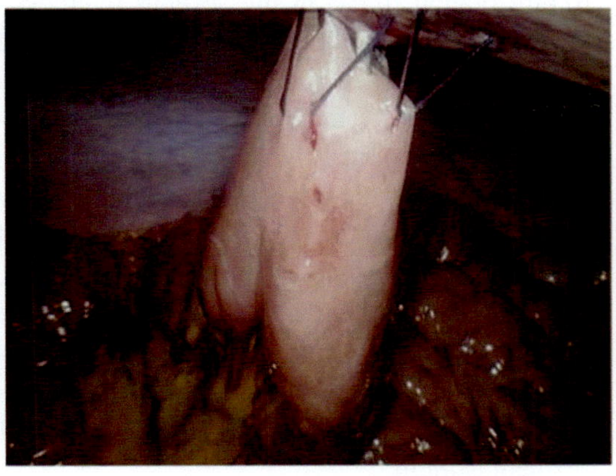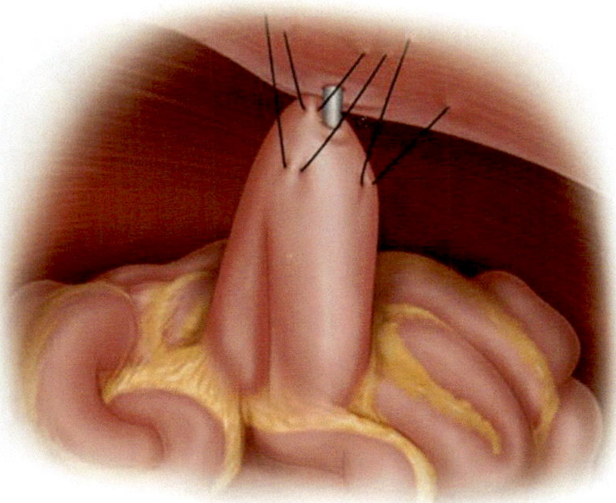

Fig. 3 A loop of jejunum is anchored to the abdominal wall with absorbable stitches placed on a diamond shape. A needle is inserted between the stitches to pass a guidewire which will allow placement of a 14F sheath and the feeding jejunostomy

Transhiatal Dissection

The bed is returned to reverse Trendelenburg position to begin the transhiatal dissection of the esophagus. A ½ inch Penrose drain is passed around the distal esophagus, and secured with a locking clip to create a mobile handle. Using the drain to aid in retraction, a transhiatal dissection is performed as high as feasible, about to the level of the inferior pulmonary vein. Periesophageal lymph nodes, including nodes anteriorly along the back of the pericardium, should be kept en bloc with the specimen. If a pneumothorax occurs at this point, make the pleural opening wide enough to avoid entrapment of air within the chest and tension physiology. If hemodynamic instability due to pneumothorax is noted several remedies can be employed. Decreasing the intra-abdominal insufflation pressure, increasing the airway pressure and taking the patient out of steep reverse Trendelenburg are useful maneuvers that resolve the problem in most cases. Placement of a chest tube is almost never required.

Creation of the Gastric Conduit

A location on the lesser curve, just cranial to the pylorus is selected to begin tubularization of the conduit. Preservation of several small draining veins along the distal lesser curve may promote better conduit perfusion. Ensure that the orogastric tube is withdrawn completely out of the stomach to avoid it being caught in the staple line. The conduit is divided from the specimen, proceeding superiorly toward the fundus. The conduit should be 4–5 cm in width. The staple line is kept as straight as possible by stretching the stomach from the tip of the fundus towards the left shoulder (Figs. 4 and 5). Stop the staple line approximately 3 cm proximal to the fundus so that the specimen and conduit can later be delivered into the chest together in the proper orientation. Finally, the Penrose drain is passed through the hiatus where it will later be retrieved via the chest. The liver retractor is removed, hemostasis is ensured and port sites are closed in the standard fashion.

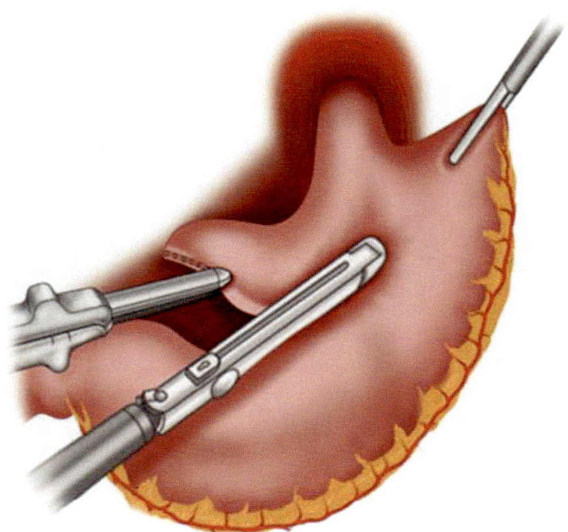

Fig. 4 The stomach is stretched at the fundus during tubularization to avoid twisting and folding. Tubularization is started just above the pylorus to allow unfolding of the lesser curvature and adequate conduit length

Positioning for the Thoracic Phase and Port Placement

The patient is positioned in the left lateral decubitus position leaning slightly forward on a bean bag, with an axillary roll and arm support and with the table flexed. At this point anesthesia should switch to single lung ventilation. The chest is entered under direct visualization with a 10 mm optical trocar in the seventh intercostal space in the posterior axillary line. Additional ports are placed as follows: A 5 mm camera port in the ninth intercostal space just posteriorly to the first port, a 10 mm port in the fourth or fifth intercostal space in the mid-axillary line, and a 5 mm port in the seventh intercostal space between the scapula and the spine (Fig. 6). Chest insufflation with CO_2 at a pressure of 8 mmHg helps exposure by flattening the diaphragm, collapsing the lungs towards the anterior mediastinum and decreasing movement of the mediastinum.

Thoracoscopic Dissection

The inferior pulmonary ligament is divided and the associated lymph nodes removed. The mediastinal pleura is incised anteriorly to the esophagus, heading superiorly to the level of the azygos vein which is divided using a vascular stapler. Next, the dissection is carried back down to the diaphragm, this time dividing the pleura posterior to the esophagus. As the dissection is carried inferiorly the transhiatal dissection performed via the abdomen is eventually encountered. Locate the Penrose drain and use this as a retraction handle. Dissect the esophagus completely out of its bed in the mediastinum, proceeding again superiorly toward the level of the

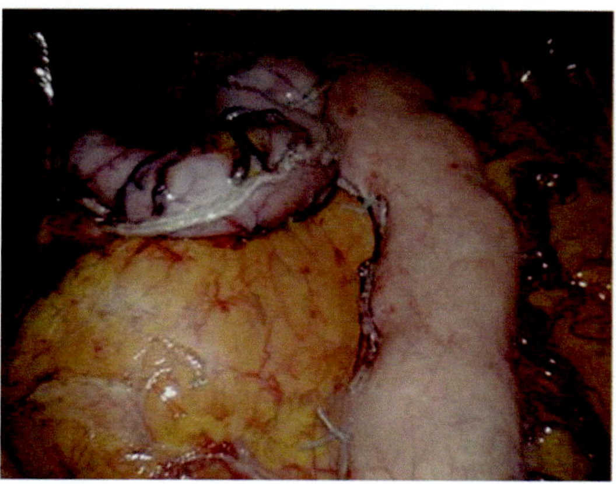

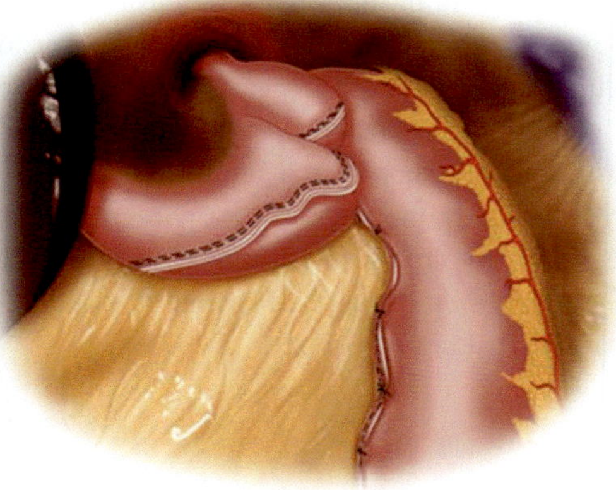

Fig. 5 The conduit is not completely divided from the specimen to facilitate transposition in the chest. A few interrupted stitches over the staple line are useful to minimize gastric injury or hematomas during retraction of the stomach

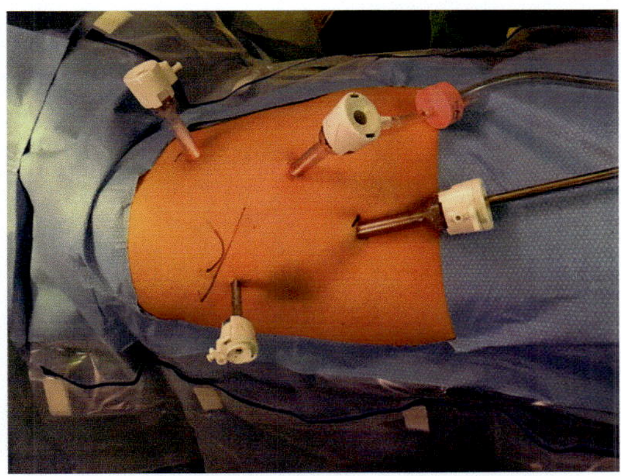

Fig. 6 Thoracic port placement

tracheoesophageal fistula. Exercise caution when using energy devices near the airway, particularly during the subcarinal node dissection. Even minor thermal injury, often not even visible during the operation, can progress over the course of several days to a full thickness injury and fistula formation. In addition, bronchial artery branches supplying the airway should be preserved to prevent ischemia. Always ensure that the bronchial cuff of the double lumen endotracheal tube is not overinflated, which can put the left mainstem bronchus at increased risk of injury.

Esophagogastric Anastomosis

The dissection of the esophagus is extended beneath the pleura around 2 cm superiorly past where the pleura was divided at the level of the azygos vein. The preserved pleura will act as a buttress for the eventual anastomosis. The esophagus is divided using a linear stapler at the level of—or above—the azygos vein, after confirming that the orogastric tube and esophageal temperature probe have been removed. Tension is minimized by placing the anastomosis no higher in the chest than necessary but at least at the level of the azygos vein to avoid redundant gastric conduit in the chest which can lead to reflux. Next, the anesthesiologist gently advances an oral anvil for the circular stapler (Orvil, Medtronic, Minneapolis, MN). The staple line is grasped on both sides to help guide the tube and keep the staple line horizontal. Once the tip of the tube can be seen, cautery is used to create a small opening just above the staple line on the medial aspect (towards the vena cava) of the staple line, allowing the end of the tube to be pulled through as the anesthesiologist guides the anvil over the back of the palate (Fig. 7). A pursestring stitch with reabsorbable suture is placed around the anvil to ensure a tight seal around the device.

azygos vein. Before reaching the azygous, the aorta will be seen to arch towards the left chest. At this level caution must be taken to identify and avoid injury to the aorta and the left mainstem bronchus. For gastroesophageal junction tumors there is no oncologic need to obtain a wide radial margin at this proximal part of the esophagus, and staying close to the esophageal wall minimizes the risk to the airway.

The thoracic duct is also at particular risk for injury during esophageal mobilization in the chest because of its inconsistent course and the fact that it is often difficult to visualize, especially in obese patients or after neoadjuvant radiation. Again, injury occurs when dissection strays outside of the periesophageal plane of dissection. Identify and clip lymphatic branches coming from the thoracic duct and arterial branches from the aorta. Prophylactic ligation of the thoracic duct itself has not consistently been shown to reduce postoperative chylothorax, but if injury to the duct or its branches is suspected the duct should be ligated just above the hiatus. Fluorescence imaging may be useful to help delineate the anatomy of the duct to aid in its preservation or ligation, though it is not routinely necessary [20].

Complete the lymphadenectomy by dissecting the subcarinal nodes, again taking care not to injure or devascularize the airway. Avoidance of injury to the airways, including the trachea and both mainstem bronchi, is vital in preventing

The distal esophagus is gently pulled upwards to deliver the specimen and the conduit into the chest. Avoid excess traction and any twisting of the conduit. The staple line of

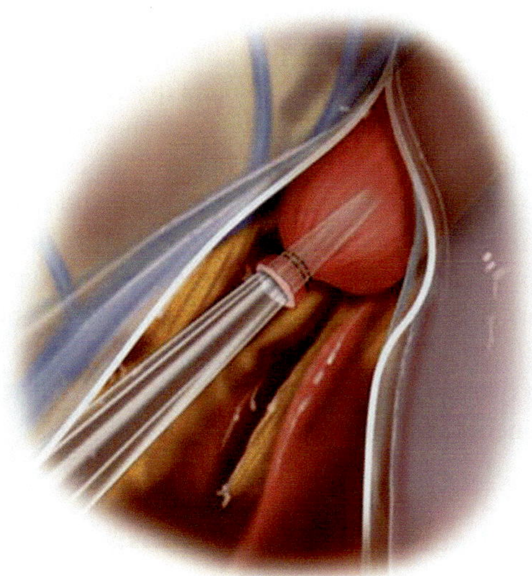

Fig. 7 The Orvil is retrieved through an opening in the esophageal stump. It is important to stay as close as possible to the esophageal stump staple line so that this is cut by the circular stapler

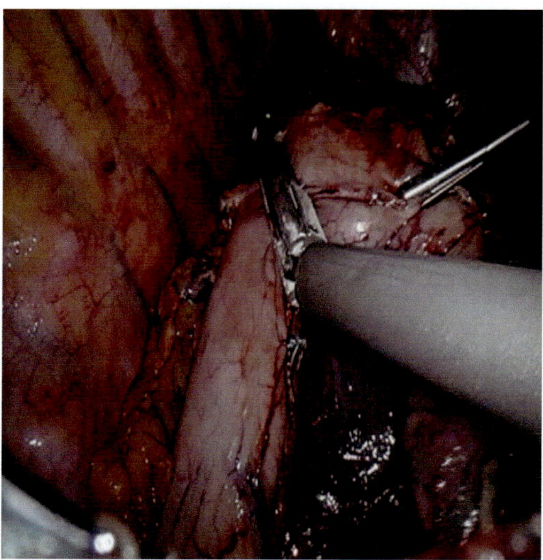

Fig. 8 The specimen is retracted towards the anterior mediastinum and the conduit is completely divided making sure the margin at the level of the hiatus is not compromised

the conduit should be oriented to the patient's right and be totally straight. At this point the conduit perfusion can be assessed using fluorescence imaging using a proprietary camera such as the Pinpoint system (Novadaq, Ontario, Canada). The speed of fluorescence appearance and any areas of demarcation can help to identify regions of poor perfusion in the conduit. If a demarcation is seen, mark the area so that the anastomosis can be created caudally where there is preserved perfusion, resecting the poorly perfused portion of the stomach after the anastomosis is performed [20].

The specimen is fully divided from the conduit using a linear stapler, taking care to maintain an adequate margin and leave enough room for insertion of the circular stapler to form an end to side esophagogastric anastomosis (Fig. 8). The specimen is removed in a retrieval bag and sent for intraoperative assessment of the proximal and distal margins. The anastomosis is performed only after the margins are confirmed to be uninvolved. The proximal tip of the conduit is grasped and opened parallel to the staple line with cautery, wide enough to allow insertion of the circular stapler. The anastomosis is performed in an area of good conduit perfusion with no tension, leaving the greater curvature vessels on the tracheal side of the anastomosis in order to protect the airways in case of leak (Fig. 9). Once the circular stapler is fired, the redundant tip of the stomach is used as a retraction handle to expose the anastomosis and place two stay sutures: One suture is placed to reinforce the area where the staple lines cross at the lateral aspect of the anastomosis. This is then further buttressed with omentum to protect the airway and aorta. The second suture is placed on the medial aspect of the anastomosis to further relieve tension. After placing these sutures, a nasogastric tube is guided into the body of the stomach under direct vision. Finally the opened proximal end of the conduit is closed with a linear stapler, making sure the anastomosis and this gastric staple line are at least 1–2 cm apart to avoid ischemia (Fig. 10). At this point the anastomosis is allowed to retract under the superior mediastinal pleura. The conduit can be tacked to the pleura with absorbable sutures. Intraoperative gastroscopy can be performed to assess the anastomosis and perform an insufflation leak test as the conduit is submerged under water. The anesthesiologist then advances a nasogastric tube under direct vision until the tip

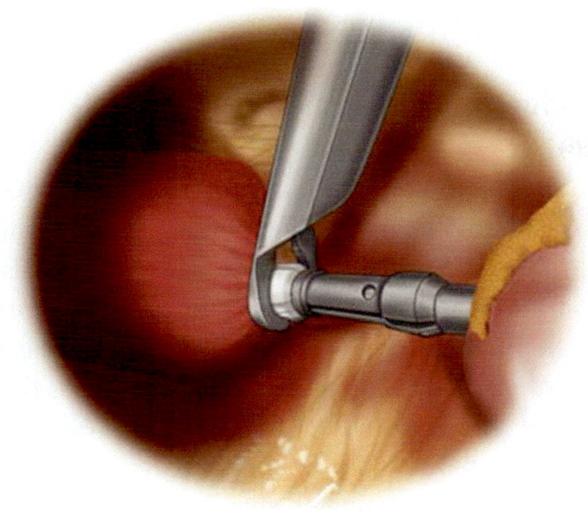

Fig. 9 The anastomosis is performed using a special grasper designed for use with the Orvil. The greater curve vessels are positioned against the airway to protect against fistula formation in the case of a leak. The preserved mediastinal pleura which will cover the eventual anastomosis is seen

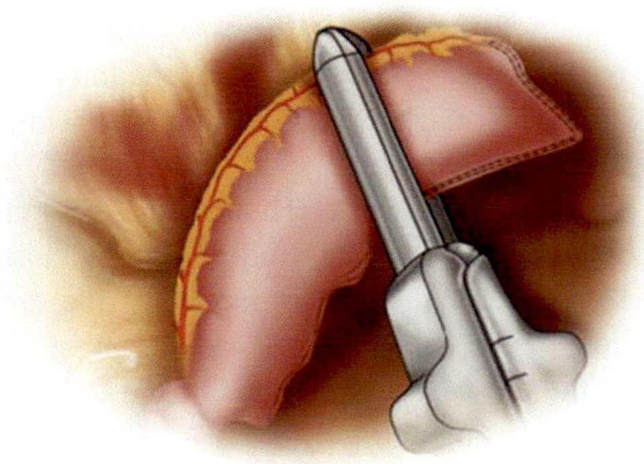

Fig. 10 Resection of opened proximal end of the conduit with linear stapler

is within the distal conduit. Lastly, the conduit can be tacked to the diaphragm at the hiatus with non-absorbable suture to help prevent against paraconduit herniation. A single straight 28 Fr chest tube is placed and the lung is re-expanded. Incisions are closed in the standard fashion.

Postoperative Care

Patients should be extubated in the operating room and monitored in the post-anesthetic care unit overnight. The nasogastric tube is kept to low intermittent suction and the patient is kept NPO. Jejunostomy feeds can be initiated on post-op day #1–2 and advanced according to protocol. The nasogastric tube is usually ready to be removed by post-op day #3 or 4, depending on the output and provided the conduit is not distended on X-ray. Contrast esophagram does not reliably identify or rule out a subclinical anastomotic leak and does not need to be routinely performed. The patient can start clear fluids on approximately post-op day #5 unless there are clinical signs of a leak such as tachycardia, atrial fibrillation, fever or rising white blood cell count. The chest tube should be removed once a chyle leak has been ruled out after initiating tube feeds, and if there are no signs of leak, typically by post-op day #3. Careful attention must be paid to the patient's fluid balance. Most patients benefit from diuresis starting on around post-op day #3, which is often continued up to discharge. Patients should ambulate 1 mile/day and use incentive spirometry at least hourly.

Any unexpected deviation from the clinical course, such as fever, cough or arrhythmia, may signal a more serious complication such as anastomotic leak or pneumonia. These should be investigated appropriately, typically with an IV and oral contrast CT scan of the chest. In the absence of complications most patients are discharged by around post-op day #7. After discharge the patient can slowly advance their diet and tube feeding can be weaned as oral calorie intake improves. The jejunostomy tube can usually be removed at the first follow-up appointment 2 weeks after discharge.

Outcomes

Several studies have compared MIE and open esophagectomy. Biere et al. randomized 115 patients at five centers to either MIE or open esophagectomy [5]. MIE was superior in terms of blood loss (200 vs 475 mL, $p < 0.001$), length of stay (11 vs 14 days, $p = 0.044$), recurrent laryngeal nerve injury (2 vs 14%, $p = 0.012$), visual analog pain scale (2 vs 3, $p < 0.001$) and several short term quality of life measures, and was inferior only in operative time (329 vs 299 min, $p = 0.002$). Takeuchi, et al. performed a propensity matched comparison of MIE and open esophagectomy in 7030 patients, performed in over 700 Japanese hospitals [4]. MIE was superior in terms of blood loss (442 vs 608 mL, $p < 0.001$), need for > 48 h ventilation (8.9 vs 10.9%, $p = 0.006$), rate of atelectasis (3.6 vs 5.1%, $p = 0.002$) and superficial infections (6.7 vs 8.7%, $p = 0.022$). MIE was inferior in terms of operative time (526 vs 461 min, $p < 0.001$), recurrent laryngeal nerve injury (10.3 vs 8.1%, $p = 0.002$) and the need for reoperation (7 vs 5.3%, $p = 0.004$) though there was no difference in anastomotic leak, pneumonia, overall morbidity, or operative and 30 day mortality. Sihag, et al. retrospectively studied the Society of Thoracic Surgeons database to compare MIE and open esophagectomy in 3740 patients [6]. MIE was superior in terms of length of stay (9 vs 10 days, $p < 0.001$), postoperative transfusions (14.1 vs 18.7%, $p = 0.002$) and wound infections (2.3 vs 6.3%, $p < 0.001$) but was inferior in terms of operative time (443 vs 312 min, $p < 0.001$), empyema (4.1 vs 1.8%, $p < 0.001$), need for reoperation (9.5 vs 4.4%, $p < 0.001$), and need for dilation prior to discharge (5.5 vs 1.9%, $p < 0.001$). Key results of these and other studies are summarized in Table 1.

Surgical Tips

Abdominal Phase

- The addition of a 5 mm port in the left upper quadrant allows both the primary surgeon and the first assistant to work with two hands, which can facilitate exposure. This is especially useful when less experienced trainees are involved, but as expertise is gained, this port can be omitted without compromising the operation.
- Minimize grasping the greater curve of the stomach, which will become the conduit. Plan grasper placement carefully for retraction during each phase of the stomach mobilization, so that the grasper doesn't have to be continually readjusted. Bluntly lift the stomach instead of grasping it when possible.
- Avoid performing transhiatal dissection until late in the abdominal phase. This avoids a pneumothorax early in the case with resulting issues with hypotension. If a pneumothorax does occur it can usually be managed without inserting a chest tube.
- The use of the Carter-Thompson fascial closure device and the Endostitch (Covidien, Dublin, Ireland) greatly facilitates the creation of the jejunostomy, which can be one of the most frustrating parts of the operation when starting out.

Thoracic Phase

- The use of CO_2 insufflation aids exposure and stabilizes the surgical field.
- Locate the previously placed Penrose drain early on after dividing the mediastinal pleura anteriorly and posteriorly. This provides a useful handle to retract the esophagus during dissection.

Table 1 Superior operative approach for selected surgical and oncologic outcomes

Outcome	Biere [5]	Takeuchi [4]	Sihag [6]	Tapias [7]	Palazzo [9]
Length of stay	MIE	ND	MIE	MIE	MIE
ICU length of stay/ventilation	ND	MIE	ND	MIE	–
Operative time	OE	OE	OE	ND	–
Blood loss/transfusion	MIE	MIE	MIE	MIE	MIE
Anastomotic leak	ND	ND	ND	ND	ND
Recurrent nerve injury	MIE	OE	–	ND	–
Superficial/wound infection	–	MIE	MIE	–	–
Pneumonia/empyema	–	MIE	OE	ND	MIE
Pain	MIE	–	–	–	–
Need for reoperation	ND	OE	OE	–	–
Margin	ND	–	–	ND	ND
Nodes removed	ND	–	–	ND	MIE
Operative/30 day mortality	ND	ND	ND	ND	ND

MIE minimally invasive esophagectomy-blue, *OE* open esophagectomy-yellow, *ND* no difference-grey

- Preserving the mediastinal pleura above the azygos vein provides an envelope of pleura to surround the anastomosis and allows anchoring the conduit to combat the effects of gravity when the patient is upright.
- It is often easiest to perform the subcarinal node dissection separately, after the esophagus is completely mobilized.
- Assess the conduit using fluorescence, color and/or Doppler signal. This will help select the ideal location for the anastomosis.

Intraoperative Trouble Shooting

- Hypotension is a common occurrence during the abdominal phase, and is typically related to patient positioning or a pneumothorax. If hypotension occurs, start by taking the patient out of reverse Trendelenburg position. If this solves the problem, gradually reintroduce reverse Trendelenburg to allow the patient time to compensate. If a pneumothorax is suspected, ensure that the pleural opening is extended widely to prevent tension physiology. Decreasing CO_2 insufflation pressure can help in both circumstances. Communicate with the anesthesia team to avoid excess administration of IV fluids, often a reflex reaction to transient hypotension, and which can be associated with cardiac and pulmonary complications postoperatively.
- Ensure that the bronchial cuff of the double lumen tube is not overinflated. If it is, the

membranous wall of the left mainstem bronchus can be stretched and prone to injury during esophageal mobilization and subcarinal node dissection.

When performing the anastomosis, double check that the conduit is not twisted. The staple line should be straight and to the patient's right (up towards the ceiling with the patient in decubitus positioning). The greater curve vessels should lie to the left and are laid to buttress between the conduit and the airway.

References

1. Luketich JD, Pennathur A, Franchetti Y, Catalano PJ, Swanson S, Sugarbaker DJ, et al. Minimally invasive esophagectomy: results of a prospective phase II multicenter trial-the Eastern Cooperative Oncology Group (E2202) Study. Ann Surg. 2015;261(4):702–7.
2. Mungo B, Lidor AO, Stem M, Molena D. Early experience and lessons learned in a new minimally invasive esophagectomy program. Surg Endosc. 2016;30:1692–8.
3. Litle VR, Buenaventura PO, Luketich JD. Minimally invasive resection for esophageal cancer. Surg Clin North Am. 2002;82(4):711–28.
4. Takeuchi H, Miyata H, Ozawa S, Udagawa H, Osugi H, Matsubara H, et al. Comparison of short-term outcomes between open and minimally invasive esophagectomy for esophageal cancer using a nationwide database in Japan. Ann Surg Oncol. 2017;24(7):1821.
5. Biere SS, van Berge Henegouwen MI, Maas KW, Bonavina L, Rosman C, Roig Garcia J, et al. Minimally invasive versus open oesophagectomy for patients with oesophageal cancer: a multicenter, open-label, randomized controlled trial. Lancet. 2012;379:1887–92.
6. Sihag S, Kosinski AS, Gaissert HA, Wright CD, Schipper PH. Minimally invasive versus open esophagectomy for esophageal cancer: a comparison of early surgical outcomes from the Society of Thoracic Surgeons National Database. Ann Thorac Surg. 2016;101:1281–9.
7. Bograd AJ, Molena D. Minimally invasive esophagectomy. Curr Prob Surg. 2021;58: 100984.
8. Tapias LF, Mathisen DJ, Wright CD, Wain JC, Gaissert HA, Muniappan A. Outcomes with open and minimally invasive Ivor Lewis esophagectomy after neoadjuvant therapy. Ann Thorac Surg. 2016;101:1097–103.
9. Straatman J, van der Wielen N, Cuesta MA, Daams F, Roig Garcia J, Bonavina L, et al. Minimally invasive versus open esophageal resection: three-year follow-up of the previously reported randomized controlled trial: the TIME trial. Ann Surg. 2017;266(2):232–6.
10. Palazzo F, Rosato EL, Chaudhary A, Evans NR, Sedecki JA, Keith S, et al. Minimally invasive esophagectomy provides significant survival advantage compared with open or hybrid esophagectomy for patients with cancers of the esophagus and gastroesophageal junction. J Am Coll Surg. 2015;220(4):672–9.
11. Nagpal K, Ahmed K, Vats A, Yakoub D, James D, Ashrafian H, et al. Is minimally invasive surgery beneficial in the management of esopahgeal cancer? A meta-analysis. Surg Endosc. 2010;24:1621–9.
12. Xiong WL, Li R, Lei HK, Jiang ZY. Comparison of outcomes between minimally invasive oesophagectomy and open oesophagectomy for oesophageal cancer. ANZ J Surg. 2017;87:165–70.
13. Kauppila JH, Xie S, Johar A, Markar SR, Lagergren P. Meta-analysis of health-related quality of life after minimally invasive versus open oesophagectomy for oesophageal cancer. Br J Surg. 2017;104:1131–40.
14. Yerokun BA, Sun Z, Yang CF, Gulack BC, Speicher PJ, Adam MA, et al. Minimally invasive versus open esophagectomy for esophageal cancer: a population-based analysis. Ann Thorac Surg. 2016;102:416–23.
15. Seesing MFJ, Gisbertz SS, Goense L, Van Hillegersberg R, Hidde K, Lagarde SM, et al. A propensity score matched analysis of open versus minimally invasive thoracic esophagectomy in the Netherlands. Ann Surg. 2017;266:839–46.
16. Harriott CB, Angeramo CA, Casas MA, Schlottmann F. Open versus hybrid versus totally minimally invasive Ivor Lewis esophagectomy: systematic review and meta-analysis. J Thorac Cardiovasc Surg. 2022;164:e233–54.
17. Maas KW, Cuesta MA, van Berge Henegouwen MI, Roig J, Bonavina L, Rosman C, et al. Quality of life and late complications after minimally invasive compared to open esophagectomy: results of a randomized trial. World J Surg. 2015;39:1986–93.
18. Nobel T, Tan KS, Barbetta A, Adusumilli P, Bains M, Bott M, et al. Does pyloric drainage have a role in the era of minimally invasive esophagectomy? Surg Endosc. 2019;33(10):3218–27.
19. Murad H, Huang B, Ndegwa N, Rouvelas I, Klevebro F. Postoperative hiatal herniation after open versus mimimally invasive esophagectomy; a systematic review and meta-analysis. Int J Surg. 2021;93:106046.
20. Turner SR, Molena D. The role of intraoperative fluorescence imaging during esophagectomy. Thorac Surg Clin. In Press.

Robotic Assisted Ivor Lewis Esophagectomy

Kunal J. Patel and Christopher D. Scott

Abstract

Robotic thoracic surgery has been increasingly adopted across the field. Many surgeons have found the articulating instrumentation, better visualization, and improved ergonomics immensely beneficial in either transitioning their practices from open to minimally invasive or enabling increased complexity in their minimally invasive practice. Robotic assisted minimally invasive esophagectomy (RAMIE) remains in the early stages of adoption. Similar to the early era of minimally invasive esophagectomy (MIE), outcomes are plagued by the growing pains of a steep learning curve. Understandably, many in the field find it difficult to justify these worse outcomes in the name of learning a new technology. However, as a new generation of surgeons is trained on the robotics platform and the outcomes become equivocal, the benefits of RAMIE, to both the patient and the surgeon, will come into sharper focus. Herein, we review the technique of a completely robotic assisted Ivor Lewis esophagectomy. We discuss the operative technique for both the abdominal and thoracic portions, including demonstration of port placement as well as 'troubleshooting' scenarios intraoperatively.

Keywords

Robotic · Ivor Lewis · Esophagectomy · Esophageal cancer · Minimally invasive esophagectomy · RAMIE · MIE

Introduction

Robotic thoracic surgery has been increasingly adopted across the field. Many surgeons have found the articulating instrumentation, better visualization, and improved ergonomics immensely beneficial in either transitioning their practices from open to minimally invasive or enabling increased complexity while remaining minimally invasive [1]. Robotic assisted minimally invasive esophagectomy) (RAMIE) remains in the early stages of adoption. Similar to the early era of minimally invasive esophagectomy (MIE), outcomes are plagued by the growing pains of a steep learning curve [2]. Understandably, many in the field find it difficult to justify these worse outcomes in the name of learning a new technology. However, as a new generation of surgeons is trained on the robotics platform and the outcomes become equivocal, the benefits of RAMIE, to both the

K. J. Patel · C. D. Scott (✉)
Division of Cardiothoracic Surgery, University of Virginia, Charlottesville, VA, USA
e-mail: cds2h@virginia.edu

patient and the surgeon, will come into sharper focus.

Operative Technique

In many regards, RAMIE is conducted very similarly to the minimal invasive esophagectomy as described elsewhere in this volume. However, there are a few key differences that the robotics platform necessitates, and we will highlight these as we move through the procedure. Our operative technique is evolved and adapted to the DaVinci Xi® system (Intuitive, Sunnyvale, CA), although much of what we discuss can be extrapolated to older systems such as the Si®, but these differences will not be discussed herein.

The patient is positioned supine on the operating table with arms tucked and a footboard for support, as we tend to utilize steep reverse Trendelenberg positioning during the abdominal portion of the procedure. We do not typically utilize the integrated Table Motion Trumpf bed for the DaVinci system, as we have not found it necessary. The standard approach with a left-sided dual lumen endotracheal tube, large bore IV access, radial arterial line, and urinary catheter is undertaken. We routinely perform a pre-operative upper endoscopy to assess for any unexpected findings in the esophagus or stomach. The pylorus is visualized but it is not our standard practice to perform any endoscopic dilations (or indeed any pyloric drainage procedure).

Abdominal Port Placement and Gastric Mobilization

The abdomen is widely prepped and draped from the nipple line to the pubis, and laterally to the furthest extent possible. Abdominal access can be obtained however the surgeon feels most comfortable; we utilize the Veress needle entry at Palmer's point. Our trocar setup includes three 8 mm robotic trocars, one 12 mm robotic trocar, an 8 mm AirSeal (Conmed, Utica, NY) trocar, and a 5 mm laparoscopic trocar for the liver retractor (Fig. 1).

Initial insufflation pressure is 15 mmHg of CO_2 with a flow of 40 L/min on Standard Insufflation Mode. In patient's without prior abdominal surgery, the initial 8 mm trocar (Arm 2—30° camera) is placed 'blindly' paramedian approximately 15 cm subxiphoid. This obviates the need for an additional laparoscopic camera set up. For patients with prior abdominal surgery, a 5 mm trocar is placed at Palmer's point after insufflation is achieved and a 5 mm 30° laparoscopic camera is introduced. Under direct visualization the remainder of the trocars are placed: laterally to the patient's left, an 8 mm trocar just above the level of the intrabdominal fat (Arm 4—tip up fenestrated grasper); splitting the difference between Arm 2 and Arm 4, an 8 mm trocar (Arm 3—vessel sealer); a 12 mm trocar in the right upper quadrant lateral to the falciform (Arm 1—cadiere forceps [with 8 mm reducer] and eventually the stapling port); in the right lower quadrant triangulated inferiorly between Arm 1 and Arm 2 is the AirSeal; and finally in the RUQ laterally just below the liver is the trocar for the liver retractor.

Once the AirSeal port is attached and ready, we convert the insufflation to AirSeal Mode (Smoke Evacuation Mode is not beneficial here). The laparoscopic snake liver retractor is inserted through the 5 mm trocar and secured to

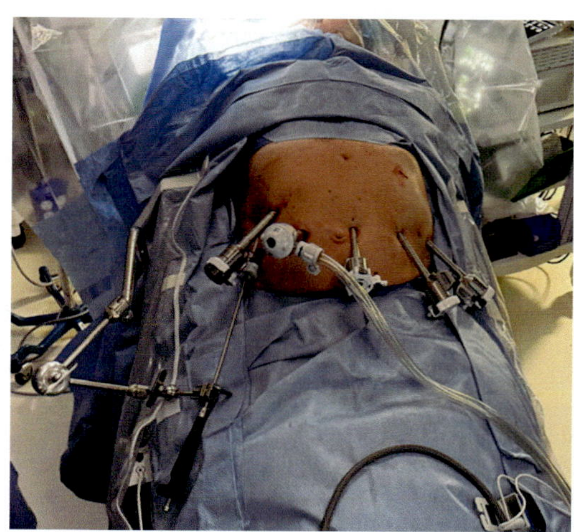

Fig. 1 Abdominal trocar placement

the bed with the retractor post. With the robot, this retractor has proven to be lower profile, and facilitates robot docking and arm clearance. One should still attempt to swing the post arm down and away from the patient as much as possible when securing the retractor though to maximize robot motion.

Once the robot is docked using the "Upper Abdomen" setting and the instruments (as listed above) are installed, we begin our gastric mobilization with the hiatal dissection. For this portion of the procedure, the bedside assistant generally is not required for any significant intra-abdominal manipulation and is limited mostly to instrument exchanges when the time for stapling arrives. We begin by opening the *pars flaccida* and identifying the right crus. The esophagus is then circumferentially mobilized from the hiatus with the dissection carried cranially towards the inferior pulmonary veins. Anyone that has ever performed benign foregut procedures with the robotic platform will know how facile it becomes to extend this dissection rather far into the mediastinum. In our experience, there is very little downside to this, especially if the anatomy is favorable, and will only expedite the thoracic portion of the case. During this dissection, the tip up grasper is used to provide counter traction, largely without needing to grab the specimen. It is quite common to violate the pleura during this dissection, particularly in the setting off post-induction therapy effects. If possible, we prefer to remain extra-pleural during this dissection to avoid any respiratory or hemodynamic issues that may result from the capnothorax, especially with the AirSeal.

After a thorough crural dissection, we turn our attention to the mobilization of the greater curve of the stomach. The gastrocolic ligament is elevated and the right gastroepiploic artery is identified. As a key step for the entirety of this procedure, and given that manual palpation is not an option, it is essential to visualize the artery and take great care to preserve it for the length of its course along the greater curve, in addition to avoiding any accidental manipulation with a robotic instrument.

The greater omentum is then divided with the vessel sealer along the greater curve of the stomach. During this dissection, a vascularized pedicle of omentum is created to use as a buttress for the anastomosis later and buffer between the anastomosis and airway. At the level of the short gastric vessels, we move the dissection closer to the stomach, as the right gastroepiploic becomes dimunitive and finish the mobilization of the fundus by dividing the gastrosplenic ligament. The remained of the greater curve is then mobilized by carrying the dissection towards the pylorus and duodenum, performing a 'partial' Kocher maneuver. Any remaining retrogastric attachments are mobilized. With the pylorus freed in this fashion, we have found that a full Kocher maneuver is rarely necessary as the pylorus will reach the hiatus without any undue tension. Additionally, as stated previously, we do not perform any pyloric drainage procedure.

The final step of our gastric mobilization is the division of the left gastric vascular pedicle. The greater curve is elevated superiorly to expose the left gastric artery and vein through the lesser sac. Gentle dissection is performed to sweep lymphatic tissue distally towards the specimen and expose the vessels. The pedicle is then transected with a single fire of the SureForm™ 45 stapler, typically a gray load (Fig. 2). We use this same stapler for the entirety of the procedure, inserted through the lone 12 mm trocar.

Conduit Creation

The final step of the abdominal portion of the procedure involves assessing and creating the gastric conduit. At this juncture, we will first assess the mobility of the pylorus for its ability to reach to the hiatus. Assuming this is the case, we can feel confident that the proximal extent of our conduit would reach the distal esophagus in the chest without tension. If it is felt that the pylorus is still tethered, additional mobilization can be undertaken at this time.

Our next step is to assess the perfusion of the gastric area likely to be included in our conduit.

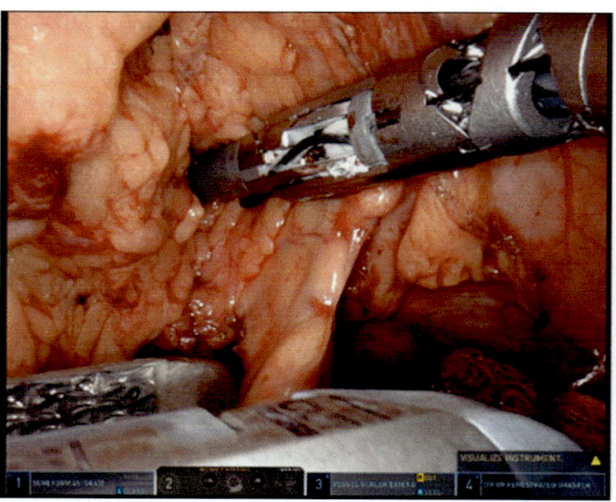
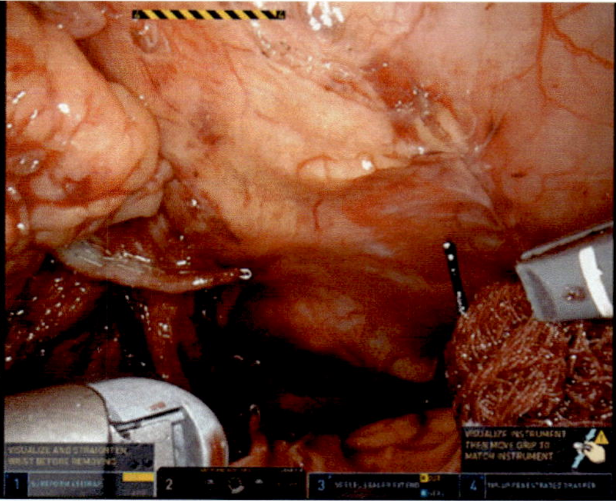

Fig. 2 Transection of the left gastric vascular pedicle is performed by first elevating the greater curve of the stomach to expose the vessels. Once the vein and artery are identified and sufficiently dissected free of extraneous tissue, a single fire of the SureForm™ 45 Gy load is used to divide the base

The Firefly™ technology incorporated into the robotic platform provides an efficient and effective visual assessment of the gastric perfusion (Fig. 3). We have our anesthesia colleagues administer 10 mg (4 mL) of indocyanine green (ICG) dye while the Firefly™ is activated on the surgeon console, and we can assess global perfusion of the stomach with the left gastric pedicle divided.

We then begin dividing the conduit with the SureForm™ 45 stapler. A starting point on the lesser curve proximal to the "crow's foot" is cleared with the vessel sealer. Any probes or suction catheters are removed to avoid mistakenly stapling them. A series of stapler fires are then used to create the conduit that is approximately 4 cm in width from the greater curve of the stomach. Our initial stapler load is a blue thickness, and with the dynamic compression of the robot, we have found this to be more than sufficient. However, one may need to upsize to a green load for certain patients if the stapler is unable to compress appropriately.

A useful retraction technique is to place the tip up grasper in Arm 4, grasp the fundus and retract cranially. Since this portion of the fundus will be incorporated in the specimen, it can be handled safely in this way. A penrose drain can be placed at the pylorus and the assistant can retract caudally, thus lengthening the stomach.

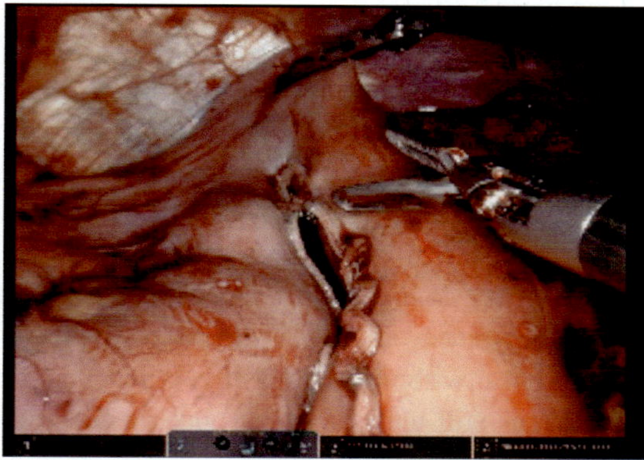
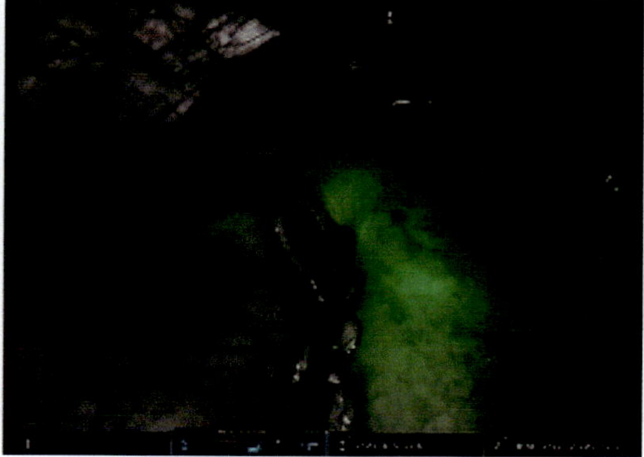

Fig. 3 The conduit is transected with a series of stapler fires from the lesser curve to the fundus. Indocyanine green and Firefly™ technology is utilized to assess conduit perfusion, particularly at the proximal extents of the conduit

This helps to minimize 'bunching' and spiraling of the conduit. We also liberally use the Firefly™ to help guide our conduit creation, particularly as we reach the proximal extent of the stomach (Fig. 3). The conduit is completely transected at the fundus. We then suture the proximal conduit to the gastric specimen using a figure-of-eight suture with a 3-0 silk. The omental flap is also incorporated into this stitch and the knot is tied loosely but securely, as we rely on this to help bring the conduit and omental flap into the chest when the specimen is mobilized.

Jejunostomy Tube Insertion

It is not our standard practice to place a jejunostomy tube in every esophagectomy patient, however there are certain patients that will clearly require and benefit from the enteral access. In these select patients, we will utilize the robot to place the feeding tube at this juncture in the case. For robotic jejunostomy tube insertion, it is often easier to port hop the camera to Arm 3 and use Arm 2 and 4 for the cadiere and needle driver, respectively. The Ligament of Treitz can be identified and subsequently the jejunum. Once the appropriate area of jejunum is selected, a barbed suture (V-lock or Stratafix) can be used to tack the lateral aspect of the jejunum to the abdominal wall. A pursestring suture can be created in the jejunum and the J tube can be inserted via seldinger technique. With the tube in place, the pursestring can be tied down. The prior barbed suture can then be continued circumferentially, creating a broad-based Stamm and fully enclosing the J tube site.

Thoracic Positioning and Port Placement

The patient is then repositioned into left lateral decubitus with the bed flexed per usual operative thoracic positioning. The anesthesia team will selectively ventilate the left lung via the dual lumen endotracheal tube. The thoracic trocar placement begins with the insertion of the 8 mm camera trocar which occurs at the 5th intercostal space along the posterior axillary line, just anterior to the latissimus dorsi. We use the blunt obturator as this insertion is performed blindly. The 30° camera is then inserted to confirm injury-free intrathoracic placement and insufflation is started at 8 mmHg CO_2 with a flow of 40 L/min on Standard Insufflation Mode. Under direct visualization, and utilizing the sharp obturators now, we place the other three robot trocars and the AirSeal trocar (Fig. 4).

The trocar placement must consider both interior and exterior landmarks for optimal functionality with minimal opportunity for instrument collisions or range of motion limitation. Exteriorly, the robot trocars will ideally be placed an approximate handbreadth apart from each other. Arm 1 (tip up fenestrated grasper) will be an 8 mm trocar that is placed posteriorly and inferiorly on the patient. Moving two handbreadths away from the camera trocar will position this trocar in the 9th or 10th intercostal space and just above the diaphragm. Arm 2 (cadiere forceps [with 8 mm reducer] and eventually the stapling port) is a 12 mm trocar placed one handbreadth inferior from the camera port and one handbreadth anterior from arm 1. This will generally be at the 7th intercostal space. The AirSeal in then triangulated between arm 2 and arm 3 as far anterior as possible without injuring the diaphragm. Lastly, arm 4 (vessel sealer, needle driver) is an 8 mm trocar that is placed at approximately the 3rd intercostal space. This is usually difficult to obtain a full handbreadth away from arm 3, but largely does not present a problem with collisions. As this port is placed high in the axilla, it is necessary to consider external landmarks here as well, specifically remaining anterior to the latissimus dorsi, and leaving enough space away from the arm for the robot to appropriately angle towards the inferior chest. Interiorly, this port placement roughly coincides with the superior aspect of the major fissure of the right lung.

The AirSeal is activated appropriately, and the robot is docked on the 'Thoracic Right' preset and the axis is slightly adjusted manually or

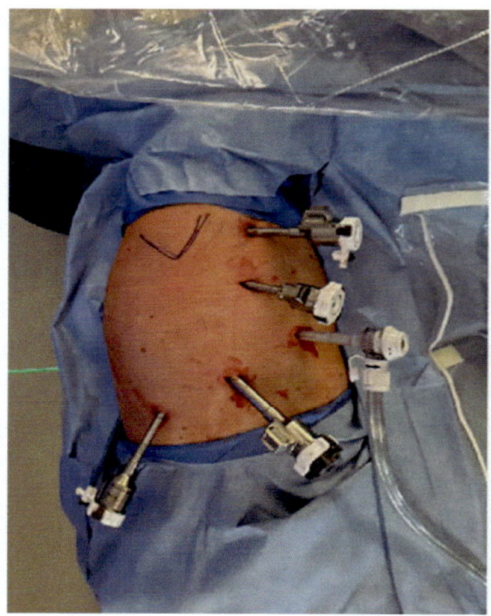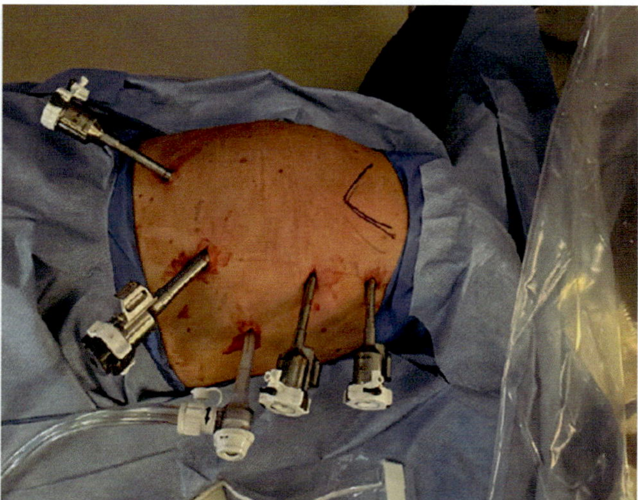

Fig. 4 Right thoracic trocar placement

if using the targeting function, approximately the level of the azygos vein is selected for target anatomy. The instruments are inserted as above and we continue the surgery with the intrathoracic esophageal dissection.

Esophageal Mobilization and Esophagogastrostomy

We begin by opening the inferior pulmonary ligament with the vessel sealer and extending the pleural incision over the esophagus to the azygous vein. This is best accomplished by using the tip up grasper (and occasionally the assistant as well) to retract the lung anteriorly to expose the posterior hilum. The azygous vein is mobilized from the underlying esophagus with the intent to pass a stapler across the vein. We then transect the azygous vein with a gray load of the Sureform™ 45 stapler.

The esophagus is then dissected from the posterior mediastinum taking care to avoid the thoracic duct and with meticulous hemostasis of the bronchial arteries supplying the mid-distal esophagus. The vessel sealer is excellent for this purpose. The final hiatal dissection is saved for last, as dissection here too early can inadvertently deliver the conduit into the chest

prematurely. A penrose drain placed around the esophagus aids in retraction and can be especially helpful when dissecting the esophagus from the airway. We also utilize this opportunity to perform regional lymph node sampling. As a technical point, we prefer the vessel sealer for the majority of the dissection because it lends to better hemostasis and (in our opinion) better lymphostasis. A key component of the intrathoracic dissection is mobilization of the esophagus from the airway. For this portion, energy dissection is used sparingly and with utmost attention. Bipolar energy dissection is used for this portion of the dissection, as it has less thermal spread than monopolar or vessel sealer energy.

Once the thoracic esophagus is mobilized several centimeters above the level of the azygous vein, the esophago-gastric specimen and gastric conduit are delivered into the chest, with particular attention given to maintaining appropriate orientation—this can be monitored by monitoring the position of the staple on the condit, which should be directly facing the surgeon. The tacking sutures are cut, and the length of the gastric conduit is assessed to assure appropriate length to the anastomotic site. At this point, 10 mg (4 mL) of indocyanine green (ICG) is administered and Firefly is used to assess the perfusion of the conduit. Commonly, the proximal conduit will be trimmed back with the stapler depending on the length. Excess length on the conduit is not desirable as it can lead to redundancy and delayed emptying.

The anastomosis is constructed with a 'modified Orringer' technique—linear stapled side-to-side esophagogastrostomy with hand-sewn closure of the common enterotomy. The proximal esophagus is grasped with a tip up grasper in Arm 1 and retracted anteriorly. The conduit can then be positioned posterior to the proximal esophagus. It is important that the esophagus is dissected at least 3 cm proximal to the intended site of the anastomosis to allow the conduit to be positioned adequately. The authors routinely perform the anastomosis at the level of the azygos vein, even with more distal tumors, to ensure proper margins and conduit length/drainage issues as discussed previously. A more proximal anastomosis is also possible, depending on the location of the tumor. Approximating sutures are placed from the lateral aspects of the esophagus to the gastric conduit (Fig. 5), after which the esophagus is transected sharply with monopolar scissors. The specimen can then be located out of the field or retrieved via a specimen bag through the assistant port if margin evaluation is warranted.

Prior to making the anastomosis, we place two more 2-0 Vicryl sutures full thickness through the posterior esophagus to the anterior conduit. These sutures facilitate the stapler positioning by keeping the esophageal lumen open. We then use the monopolar scissors to open the anterior conduit (Fig. 6). A generous opening is necessary to facilitate the stapler. The gastrotomy does not need to be a large distance away from the proximal conduit as the stapled anastomosis only utilizes approximately 30 mm of the stapler length. A blue load stapler is used to create the posterior anastomosis (Fig. 7). It is paramount to plan the site of the gastrotomy far enough from the conduit staple line to preserve blood flow to the anastomosis.

The completion of the anastomosis is performed with two six inch 3-0 absorbable Stratafix™ (Ethicon, USA) sutures in a single layer running fashion. We run these barbed sutures from each corner of the anastomosis towards the center, with some overlap, prior to tying the sutures to each other (Fig. 8). Before tying these sutures, we will have the anesthesia team pass a nasogastric tube past the anastomosis into the conduit. We do not standardly buttress the anastomosis, but if deemed necessary, additional sutures can be placed. The final step of the anastomosis is to wrap the omental flap around the staple line and anastomosis, preferentially creating a buffer between the airway and the conduit (Fig. 9). A single chest tube is

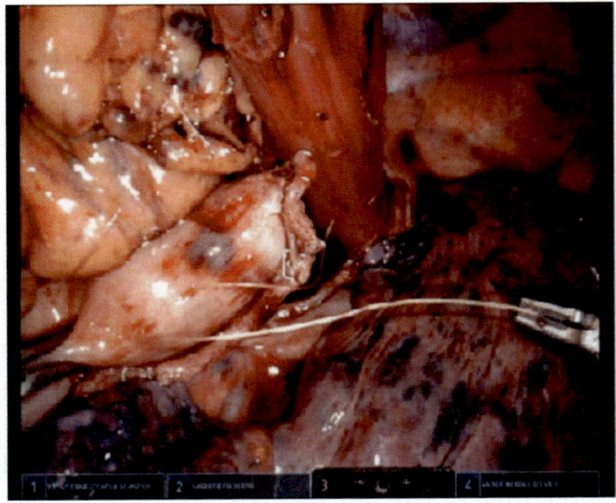 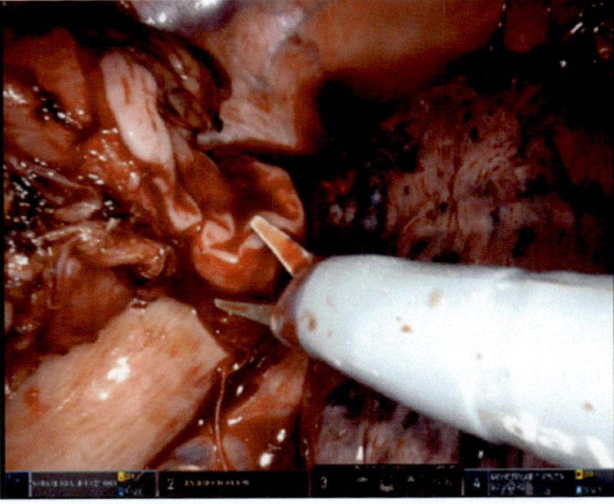

Fig. 5 Prior to transecting the proximal esophagus, two lateral tacking sutures are placed using a 2-0 Vicryl at the 3- and 9-o'clock positions (left). The esophagus is transected with the monopolar scissors 1–2 cm proximal to the tacking sutures to create an overlap between the conduit and esophagus (right)

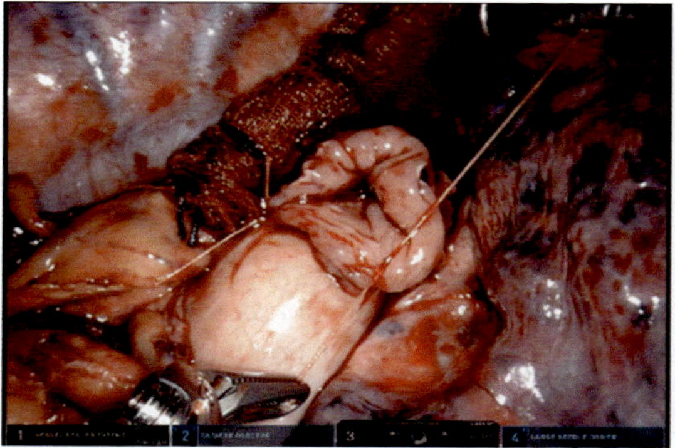

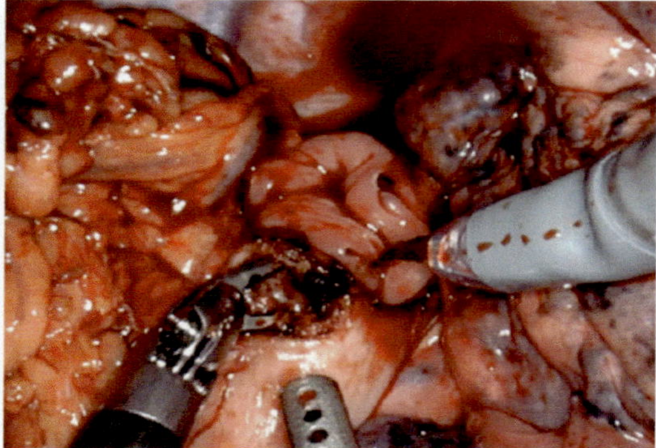

Fig. 6 The location of the gastrotomy is carefully chosen at a distance sufficiently far from the conduit staple line, but not so far as to create an excessively large "dog ear" behind the anastomosis. Two more traction sutures on placed between the esophagus and conduit (left) and the gastrotomy is created with the monopolar scissors to create a reasonable size match (right)

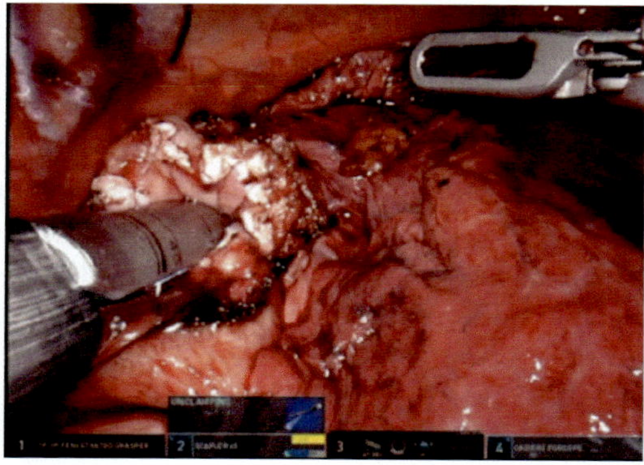

Fig. 7 A blue load of the linear stapler is utilized to create the posterior anastomosis. The larger arm of the stapler is placed within the conduit with the slimmer arm in the esophagus. Gentle tension on the esophagus is used to ensure there is no retraction of the tissue, and the stapler is only advanced to about 30 mm to create an appropriately sized esophago-gastrostomy

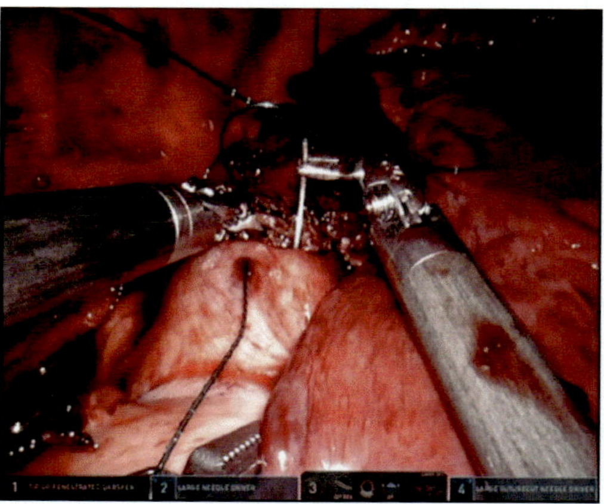

Fig. 8 Running 3-0 barbed sutures are used to close the anterior anastomosis in a single layer with full thickness bites. Occasionally, at surgeon discretion, the anastomosis can be reinforced with Lembert-type sutures

placed posteriorly, directed towards the apex of the chest in close proximity to the conduit without contacting it. The specimen is placed into a 15 mm extraction bag and removed through the AirSeal port (which needs to be enlarged) and sent for routine pathologic analysis. The lung is then inflated under direct visualization, the trocar sites are closed, and the procedure is thus concluded.

Postoperative Care

Our standard postoperative pathway sees our patients extubated in the operating room and transferred directly to the surgical ICU for overnight monitoring. They remain NPO with the nasogastric tube to low continuous wall suction until evaluation of the anastomosis on post-operative day #5. If a jejunostomy tube was placed at the time of surgery, we will begin trickle tube

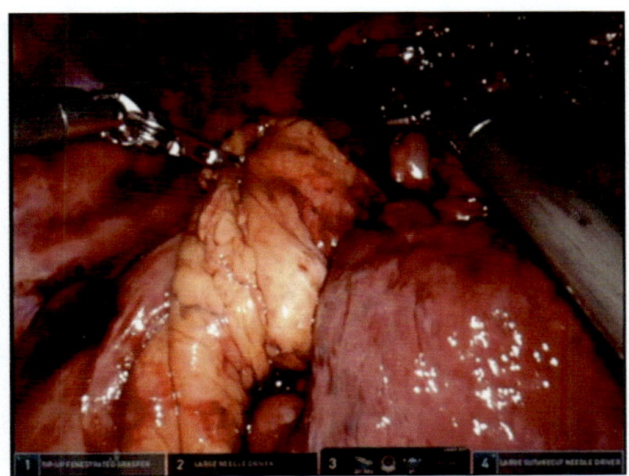

Fig. 9 An omental flap is a useful and relatively easy adjunct to reinforce the staple lines and anastomosis and create a buffer between the conduit and airway

feeds on post-operative day #2 and advance to goal as tolerated. On day #5, we routinely obtain a contrast esophagram, which in conjunction with clinical markers of progress (*e.g.* absence of fevers, white blood cell count, chest tube output, etc.) are used as a milestone for removing the nasogastric tube, and subsequently the chest tube. The esophagram also helps us evaluate gastric emptying, which occasionally prompts us to perform an endoscopic pyloric procedure if necessary.

Discharge home usually occurs on postoperative day #7 on our normal pathway with the patient on a soft diet. The nutrition team at our institution maintains close contact with our post-esophagectomy patients and will generally manage the cessation of tube feeds if patients are tolerating their diet and maintaining caloric intake. This enables us to remove the jejunostomy tube at the routine post-operative visit 3–4 weeks after discharge.

Intraoperative Troubleshooting

Port Placement

Typically, external collisions are uncommon during the abdominal portion of the procedure, given the working domain and extra space created with insufflation. While it is possible to place all four robotic trocars across the abdomen at the same level in a straight line, the authors find that moving Arm 1 superiorly a few centimeters is helpful in creating additional space for the assistant port. This allows the assistant port to move higher on the abdomen and increase their reach into the mediastinum, while avoiding Arm 1 and 2. When placing the Arm 1 trocar, the falciform is identified and the port is placed just below this level.

When placing the trocars for the thoracic portion, the spacing is optimized by placement of Arm 4 high enough in the chest. This decision need be made prior to placing the first trocar so that spacing can be optimized. This trocar is typically placed in the 3rd intercostal space. It is important to understand the relationship of this trocar and the right shoulder/arm. When positioning, it is helpful to adduct the right arm as much as possible. Prior to making the incision for this port, an empty trocar can be used to simulate the motion of the instrument to ensure there are no collisions with the right shoulder/arm.

Capnothorax

Commonly, we are operating on patients in the neoadjuvant setting. Given the location of the tumors abutting the pleural spaces and the resultant inflammatory effects of induction therapy, it is common and often necessary to enter/resect the pleura. Typically, the creation of a capnothorax can be adequately managed with routine anesthesia maneuvers. If difficulties with ventilation persist, the CO_2 pressure can be reduced. It also important to ensure that a tension physiology is not created, as a small rent in the pleura can lead to tension as the airseal maintains a steady pressurization that can trap air in the pleural space. If a difficult mediastinal dissection is anticipated, and/or the patient's pulmonary reserve is compromised, the authors prefer to save this step for later in the case so as to minimize physiologic decompensation.

Outcomes

Some of the beneficial endpoints of MIE versus open esophagectomy (reduced pain and blood loss, shorter length of stay, fewer respiratory complications, etc.) are already being replicated or surpassed by RAMIE [2–8]. We would anticipate that as experience and techniques evolve, essential endpoints such as leak rates and oncologic outcomes will similarly equilibrate, as this is the predictable evolution of any widely adopted technology. Indeed, a recent multicenter trial comparing RAMIE to MIE demonstrated equivalent (and acceptable) leak rates (12.2 vs. 11.3%), however other international studies have been far more varied, with complication rates close to 30% [6, 9]. Several factors were cited for the noticeably high leak rate at the varying centers, most prominently anastomotic technique with handsewn performing by far the worst. However, surgeon experience and practice environments (academic versus private) will also make a difference. In addition to this study, other single center experiences have demonstrated acceptably low leak rates with circular (4–10%) and linear (8%) stapling techniques, including the technique we describe here (8.1%) [7, 8, 10–12].

As a final comment, an underappreciated and under-investigated aspect of the robot is the ergonomic benefits afforded the operative surgeon [13]. While surgeon health and wellness has not been a main consideration, in the presence of equivocal patient outcomes with robotic technology, the surgeon's wellbeing may stand to benefit as well. The Ivor Lewis esophagectomy, in all its current iterations is a demanding procedure, mentally and physically. If the robotics platform can improve upon this, there lies a benefit that cannot be adequately quantified.

References

1. Mazzei M, Abbas AE. Why comprehensive adoption of robotic assisted thoracic surgery is ideal for both simple and complex lung resections. J Thorac Dis. 2020;12:70–81. https://doi.org/10.21037/jtd.2020.01.22.

2. Young A, Alvarez Gallesio JM, Sewell DB, Carr R, Molena D. Outcomes of robotic esophagectomy. J Thorac Dis. 2021;13:6163–8. https://doi.org/10.21037/jtd-2019-rts-07.

3. Yoshimura S, et al. Quality of life after robot-assisted transmediastinal radical surgery for esophageal cancer. Surg Endosc. 2018;32:2249–54. https://doi.org/10.1007/s00464-017-5918-x.

4. Sugawara K, et al. Long-term health-related quality of life following robot-assisted radical transmediastinal esophagectomy. Surg Endosc. 2020;34:1602–11. https://doi.org/10.1007/s00464-019-06923-7.

5. Cerfolio RJ, Bryant AS, Hawn MT. Technical aspects and early results of robotic esophagectomy with chest anastomosis. J Thorac Cardiovasc Surg. 2013;145:90–6. https://doi.org/10.1016/j.jtcvs.2012.04.022.

6. Yang Y, et al. Robot-assisted versus conventional minimally invasive esophagectomy for resectable esophageal squamous cell carcinoma: early results of a multicenter randomized controlled trial: the RAMIE trial. Ann Surg. 2022;275:646–53. https://doi.org/10.1097/sla.0000000000005023.

7. van der Sluis PC, et al. Robot-assisted minimally invasive esophagectomy with intrathoracic anastomosis (Ivor Lewis): promising results in 100 consecutive patients (the European experience). J Gastrointest Surg. 2021;25:1–8. https://doi.org/10.1007/s11605-019-04510-8.

8. Babic B, et al. Robot-assisted minimally invasive esophagectomy (RAMIE) versus hybrid minimally invasive esophagectomy: propensity score matched short-term outcome analysis of a European high-volume center. Surg Endosc. 2022;36:7747–55. https://doi.org/10.1007/s00464-022-09254-2.

9. Kingma BF, et al. Worldwide techniques and outcomes in robot-assisted minimally invasive esophagectomy (RAMIE): results from the multicenter international registry. Ann Surg. 2022;276:e386–92. https://doi.org/10.1097/sla.0000000000004550.

10. Capovilla G, et al. End to side circular stapled anastomosis during robotic-assisted Ivor Lewis minimally invasive esophagectomy (RAMIE). Dis Esophagus. 2022;35. https://doi.org/10.1093/dote/doab088.

11. Zhang H, et al. Robotic side-to-side and end-to-side stapled esophagogastric anastomosis of Ivor Lewis esophagectomy for cancer. World J Surg. 2019;43:3074–82. https://doi.org/10.1007/s00268-019-05133-5.

12. Wang F, et al. Intrathoracic side-to-side esophagogastrostomy with a linear stapler and barbed suture in robot-assisted Ivor Lewis esophagectomy. J Surg Oncol. 2019;120:1142–7. https://doi.org/10.1002/jso.25698.

13. Wee IJY, Kuo LJ, Ngu JC. A systematic review of the true benefit of robotic surgery: ergonomics. Int J Med Robot. 2020;16: e2113. https://doi.org/10.1002/rcs.2113.

Minimally Invasive McKeown Esophagectomy

Yehonatan Nevo and Lorenzo Ferri

Abstract

Minimally invasive McKeown esophagectomy (MIE) has several potential benefits over the open approach, including: reduced post-operative pain, lower rates of pulmonary complications, and faster recovery with shorter length of stay. MIE also results in less blood loss, reducing the need for blood transfusions. MIE is a demanding procedure but with the right training and proctoring can be safely adopted into practice without compromising the surgical or oncological quality.

Keywords

Esophagectomy · Minimally-invasive · Three-hole · Thoracoscopic · Laparoscopic · Lymphadenectomy

Y. Nevo (✉)
Upper Gastrointestinal Surgery Service, Department of Surgery, Sheba Medical Center, Ramat-Gan, Israel
e-mail: yehonatan.nevo@sheba.health.gov.il

L. Ferri
Division of Thoracic and Upper Gastrointestinal Surgery, McGill University Health Center, Montreal, QC, Canada
e-mail: lorenzo.ferri@mcgill.ca

Introduction

Minimally invasive McKeown esophagectomy (MIE) has several potential benefits over the open approach, including: reduced post-operative pain, lower rates of pulmonary complications, and faster recovery with shorter length of stay. MIE also results in less blood loss, reducing the need for blood transfusions. MIE is a demanding procedure but with the right training and proctoring can be safely adopted into practice without compromising the surgical or oncological quality [1–11].

Preoperative Considerations

- *Pain Management*: We routinely use thoracic epidural catheter, although paravertebral analgesia has recently emerged as a safe alternative while avoiding the thoracic epidural associated-side effects including hypotension. Intercostal (IC) nerve blocks using long-acting liposomal local anesthetics is another alternative to epidurals in minimally invasive thoracic surgery patients, though it's efficacy in MIE is yet to be proven.
- *Single-lung ventilation*: Excellent single-lung ventilation is vital to maintain good exposure during thoracoscopy. Although positive pressure capnothorax especially in the prone position, can obviate the need for

a double lumen tube, our preference is for single-lung ventilation. Because of the short right mainstem bronchus, we prefer a double-lumen tube rather than a right sided bronchial blocker for lung isolation.

- *EGD with endoscopic pyloromyotomy*: An on-table esophagogastroduodenoscopy (EGD) is routinely performed to verify the lesion and confirm its location prior to beginning the procedure. Particular attention is devoted to the extent of involvement in the lesser and greater curvatures, which may alter the conduit. Endoscopic pyloromyotomy is done using an ITknife2™ (model KD-611L, Olympus) with cutting the pyloric mucosa and muscularis propria in three different areas, ensuring that the lip of tissue between the duodenal bulb and pre-pyloric antrum is completely eliminated and the pyloric channel is completely open (Fig. 1). We have previously demonstrated the utility and effectiveness of this novel technique of pyloric drainage.

- *Enhanced Recovery Pathway*: Establishing and following an enhanced recovery pathway (ERP) provides standardized and evidence-based perioperative management for the esophagectomy patient. We have shown that ERPs are cost-effective, with decreased complications and shortened postoperative length of stay. Key elements of the pathway include extubation immediately after the operation, avoidance of routine ICU care, early removal, or complete avoidance of the nasogastric (NG) tube, early oral feeding, and diligent chest physiotherapy with frequent ambulation. Prehabilitaiton is an important element of ERP's. Preoperative conditioning intervention including exercise, nutrition, and physcological prehabilitation help prevent functional impairment before and after surgery, as well as improve quality of life. Patients receive teaching from a nurse-educator at the pre-operative clinic, and are provided with a comprehensive information booklet that reviews all procedures in an easy-to-understand language with illustrations.

Operative Technique

Thoracoscopy

After completion of intraoperative EGD including endoscopic pyloromyotomy, the patient is positioned in the hybrid left lateral-prone position (Fig. 2). Patients are placed in the left semi-prone position, and the operating table is then rotated to create the left lateral decubitus position. The left leg (lower leg) is flexed gently at the knee and the upper leg remains in extension, with adequate padding between the legs. The arms are well padded and supported on arm boards. A vacuumed beanbag is used to secure the patient, in addition to the use of tape or Velcro.

We employ a four-port thoracoscopy using 12 mm trocars (Fig. 3). Our trocar placements are the following:

1. Third intercostal space, anterior axillary line
2. Fifth intercostal space, posterior axillary line

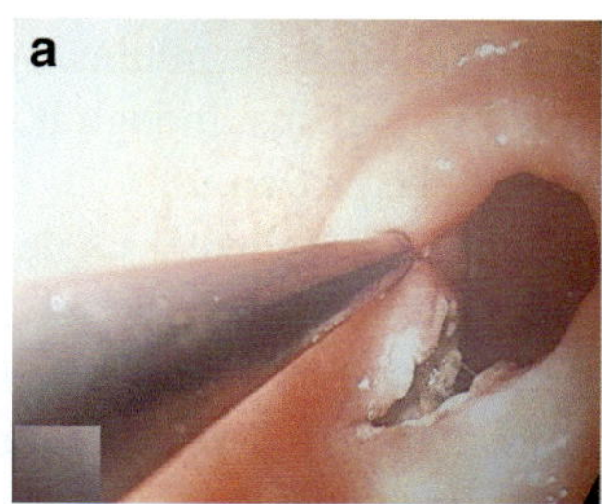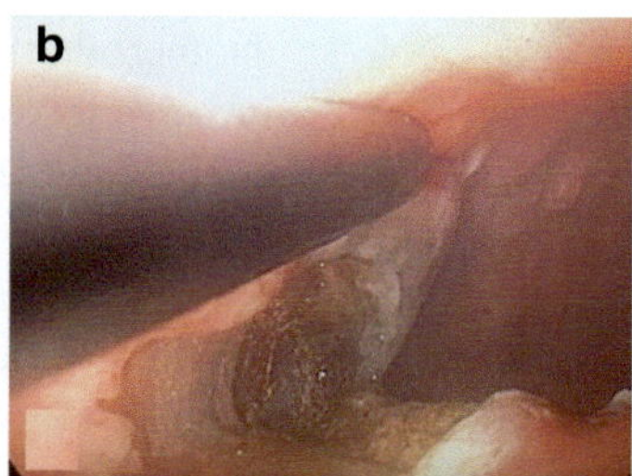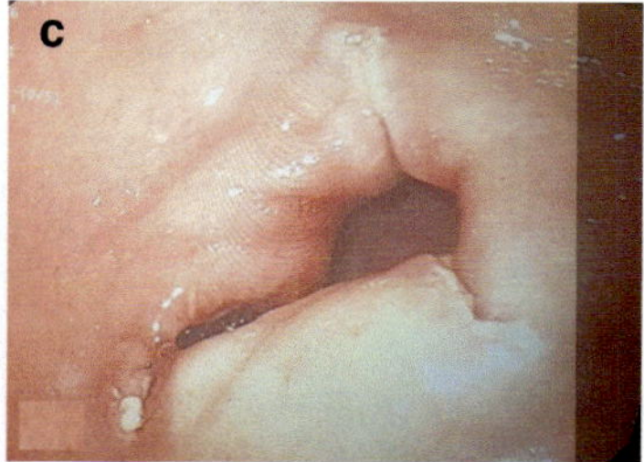

Fig. 1 **a** The endoscopic Myotomy is performed by using ITknife **b** The muscularis propria is adequately cut and the pyloric channel is completely open **c** Pyloromyotomy in three different areas

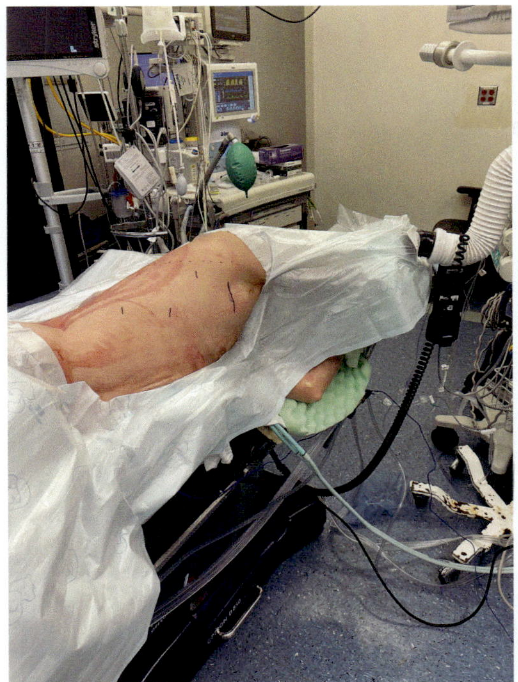

Fig. 2 Hybrid left lateral-prone positioning for thoracoscopy

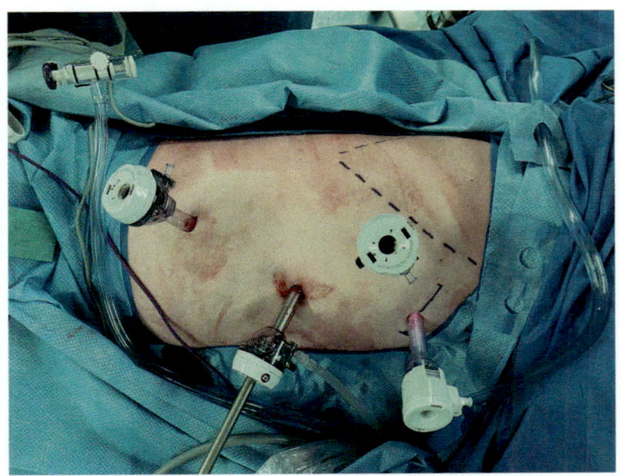

Fig. 3 Thoracoscopy trocar placement

3. Seventh intercostal spaces mid axillary line
4. Ninth intercostal spaces posterior axillary line.

The first port is inserted using an optical trocar and artificial pneumothorax is achieved using carbon dioxide at a pressure of 8–10 mmHg to collapse the right lung and expand the mediastinum. The subcarinal dissection is performed by initially rotating the table to almost prone position. The azygous vein is circumferentially dissected and divided with a linear stapler device and the pleura is divided anteriorly and posteriorly along the length of the esophagus with hook cautery. The mobilization of the thoracic esophagus is performed from the thoracic inlet to the diaphragm, and subcarinal mediastinal lymph node dissection is completed (Fig. 4). Further dissection is completed with a harmonic scalpel, and a Penrose drain is used to encircle the esophagus to provide countertraction. The thoracic duct is clipped behind the lower esophagus and resected together with the esophagus.

Dissection with energy devices near the trachea is performed with great care, as inadvertent injury may result in airway fistulization. The supracarinal dissection is performed by placing the patient in the left lateral decubitus position. The pleura is incised along the posterior edge of the esophagus up to the right subclavian vein. The dorsal and left sides of the upper esophagus are dissected along with the thoracic duct. Dissection along the left and right recurrent laryngeal nerve (RLN) is then performed. The anterior part of the upper esophagus is dissected from the trachea, and the upper esophagus is circumferentially dissected along with the surrounding nodes. The thoracic duct is clipped at the level of the arch of the aorta.

Once the esophagus is fully mobilized from the thoracic inlet to the diaphragm, with all nodal tissue swept into the specimen, it is divided at a level proximal to the tumor, usually cephalad to the azygous vein, consequently also dividing the vagus below the bifurcation of the recurrent laryngeal nerves with electrocautry. The proximal and distal margins are secured to a common umbilical tape to facilitate retrieval via the neck and laparoscopy. The chest is copiously irrigated and a large-capacity 19-French closed suction Jackson-Pratt (JP) drain is inserted in lieu of a chest tube (Fig. 5) The trocar sites are closed in layers, and the double-lumen endotracheal tube is exchanged for a single-lumen tube to enhance mobility of the airway during the cervical portion of the operation.

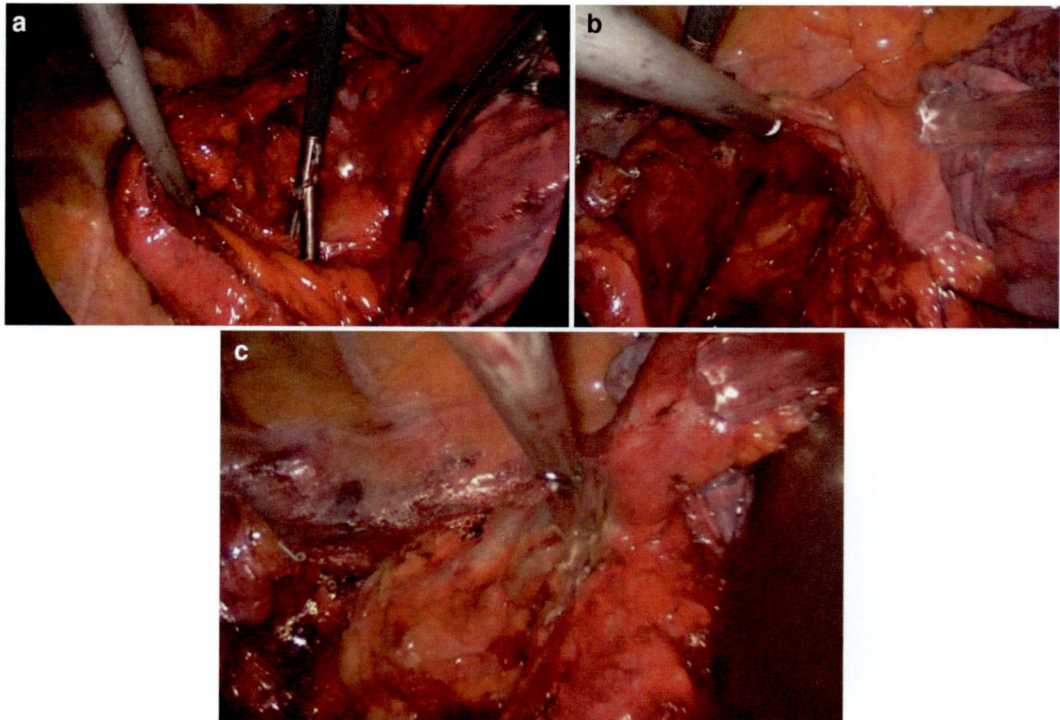

Fig. 4   **a** Esophageal mobilization **b**, **c** Subcarinal dissection

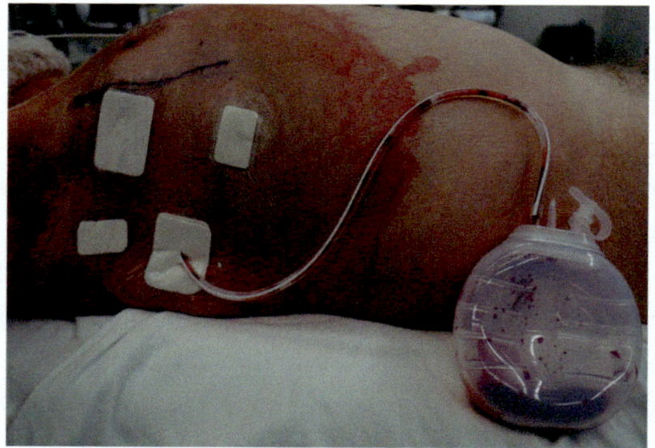

Fig. 5   Use of large-capacity Jackson-Pratt drains in lieu of chest tubes

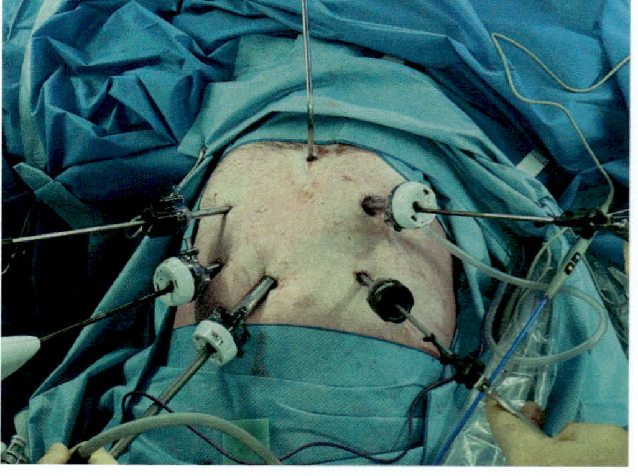

Fig. 6   Laparoscopy trocar placement

Laparoscopy

The patient is repositioned in the supine, split-leg position for laparoscopy. The neck is extended, with a roll placed between the scapula. A five-port laparoscopy is employed (Fig. 6). A 12-mm optiview port is placed in the left upper quadrant mid-clavicular line, a 12-mm port is placed supraumbilically for the camera, a 5-mm port on the left, mid-point between the umbilical and left upper quadrant ports, for operating instruments, a 5-mm incision in the epigastrium for the Nathanson liver retractor, and a 5-mm operating port in the right upper quadrant at the midclavicular line and a 12-mm port on the right, mid-point between the umbilical and the right upper quadrant ports for operating instruments. A 10-mm, 30° camera is employed.

The gastrohepatic omentum is opened and the right and left crura are circumferentially dissected without complete division of the phrenoesophageal membrane, in order to preserve pneumoperitoneum.

We perform a complete D2 celiac lymph node dissection by skeletonizing the splenic artery, the hepatic artery, and the splenic vein (Fig. 7). The left gastric pedicle is dissected, skeletonized, clipped, and divided. We do not staple the left gastric pedicle, as it may provide an inadequate lymph node dissection. All lymph node–bearing tissue is included with the specimen (Fig. 8). We proceed along the entire celiac axis down to the aorta to include the periceliac lymph nodes en bloc with the specimen.

The greater curve is dissected after creation of a window in the gastrocolic omentum, and the lesser sac is entered. Dissection proceeds 5 cm from the greater curvature, with extreme caution taken to preserve the gastroepiploic arcade, the dependent blood supply to the future conduit

(Fig. 9). The retrogastric attachments are freed and dissection is carried up to the left esophageal hiatus. A Kocher maneuver is completed, with adequate mobilization of the pylorus ensured by testing its extension to the caudate lobe or right crus. After ensuring satisfactory hemostasis, the esophageal hiatus is completely mobilized and the phrenoesophageal membrane is divided.

An accessory incision 5 cm in length is constructed in the upper midline, with insertion of a wound protector (Fig. 10). A 4-cm gastric conduit is fashioned with sequential firings of the GIA™ stapler (generally three firings) and oversewing of the staple line (Fig. 11). Extracorporeal construction is a useful adjunct in the creation of an excellent conduit and greatly facilitates assessment and revision of the distal margin, should this be necessary.

Cervical Phase

A 4- to 5-cm cervical collar incision is made, the platysma is incised, and subplatysmal planes are generated. The omohyoid muscle and middle thyroid vein are divided for optimal exposure.

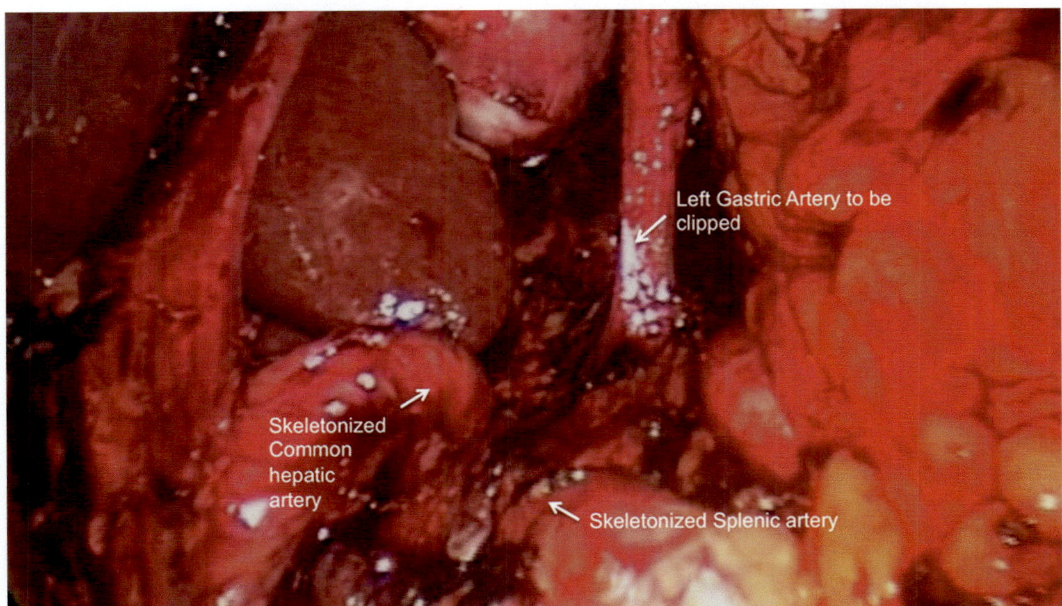

Fig. 7 D2 dissection and dissection of the left gastric pedicle to be divided

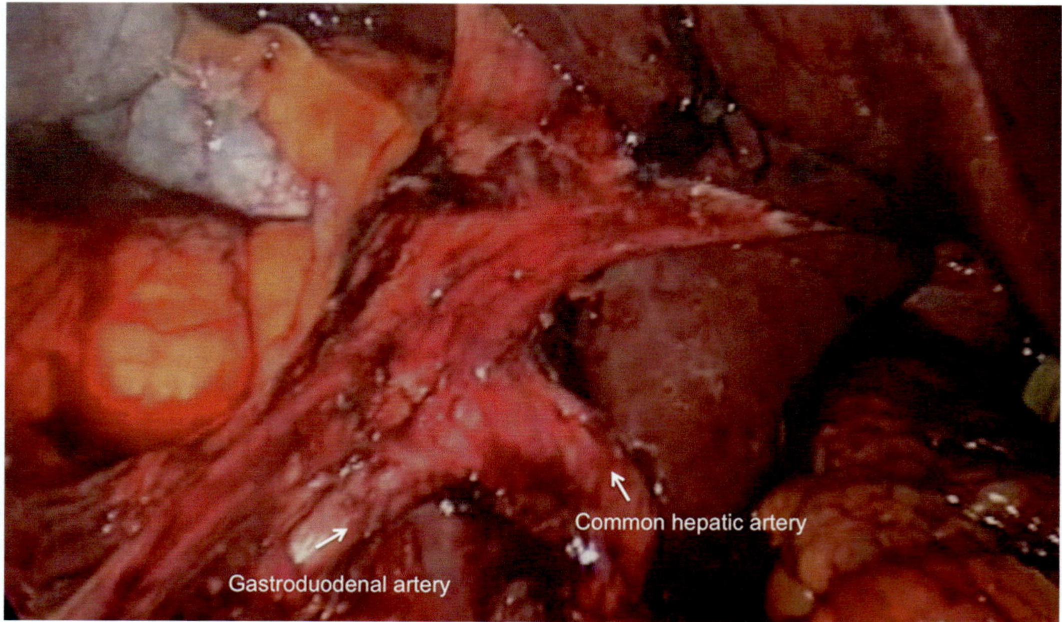

Fig. 8 Completed D2 dissection demonstrating skeletonized hepatic and gastroduodenal arteries

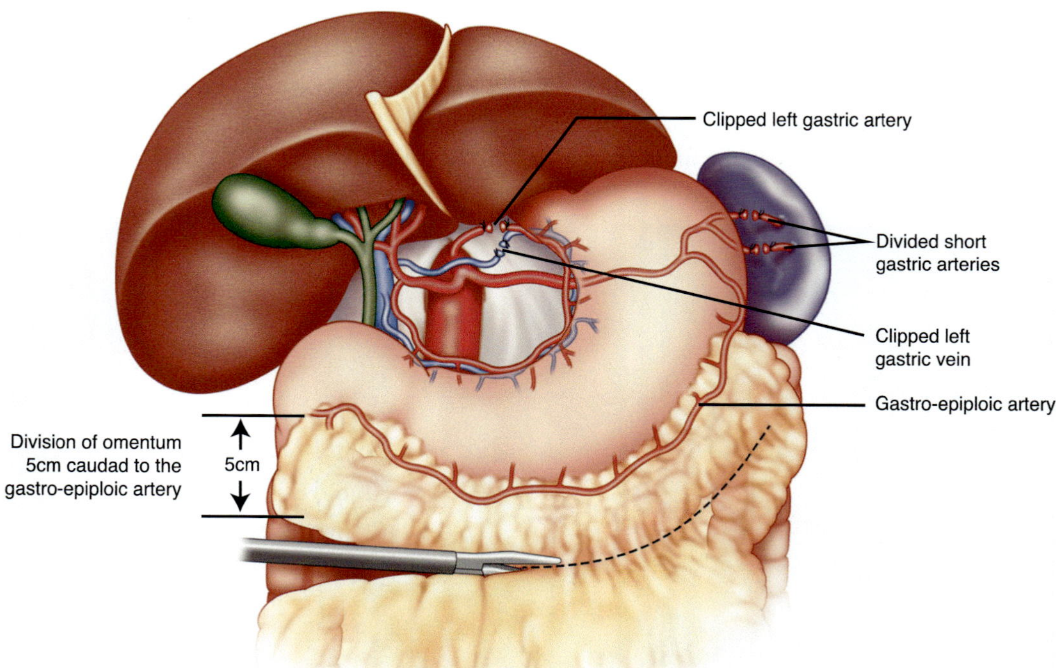

Fig. 9 Dissection along the greater curve of the stomach

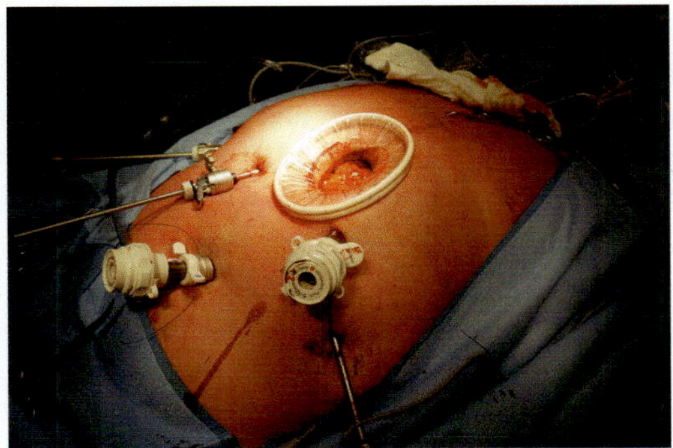

Fig. 10 Accessory incision

Blunt dissection and lateral mobilization are completed in order to deliver the esophagus into the wound. Identification of the left recurrent laryngeal nerve is paramount to its preservation, and lymph nodes along this structure are resected (Fig. 12). The proximal margin is revised in the neck, and stay sutures of 4-0 silk are placed at four corners to facilitate the eventual anastomosis (Fig. 13).

The conduit is introduced into an endoscopic camera bag in preparation for guidance to the neck (Fig. 14). The proximal end is secured with a Foley catheter, which is also attached to the umbilical tape at the cervical esophagus. The surgeon then gently guides the conduit in the posterior mediastinal orthotopic position, using the accessory incision and delivering the conduit into the neck while always maintaining orientation to prevent conduit torsion.

The cervical anastomosis can be completed with a stapling device (side to side or end to side) or, as we prefer, through a hand-sewn anastomosis (Fig. 15). Our preference is to use single-layer running suture with incorporation of the muscular layer and small bites of mucosa. A JP drain is inserted in the neck near the anastomosis. Fascia for the abdominal incisions is closed with 1 polydioxanone suture (PDS). The platysma at the collar incision is approximated with 2-0 Vicryl sutures. Skin closure is completed with 4-0 Monocryl sutures.

We do not routinely employ a jejunostomy under most circumstances because the associated complication rate surpasses our rate of anastomotic leak.

Perioperative Care

In the postoperative part of our ERP the following daily objectives are included: removal of the NG tube (we recently omitted the use of routine NG tube placement entirely) and foley catheter on day 1. Sips of water are allowed on day

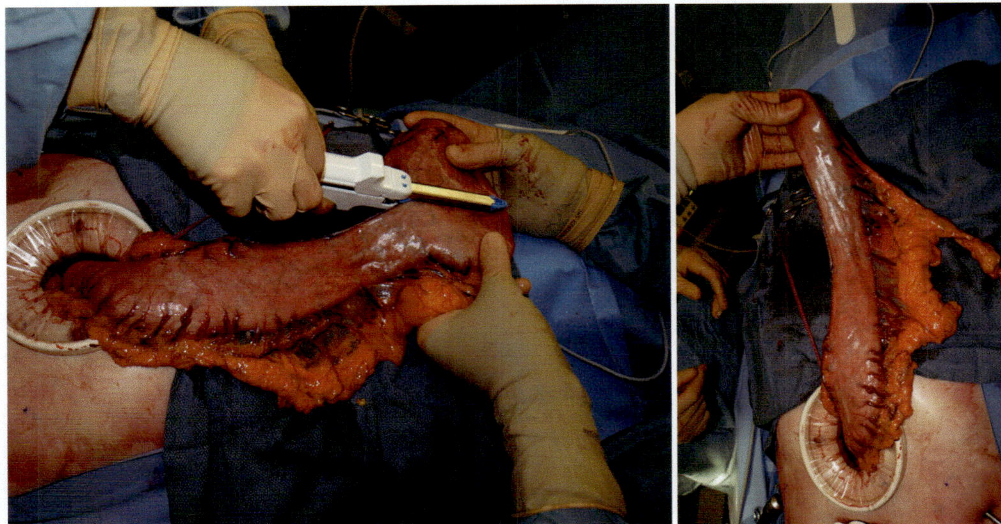

Fig. 11 Construction of gastric conduit

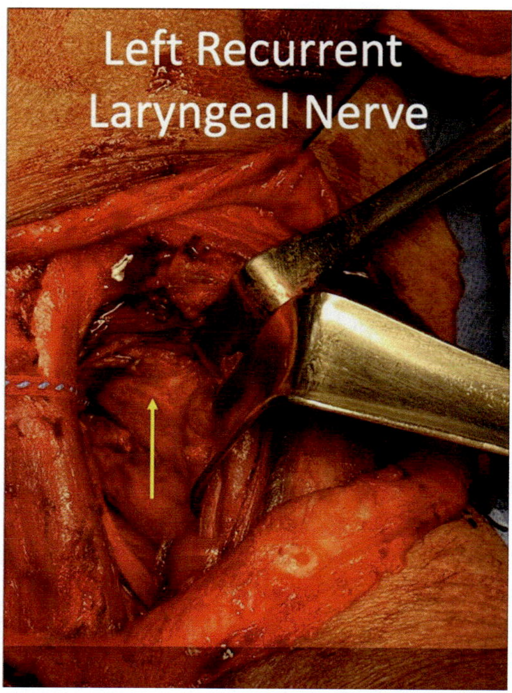

Fig. 12 Dissection of cervical esophagus with visualization and preservation of recurrent laryngeal nerves

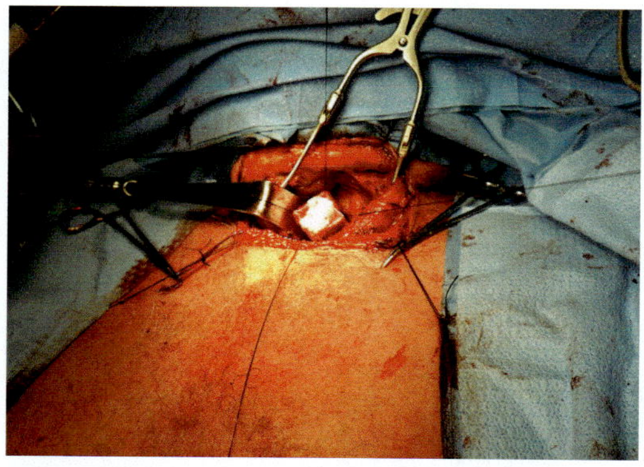

Fig. 13 Prepared cervical esophagus with stay sutures

2 with gradual progression to a liquid diet. We do not perform a routine barium esophagogram based on review of our experience showing minimal impact on the clinical course, and remove the 19-French JP drain on day 5. The epidural catheter is also removed on day 5.

The planned discharge date is day 6, although patients can leave earlier if appropriate. Each patient is assessed daily and is deemed fit for discharge if he meets the following criteria: sufficient liquid oral intake, adequate oral analgesia using both opioid and non-opioid analgesics, vital signs within normal limits and inflammatory parameters not trending up. A dedicated nurse-coordinator follows the patients routinely after surgery and contacts them after discharge; patients can also contact the nurse directly if ad-hoc issues arise at home.

Technical Pitfalls and Complications

Bleeding

Serious hemorrhage during esophageal surgery is reported to occur in up to 4% of surgeries. The extent of bleeding and repair largely depends on the vessel injured. Excellent anatomical knowledge and awareness of the trajectory of all major vessels is critical during esophageal dissection. The esophagus is in proximity to several major vessels, including the aorta, pulmonary veins, and pulmonary arteries; their inadvertent injury will result in catastrophic hemorrhage. Furthermore, if the feeding vessels to the esophagus originating from the aorta are not adequately controlled during mobilization, significant bleeding can result.

Splenic Injury

Splenectomy rates during esophagectomy are reported to be between 4 and 9%. Injury is primarily due to excessive tension on the short gastric vessels during gastric mobilization, which results in a splenic capsular tear. If possible, splenic salvage techniques for arresting the hemorrhage are attempted prior to splenectomy. The increasing use of laparoscopy has decreased splenic injury rates, owing to decreased tension on the short gastric vessels.

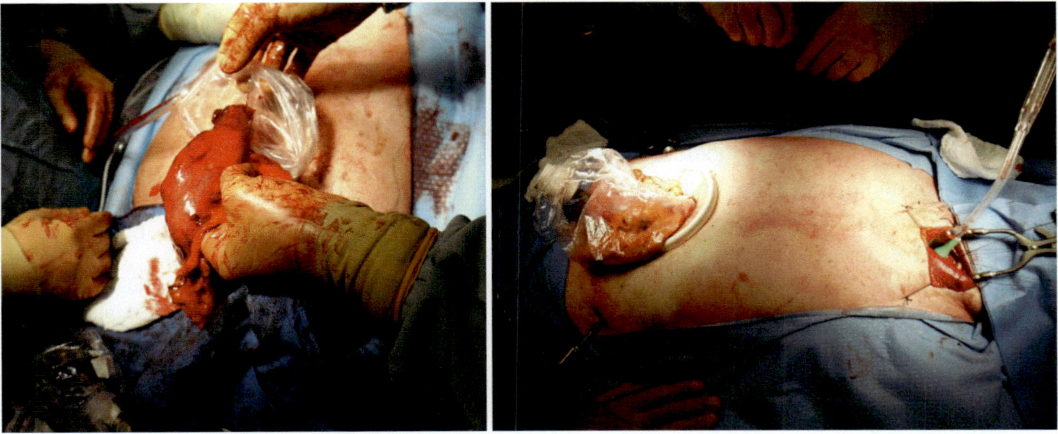

Fig. 14 Insertion of conduit in camera bag in preparation for guidance to neck

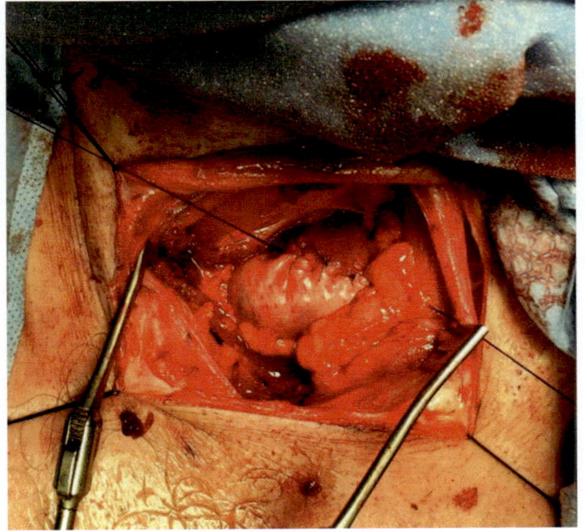

Fig. 15 Construction of cervical anastomosis

Airway Injury

The trachea, the carina, and the right and left bronchi are all susceptible to injury during esophageal mobilization. The thin-walled membranous portion of the airway that abuts the esophagus is particularly vulnerable to cautery or blunt injury. Injuries proximal to the endotracheal tube usually will not result in an unstable physiological status, as air does not escape into the thoracic cavity. These injuries are primarily repaired with absorbable sutures in an interrupted fashion, with further buttressing with muscle or a fat pad. Injuries that are distal to the endotracheal tube may result in significant hemodynamic instability (although this is limited for double-lumen tubes). Repair options include advancing the tube past the injury, if possible, and swift repair of the opening.

Nerve Injury

The recurrent laryngeal nerve is vulnerable to injury during dissection at the thoracic inlet and during the cervical portion of the three-hole esophagectomy. Careful dissection and clear visualization of the nerve avoids its inadvertent injury.

Conduit Necrosis

One of the most dreaded complications is the loss of the gastric conduit due to inadvertent injury to the right gastroepiploic arcade. The rate of gastric conduit ischemia is approximately 3%, with higher rates reported for colonic and jejunal conduits. Conduit ischemia can be addressed by gentle handling of the conduit, careful dissection (especially at the pyloro-antral region), and verification of the artery trajectory during dissection of the greater curve.

Other Postoperative Complications

A complete discussion of postoperative complications is beyond the scope of this chapter. Early postoperative complications include chylothorax, delayed conduit necrosis, and anastomotic leak. Respiratory complications (atelectasis, pneumonia) are among the most common and morbid for the post-esophagectomy patient and are best avoided with early ambulation, incentive spirometry, and excellent chest physiotherapy. Cardiac complications such as atrial fibrillation and supraventricular tachycardia may occur in isolation in the postoperative period, but they often herald another complication such as an anastomotic leak or pneumonia, so their occurrence should prompt a thorough work-up.

References

1. Lee L, Sudarshan M, Li C, Latimer E, Fried GM, Mulder DS, et al. Cost-effectiveness of minimally invasive versus open esophagectomy for esophageal cancer. Ann Surg Oncol. 2013;20:3732–9.
2. Li C, Ferri LE, Mulder DS, Ncuti A, Neville A, Lee L, et al. An enhanced recovery pathway decreases duration of stay after esophagectomy. Surgery. 2012;152:606–14.
3. Luketich JD, Pennathur A, Awais O, Levy RM, Keeley S, Shende M, et al. Outcomes after minimally invasive esophagectomy: review of over 1000 patients. Ann Surg. 2012;256:95–103.
4. Raymond D. Complications of esophagectomy. Surg Clin North Am. 2012;92:1299–313.
5. Sudarshan M, Ferri L. A critical review of minimally invasive esophagectomy. Surg Laparosc Endosc Percutan Tech. 2012;22:310–8.
6. kammili A, Cools-Lartigue J, Mulder D, Feldman LS, Ferri LE, Mueller CL. Transition from open to minimally invasive en bloc esophagectomy can be achieved without compromising surgical quality. Surg Endosc. 2021;35(6):3067–76. https://doi.org/10.1007/s00464-020-07696-0. Epub 2020 Jun 15. PMID: 32556773.
7. van den Berg JW, Tabrett K, Cheong E. Paravertebral catheter analgesia for minimally invasive Ivor Lewis oesophagectomy. J Thorac Dis. 2019;11(Suppl 5):S786–93.
8. Nevo Y, Calderone A, Kammili A, Boulila C, Renaud S, Cools-Lartigue J, Spicer J, Mueller C, Ferri L. Endoscopic pyloromyotomy in minimally invasive esophagectomy: a novel approach. Surg Endosc. 2021.
9. Low DE, Allum W, De Manzoni G, et al. Guidelines for perioperative care in esophagectomy: enhanced recovery after surgery (ERAS®) society recommendations. World J Surg. 2019;43(2):299–330.
10. Nevo Y, Arjah S, Katz A, Ramírez García Luna JL, Spicer J, Cools-Lartigue J, Mueller C, Feldman L, Ferri L. ERAS 2.0: continued refinement of an established enhanced recovery protocol for esophagectomy. Ann Surg Oncol. 2021;28(9):4850–8.
11. Allen SK, Brown V, White D, King D, Hunt J, Wainwright J, Emery A, Hodge E, Kehinde A, Prabhu P, Rockall TA, Preston SR, Sultan J. Multimodal prehabilitation during neoadjuvant therapy prior to esophagogastric cancer resection: effect on cardiopulmonary exercise test performance, muscle mass and quality of life-a pilot randomized clinical trial. Ann Surg Oncol. 2021.

Colonic Interposition After Esophagectomy

Michele Valmasoni and Stefano Merigliano

Abstract

Reconstruction after esophageal cancer esophagectomy represents a complex clinical and surgical question. Patients facing this procedure are fragile with many comorbidities and often a history of chemoradiation and previous surgery. The two main esophageal substitutes are the gastric and colonic conduit, both of which require complex surgical procedures that must be carried out with expertise and knowledge to be successful. In this chapter, we describe our experience with the use of colon interposition.

Keywords

Esophageal cancer · Esophagectomy · Laparotomy · Colon conduit · Colonic interposition

M. Valmasoni · S. Merigliano (✉)
University of Padova School of Medicine, Padova, Italy
e-mail: stefano.merigliano@unipd.it

M. Valmasoni
e-mail: michele.valmasoni@unipd.it

Introduction

The colon was historically the first bowel segment to be used as a substitute for the esophagus; the first colonic interposition after esophagectomy was performed successfully by Von Hacker in 1914. However, after the 1960s, the stomach replaced the colon as the conduit of choice because its vascularization is more reliable, the functional results are better, and the substitution is technically easier, requiring only one anastomosis. Today, after esophagectomy for cancer, the colon is used only when the stomach is not available or is not anatomically suitable [1–17].

Indications

Colonic interposition is indicated whenever the stomach is not available due to a history of gastric surgery, the necessity of extended gastric resection for oncological reasons, vascular impairment, or other gastric pathology such as caustic burns. Colon interposition can also be a solution for reconstructions that require a longer conduit after pharyngo-laryngo-esophagectomy. Colon is the bowel of choice after previous gastric conduit failure.

Contraindications to the use of the colon include a history of colon surgery, the presence of significant colon pathology (e.g. diverticula and tumors) or alteration to its vascular integrity.

Preoperative Evaluation

The patient's preparation includes oncological staging and typical preoperative studies necessary for major surgery (with particular attention to the presence of diabetes, cardio-vascular, and pulmonary pathology). The need to perform a thoracotomy for esophagectomy and reconstruction at the same time requires a careful assessment of the functional respiratory reserve. Nutrition is very important and if the oncological timing allows it, it is preferable to obtain the best possible nutritional status before proceeding with surgery.

The preoperative evaluation of the colon is fundamental and should be performed with a colon computed tomography, or alternatively with contrast enema, to rule out the presence of colon pathology and evaluate the length of the colon. We do not routinely perform endoscopy and angiographic study is performed only in the presence of particular indications (e.g. history of vascular pathology, symptoms suggestive of intestinal vascular insufficiency, previous abdominal surgery, advanced age).

Patient Position

If esophagectomy is required, a right thoracotomy is performed in the left lateral decubitus. We use the same position even if the resection is performed with minimally invasive technique.

For reconstruction, the patient is placed on the operating bed in a prone position, with the legs closed and the arms along the body. The neck should be extended as much as possible, eventually using a roller under the shoulders to accentuate the extension of the head. The head must then be rotated to the right to allow a clear operating field on the left cervical side.

The preparation of the surgical field goes from the jaw to the pubis; the cervical field can be temporarily protected during the abdominal step with a sterile drape. However, it is important to have contemporary access to the two anatomical districts (the abdomen and the neck).

Preparation of the Left Colon

A median xiphopubic incision allows easy access to the abdominal cavity and an abdominal retractor allows for correct field exposure.

Initial exploration of the peritoneal cavity: any adhesions are lysed very carefully, avoiding injuries to the colon and its mesentery. If, in the initial evaluation, the residual stomach (when present) is sufficient for a distal colon-gastric anastomosis, it is important to pay attention to preserve the gastro-epiploic arch. If the remaining stomach is not sufficient, it is better to complete the gastrectomy.

The greater omentum (if present) is moved upwards and the gastro-colic ligament is sectioned along the whole transverse colon to access the transverse mesocolon. In this phase, if the vascularization of the omentum is not satisfactory, it is better to remove it; otherwise, we suggest preserving it, because it could be useful for wrapping the intra-abdominal anastomoses.

The colon is then completely mobilized, releasing and lowering the splenic and hepatic flexures completely and continuing the dissection to the left until the colon-sigmoid junction, and to the right until the cecum. Particular attention should be paid to the anatomical plane identified by the Gerota fascia in the left and right parietal-colic grooves, to avoid entering the mesocolon with the risk of damage to the vasculature or vice versa to open the renal capsule.

When the colon is completely mobilized, its mesentery is tensioned with a cautious maneuver by pulling the colon vertically to be able to evaluate the entire vascular anatomy. The use of trans illumination makes it easy to visualize vasculature in most cases (Fig. 1).

The left, middle, and right colic vessels, as well as the marginal colic vessels, must be identified with certainty; their integrity must be checked (paying attention to the Griffiths point) and we recommend checking the anatomy of the sigmoid vessels too (Fig. 2).

At this point, it is necessary to measure the colon segment necessary for reconstruction. We use a large thread or umbilical tape, starting to

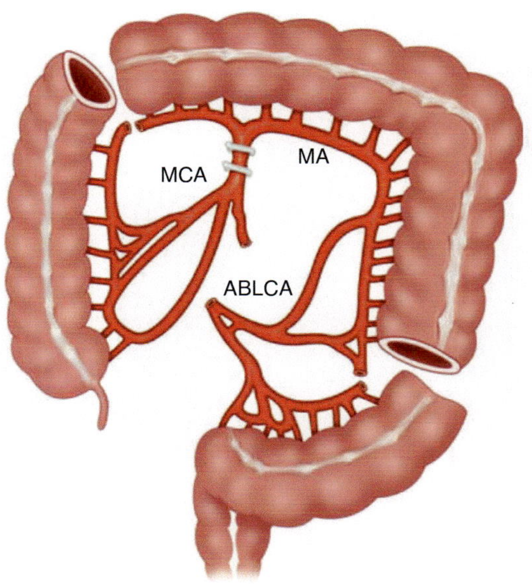

Fig. 1 Vascular anatomy of the left colon. *MCA* middle colic artery, *MA* marginal artery, *ABLCA* Ascending branch of left colic artery (Drawing by Gonzalo Etchepareborda)

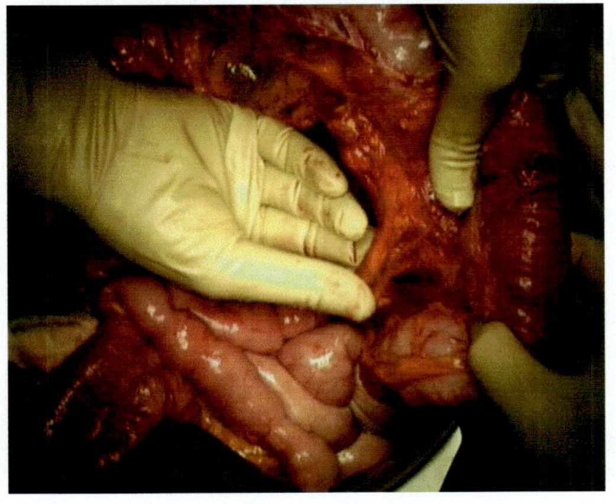

Fig. 2 Checking the left colic vessels, after complete colon mobilization

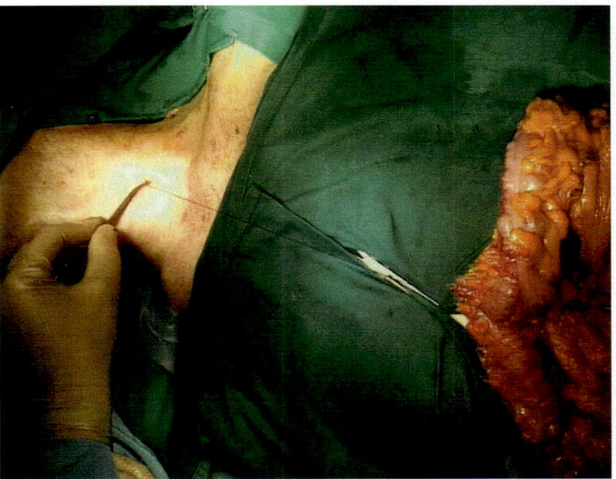

Fig. 3 Measuring the needed conduit length from the left colic pedicle to the neck

Once the necessary length has been identified, the mesocolon is opened near the middle colic vessels and the marginal arch, at the identified section point. Before proceeding with ligation of the vessels, it is necessary to verify the effectiveness of residual vascularization by placing vascular clamps at the base of the medium colic pedicle (carefully preserving the V-shaped right-left bifurcation) and the marginal arch near the point of the section. After a few minutes, we proceed to a touch evaluation of the arterial flow and a visual evaluation of the venous outflow (Figs. 4 and 5). Some authors use a Doppler probe for added security and in recent years the use of indocyanine green enhanced near-infrared fluorescence is gaining popularity for the perfusion assessment of the conduit.

When the medium colic vessels and the marginal arch are ligated, the colon is sectioned with a linear stapler; we always prefer to secure the staple line with some hand stitches (Figs. 6 and 7).

measure from the origin of the left colic vessels, following the marginal arcade (and not the colon), passing the middle colic vessels and beyond to obtain a sufficient length. During this measurement, it is important to consider the transposition pathway, because the retrosternal and subcutaneous routes are longer than the posterior mediastinal path (Fig. 3).

Cervicotomy

A left cervical incision is made. It needs to be sufficiently wide, to allow a good vision and an easy mobilization of the esophagus or of the esophageal stump that had been stitched to the skin in a terminal esophagostomy (the cervical esophageal segment has to be maintained as long as possible during the esophagectomy).

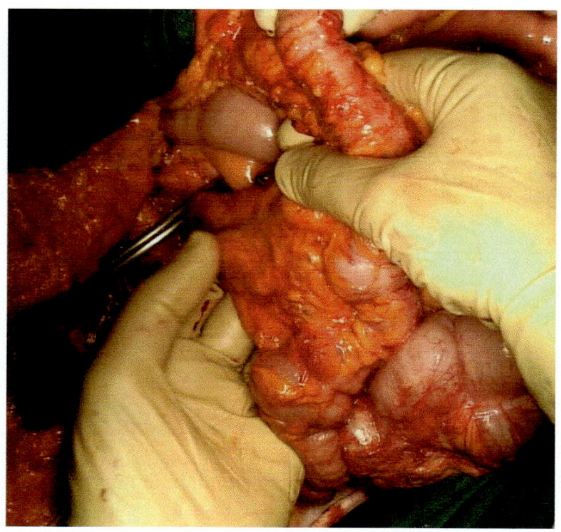

Fig. 4 After closing with a clamp the base of the middle colic pedicle and the marginal arch coming from the right, it is important to check if the vascularization from the left colic vessels is valid

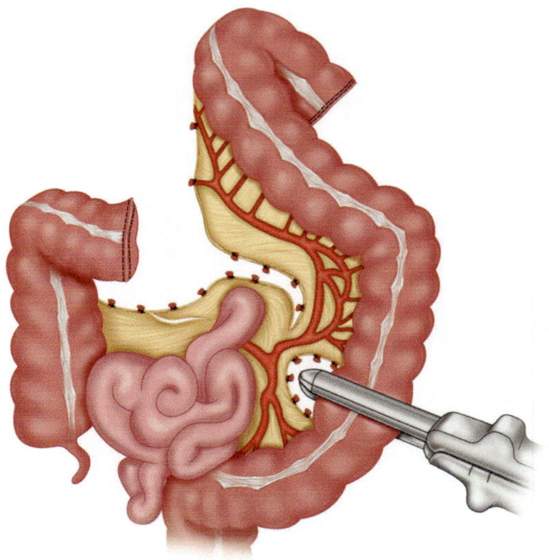

Fig. 6 Division of the colon with a linear stapler (Drawing by Gonzalo Etchepareborda)

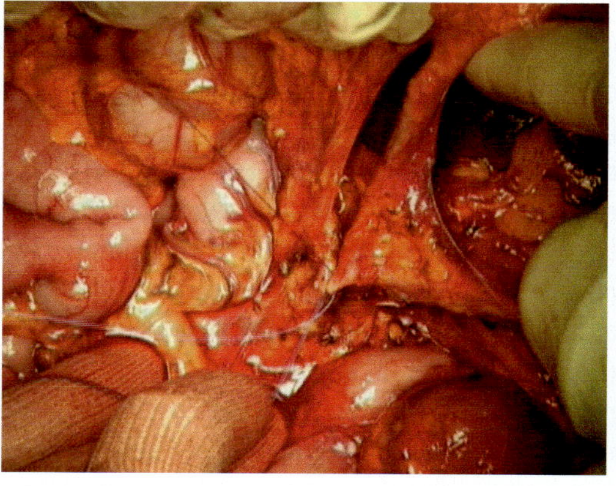

Fig. 5 Ligation of the middle colic artery, paying attention to preserve the V-shape left–right bifurcation

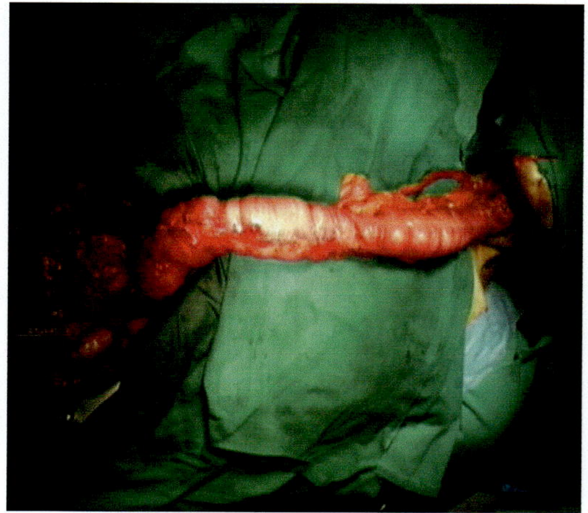

Fig. 7 The isolated colonic conduit ready to be transposed to the neck

If the esophagus was mobilized in the thorax during the same operation, we attach a large sponge or tube to the abdominal esophagus to bring the sponge along the posterior mediastinal pathway while recovering the esophagus through the cervicotomy. We prefer to fix the colon to the sponge and not to the esophagus for transposition, because of the risk of esophagus rupture during pull-up.

If the posterior mediastinal pathway is not available, we proceed to the deep cervical fascia incision to gain access to the retrosternal space.

We remove the sternal head of the left clavicle, to ensure sufficient passage of the colon while avoiding compression, which can cause local ischemia. In our experience, it is only rarely necessary to perform a sternal split.

In the very rare case of a previous sternotomy, the conduit can be transposed to the neck using a subcutaneous route.

Colon Conduit Pull-Up

Posterior Mediastinum Route

This way is anatomically preferable, but not always possible. If esophagectomy was performed with previous surgery, mediastinal adhesions render this path unusable.

Before proceeding to colon transposition, it is necessary to isolate the diaphragmatic crus to make it wide enough to allow an easy passage of the colon. If necessary, a partial section of the right diaphragmatic pillar can help, taking care not to enlarge the hiatus too much to avoid the onset of visceral hernias.

The colonic segment is wrapped with a suitable length sterile plastic bag (for example, the one used to cover the laparoscopic camera), to guarantee vascular protection during the pull-up, and then fixed to the sponge previously pulled in the posterior mediastinum. With a careful traction of the sponge from the neck, the colon is pulled up, helping the transdiaphragmatic passage with the hands, until a sufficient portion of the colon reaches the left lateral cervical space. Once the plastic bag has been removed from the neck, the esophagus is dissected to measure for the anastomosis.

The esophago-colic, termino-lateral anastomosis is hand sewn with two semi-continuous 4/0 or 3/0 polydioxanone (PDS) sutures and a second layer of single stitches. Once the posterior wall of the anastomosis is completed, a nasogastric tube is accompanied by the anastomosis and pushed into the colonic conduit.

Retrosternal Route

Before pulling the colonic conduit to the neck through the retrosternal route, it is necessary to remove the xiphoid process and detach the medial insertions of the diaphragm to access the retrosternal space; then, with blunt hand dissection, a retrosternal tunnel is prepared up to the neck, avoiding if possible opening the pleurae (Fig. 8). At this stage, it is important

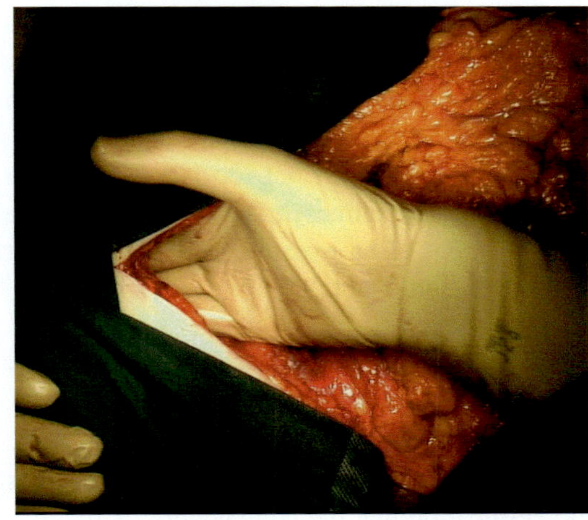

Fig. 8 Blunt hand dissection to prepare the retrosternal route

that hemostasis is satisfactory before proceeding because it can be difficult to stop bleeding after transposition of the colon. Remember to close the diaphragmatic hiatus to avoid visceral hernias.

The colonic segment is then accompanied through the retrosternal pathway with long ring forceps and recovered at the neck to perform the anastomosis (Fig. 9).

Subcutaneous Route

The subcutaneous route remains the last chance when the retrosternal pathway is not available, for example, for a previous sternotomy or

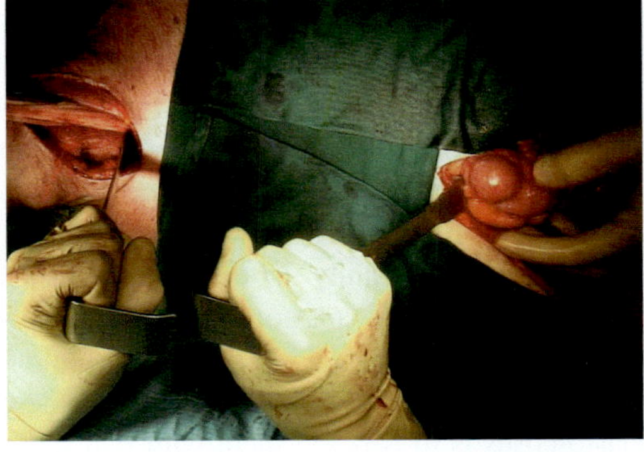

Fig. 9 Colon pull-up with a sponge trough the retrosternal route

irradiation. Removal of the xiphoid process is particularly important to avoid colon trauma. The subcutaneous tunnel must be large enough to allow an agile passage of the conduit without compressing it but not too large to prevent redundancy. Sometimes it is necessary to stage the placement of an expander if the skin is not sufficiently compliant.

Abdominal Anastomoses

After cervical esophageal-colic anastomosis and verification that the colic conduit is rectilinear and there is no traction on the anastomosis, intra-abdominal anastomoses are performed.

The transposed colon must be interrupted in the abdomen to have two sufficiently long portions to perform the proximal anastomosis (colon-gastric or colon-jejunal) and the distal colon-colic anastomosis. Particular care must be taken to isolate the needed colon tract, by interrupting the vasa recta for a sufficient length while preserving the marginal arch scrupulously. We recommend always removing a small portion of the isolated colon to avoid ischemia of the anastomoses.

If a suitable gastric residue is present, a terminolateral colon-gastric anastomosis can be performed on the posterior surface of the stomach (hand sewn or with a circular stapler, introduced through a gastrotomy, or semi-mechanical with a linear stapler).

In the absence of a gastric stump, a terminolateral colon-jejunal anastomosis is necessary on a Roux-en-Y jejunal loop. This second option allows for easier reconstruction and ensures greater control over bile reflux.

Before performing the proximal anastomosis, the nasogastric tube previously positioned in the colonic conduit is always positioned through this anastomosis.

The colon continuity is then reestablished with the colon-colic anastomosis (termino-terminal or latero-lateral) laid in front of the colon-jejunal anastomosis. Our preference for these anastomoses is to perform them with two semi-continuous double layer sutures (Fig. 10).

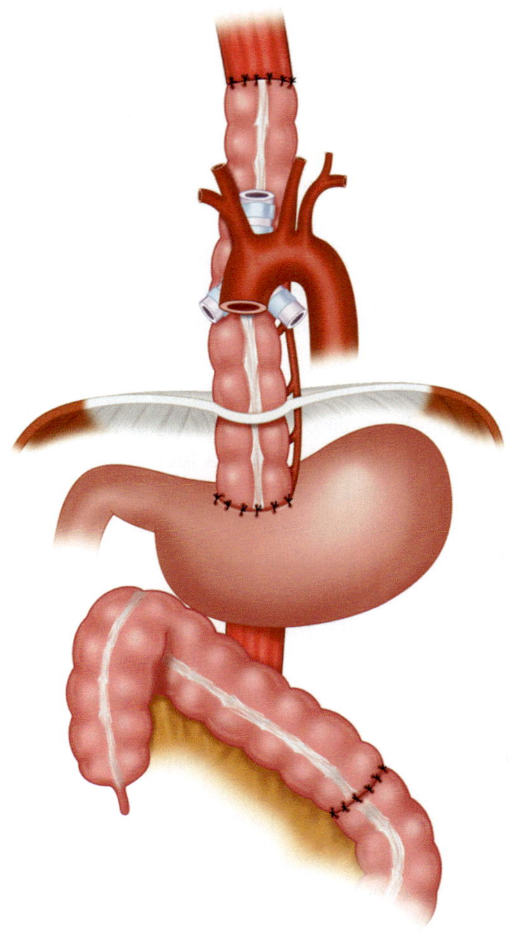

Fig. 10 Status after using the left colon for colonic interposition (Drawing by Gonzalo Etchepareborda)

We recommend performing a nutritional jejunostomy.

Right Colon: Technical Differences

The dissection of the colon occurs in a way similar to that described for the left colon; in this case, however, a sufficient mobilization of the cecum and the last ileal tract is necessary. The ileocolic, right colic, and ileal vessels should be exposed and clamped with vascular clamps to verify that the flow of the middle colic vessels is adequate (Fig. 11).

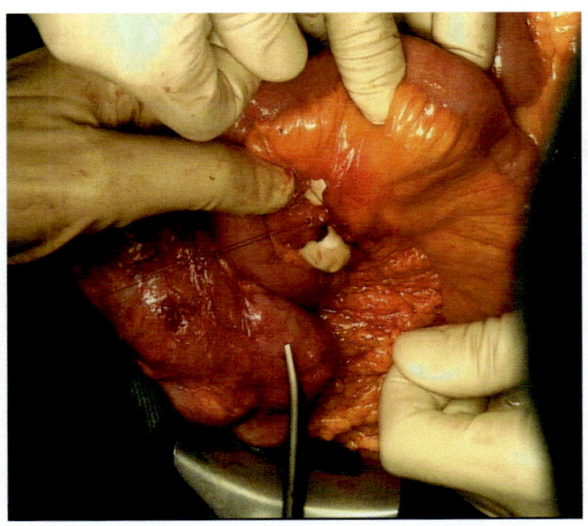

Fig. 11 Right colonic conduit preparation: isolation of the last ileal tract

Measurement of the necessary length of the colon takes place as already described, starting from the middle colic pedicle. After ligation of the right ileocolic and colic vessels, and if necessary, the ileal vessels, the colon is transected from the last ileal tract to the measured length. An appendectomy is always performed. The colon conduit is transposed to the neck as previously described (Fig. 12).

An end-to-end or end-to-side esophagus-ileal anastomosis is performed with semi-continuous and double-layered 4/0 or 3/0 absorbable monofilament sutures.

Abdominal anastomoses are performed in a similar way to the previous description, with the distal one being an ileo-colic anastomosis (Fig. 13).

Some authors prefer to use the right colon because the dimension of the terminal ileus is

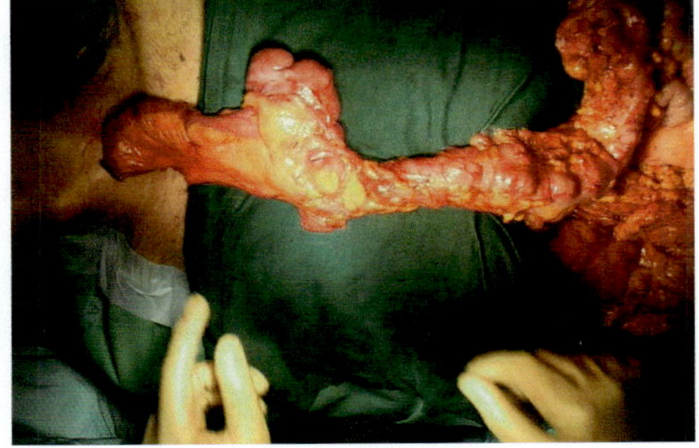

Fig. 12 The ileo-colic conduit ready to be transposed

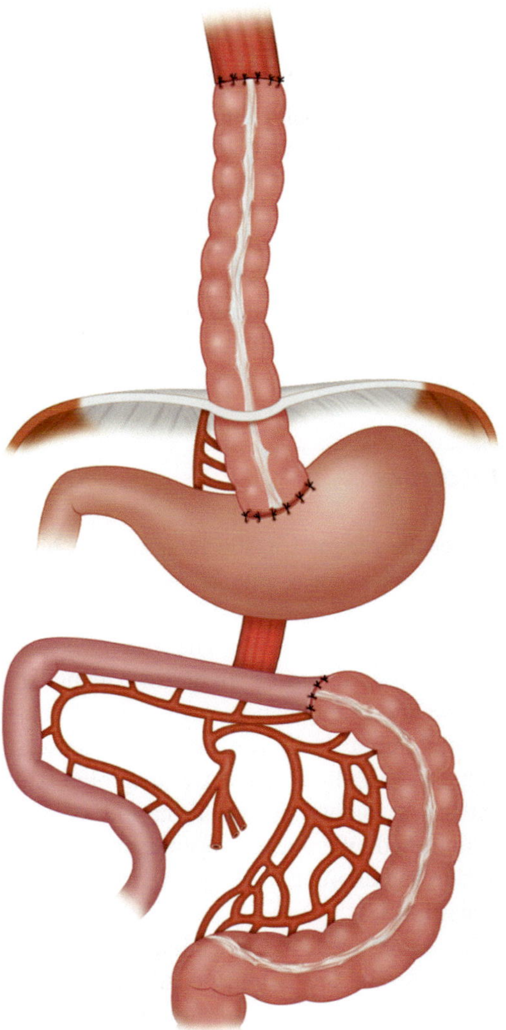

Fig. 13 Status after using the right colon for colonic interposition (Drawing by Gonzalo Etchepareborda)

similar to the cervical esophagus, but the clinical results are better for the interposition of the left colon with a significantly lower incidence of postoperative necrosis or ischemia.

Postoperative Care

In the early postoperative days, it is important to maintain adequate volume (avoiding fluid overload) and blood pressure, possibly without using vasoconstrictors medications, to avoid reduced microcirculation and the risk of anastomotic ischemia.

We consider early extubation to be important, as well as mobilization of the patient and an effective use of incentive spirometer. For this reason, postoperative pain control must be optimal.

We maintain the nasogastric tube until contrast swallowing or endoscopic check of anastomosis, which usually occurs in 7–8 days. The patient then gradually resumes oral feeding while decreasing nutritional intake through the jejunostomy.

is indicated only in the presence of symptoms that have an impact on quality of life, since corrective surgery is not easy and potentially dangerous for the survival of the colonic conduit.

Cancer of the transposed colon is a rare event, but if the patient develops dysphagia during follow-up, an endoscopy is mandatory.

Regarding long-term quality of life, the results are very satisfactory and, in some ways, superior to gastric transposition, since there are usually no problems related to acid or biliary reflux.

Outcomes

The results reported in the literature are highly variable, with a leak rate of 0–15%, a conduit necrosis rate of 0–10%, and a postoperative mortality rate of 0–16%. The risk of leakage has been reported to be higher in patients who underwent chemoradiation.

Anastomotic leaks can be treated conservatively if promptly diagnosed, if the colon is not ischemic at endoscopy, and if the risk of sepsis is controlled. We suggest opening the cervical incision and draining the leak externally to avoid mediastinitis.

The most severe complication is represented by necrosis of the colonic conduit; this event often requires immediate surgery to save as much bowel as possible for future reconstruction. In this case, the prevention of sepsis and adequate nutrition are critical to patient survival.

Dysphagia, reflux, and dumping syndrome may be common in the postoperative period, but these symptoms usually resolve within a few months without specific therapies.

Anastomotic stenosis is described in 0–40% of cases and often can be successfully treated with endoscopic dilations; only a low percentage of cases require reoperation.

In the long run, colonic kinking can occur due to relaxation and redundancy (0–40% of cases in the literature). We believe that surgery

Surgical Tips

- When sectioning the esophagus, we perform a knife section of the esophageal muscular layers to obtain a longer mucosal cylinder useful for easier anastomosis.
- After performing the termino-lateral esophago-colon anastomosis in the neck, it is sometimes useful to approximate the terminal end of the colonic conduit to the esophagus, with some stitches, to avoid the formation of a "cul de sac" that can impair deglutition.
- We recommend resection of the clavicular head even if the passage seems to be large enough when using the retrosternal route.
- Pay particular attention to preserve the V-shaped left–right bifurcation of the middle colic vessels; if necessary, perform a tangential resection of the superior mesenteric vessels.
- If the vascularization of the colon conduit vascularization is dubious after the pull-up (congested mucosa, swelling) perform only half of the esophago-colon anastomosis and a temporary cutaneous stoma to check the colonic trophism.
- Some stitches between the colon conduit and the diaphragm crus can help reduce redundancy, but they must be placed after the esophago-colon anastomosis has been performed to avoid tension to the anastomosis.

References

1. Mansour KA, Bryan FC, Carlson GW. Bowel interposition for esophageal replacement: twenty-five-year experience. Ann Thorac Surg. 1997;64(3):752–6.
2. Joosten JJ, Gisbertz SS, Heineman DJ, Daams F, Eshuis WJ, van Berge Henegouwen MI. The role of fluorescence angiography in colonic interposition after esophagectomy. Dis Esophagus. 2022;1–7.
3. Cerfolio RJ, Allen MS, Deschamps C, Trastek VF, Pairolero PC. Esophageal replacement by colon interposition. Ann Thorac Surg. 1995;59(6):1382–4.
4. Larson TC, Shuman LS, Libshitz HI, McMurtrey MJ. Complications of colonic interposition. Cancer. 1985;56(3):681–90.
5. Fürst H, Hartl WH, Löhe F, Schildberg FW. Colon interposition for esophageal replacement. Ann Surg. 2000;231(2):173–8.
6. Fürst H, Hartl WH, Löhe F, Schildberg FW. Colon interposition for esophageal replacement: an alternative technique based on the use of the right colon. Ann Surg. 2000;231(2):173–8.
7. Peters JH. Arterial anatomic considerations in colon interposition for esophageal replacement. Arch Surg. 1995;130(8):858–63.
8. Bakshi A, Sugarbaker DJ, Burt BM. Alternative conduits for esophageal replacement. Ann Cardiothorac Surg. 2017;6(2):137–43.
9. Fisher RA, Griffiths EA, Evison F, Mason RC, Zylstra J, Davies AR, et al. A national audit of colonic interposition for esophageal replacement. Dis Esophagus. 2017;30(5):1–10.
10. Yildirim S. Colonic interposition versus gastric pull-up after total esophagectomy. J Gastrointest Surg. 2004;8(6):675–8.
11. Davis PA. Colonic interposition after esophagectomy for cancer. Arch Surg. 2003;138(3):303–8.
12. Freeman NV, Cass DT. Colon interposition: a modification of the Waterston technique using the normal esophageal route. J Pediatric Surg. 1982;17(1):17–21.
13. Thomas P, Fuentes P, Giudicelli R, Reboud E. Colon interposition for esophageal replacement: current indications and long-term function. Ann Thorac Surg. 1997;64(3):757–64.
14. Chang AC. Colon interposition for staged esophageal reconstruction. Oper Tech Thorac Cardiovasc Surg. 2010;15(3):231–42.
15. Thomas PMD, Fuentes PMD, Giudicelli RMD, Reboud EMD. Colon interposition for esophageal replacement: current indications and long-term function. Ann Thorac Surg. 1997;64(3):757–64.
16. Wolff WI. Colonic interposition as esophageal replacement. Am J Surg. 1966;111(5):698–703.
17. Cense HA, Visser MRM, van Sandick JW, de Boer AGEM, Lamme B, Obertop H, et al. Quality of life after colon interposition by necessity for esophageal cancer replacement. J Surg Oncol. 2004;88(1):32–8.

Perioperative Care and Management of Post-operative Complications

Darren S. Bryan and Mark K. Ferguson

Abstract

As perioperative management of patients undergoing esophageal resection becomes more nuanced, the importance of a patient-centered approach to care is increasingly apparent. Predictors of adverse outcomes after esophagectomy include low spirometry and DLCO, extremes of body mass index, advanced age, frailty, sarcopenia, and neo-adjuvant therapy. Perioperative care plans as part of enhanced recovery after surgery (ERAS) pathways include interventions designed to minimize the adverse impact of surgery on the patient, reduce postoperative complications, shorten the duration of hospital stay, and decrease costs. Despite improved risk stratification and interventions focused on modifiable risk factors, adverse outcomes continue to have a negative impact on hospital length of stay, morbidity, and mortality. The most common postoperative complications are pneumonia, atrial fibrillation, anastomotic leak and chyle leak. Early identification and timely intervention are essential to minimize the effects of these potentially devastating complications.

Keywords

Esophagectomy · Esophageal cancer · Preoperative preparation · Enhanced recovery · Complications · Postoperative care

Introduction

Esophageal resection is associated with high rates of post-operative complications [1, 2]. While outcomes have improved over time with advances in surgical techniques and a greater understanding of important points of perioperative care, esophageal resection remains well within the domain of "high risk" surgery [3]. Complications are related to the inherent morbidity of esophageal surgery, as well as common comorbidities associated with esophageal malignancy. For these reasons, an emphasis is placed on the identification of appropriate candidates for resection, the implementation of perioperative care regimens directed at predefined post-operative goals (e.g. nutritional intake, physical activity, pain management), and a focus on minimizing operative morbidity and mortality. To these ends, enhanced recovery after surgery (ERAS) programs have been implemented across surgical specialties, generally showing

D. S. Bryan · M. K. Ferguson (✉)
Section of Thoracic Surgery, The University of Chicago, Chicago, IL, USA
e-mail: mferguso@bsd.uchicago.edu

D. S. Bryan
e-mail: dbryan@bsd.uchicago.edu

© The Author(s), under exclusive license to Springer Nature Switzerland AG 2023
F. Schlottmann et al. (eds.), *Esophageal Cancer*,
https://doi.org/10.1007/978-3-031-39086-9_19

decreased morbidity, decreased costs of treatment, and improved lengths of stay [4–9]. ERAS programs for esophagectomy have been demonstrated to be feasible and safe. Multiple studies have shown no increases in perioperative surgical or medical complications, and unchanged mortality with shorter lengths of stay [9–13]. When complications arise, early identification and management are important for positive outcomes.

Preoperative Management

Patient deconditioning is a common feature of esophageal cancer and must be evaluated as part of treatment planning. Sarcopenia, a state of dysregulated energy metabolism that results in a reduction of skeletal muscle mass, is present in up to 75% of patients with esophageal cancer and is associated with adverse outcomes including induction therapy toxicity, an increase in post-operative complications, and worse overall survival [14–17]. Sarcopenia is driven by nutritional deficiencies in the setting of an inflammatory state, increased tumor-related metabolic demands, malignant dysphagia, and induction therapy. Multimodal prehabilitation, focusing on patient education, exercise, nutrition, and modifiable risk factors, shows promise in the ability to limit disease- and treatment-related sarcopenia. When initiated before induction therapy for esophageal cancer, prehabilitation has been shown to limit skeletal muscle loss and to be associated with decreased visceral obesity and a lower risk of postoperative complications [17].

Patient Education

Patient engagement in the care process, starting at the initial point of contact in the clinic, is of vital importance. Patients and their support systems should be recruited as integral components of the care team, and the physician–patient relationship conceptualized as a two-way street with each party contributing to the partnership. Brief consultations often fall short of appropriately

informing patients of what an esophageal operation entails and adequately emphasizing the importance of the patient's role in their own preparation and recovery. Thus, the importance of an early start to patient education with a unified, multidisciplinary, and coherent message cannot be overstated. Education should be tailored to the patient and support network, with frequent checks for understanding. Motivated patients who are engaged in their care and participate in a shared decision-making process are more likely to be satisfied in their care, and more likely to adhere to therapy [18–20]. Examples of materials that are useful in this process include decision making aids, printed handouts, informative videos, question and answer sessions, and consultation with patient advocacy and survivor groups.

Smoking Cessation

Cigarette smokers have an increased risk of pulmonary and wound healing complications, which are mitigated in part by smoking cessation [21, 22]. Although the required duration of abstinence from smoking to achieve a reduction in complications is not established, greater than eight weeks is preferable [21–23]. A meta-analysis of randomized controlled trials demonstrated a 41% reduction in both total and pulmonary complications for past smokers compared to current smokers. Each week of cessation increased the magnitude of the effect by 19% [22]. Smoking cessation is best achieved with the combination of behavioral intervention (clinician consultation and continued intervention with support groups or toll-free number support) and medication including nicotine replacement therapy, and should be done in conjunction with the patient's primary care team.

Exercise

Exercise regimens as a component of prehabiliation programs have been shown to reduce morbidity, postoperative pain, and hospital length of stay after esophageal surgery [24, 25]. Although the regimens used in these studies are heterogeneous, they demonstrate that both pre-and post-operative pulmonary exercises such as incentive spirometry and walking therapy are effective and easily implemented, with goals that enable measurement of progress.

Carbohydrate Loading

Traditionally, patients have been restricted to 'nothing by mouth' after midnight on the night prior to surgery, however prolonged fasting aggravates the surgical stress response, increases insulin resistance, exaggerates protein losses, and impairs gastrointestinal function [26–29]. It also increases the time to resolution of negative protein balance and anabolism. From a patient-centered standpoint, fasting results in unnecessary symptoms such as thirst, hunger, headaches and anxiety. Current guidelines recommend that clear liquids can be ingested up to 2 h before procedures [30]. Preoperative carbohydrate loading with a high-calorie (12.5% carbohydrate, 400 mL) clear drink 2 h before surgery has been shown to decrease insulin resistance, improve gastric emptying, and may reduce duration of hospital stay [31]. Importantly, it has not been shown to increase the risk of perioperative aspiration.

Assessment of Risk for Postoperative Nausea and Vomiting

Postoperative nausea and vomiting (PONV) in esophagectomy patients can delay oral intake and ambulation and increase the risk of aspiration. Routine pre-operative screening helps to identify patients at risk. The Apfel simplified score is a useful quick screen for PONV which assigns a single point to female gender, patients with a history of PONV or motion sickness, non-smoking status, and predicted postoperative opioid use (Table 1) [32]. Patients with an Apfel score ≥ 2 have a greater than 39% chance of postoperative nausea and vomiting and should

Table 1 Apfel risk scoring system for postoperative nausea and vomiting (PONV). A point is assigned for female gender, a history of PONV or motion sickness, non-smoking status, and predicted postoperative opioid use; the sum is the Apfel score [32]

Apfel score	Risk of PONV (%)
0	10
1	21
2	39
3	61
4	79

be considered for prophylaxis, such as the application of a scopalamine patch in the preoperative holding area. The use of low dose propofol (<20 mcg/kg/min) and intraoperative ondansetron reduce PONV and should be considered for all patients in the absence of a contraindication [33].

Predictors of Perioperative Complications

Postoperative complications in patients undergoing esophageal resection are common, occurring in up to 60% of cases (Table 2) [2, 34]. Great emphasis has been placed on identifying patients at increased risk for specific postoperative complications after esophagectomy, providing means to mitigate risk.

Pulmonary

The most common complications after esophagectomy are pulmonary, with pneumonia occurring in 14.6% [2]. Post-operative pulmonary complications are associated with a ten-fold higher rate of postoperative mortality and a substantially shortened life expectancy [35–39]. Predictors of postoperative pulmonary complications include low forced expiratory volume in the first second (FEV1), administration of preoperative radiation, extremes of BMI, poor performance status, and advanced age [38–41]. Given the prevalence and impact of pulmonary

Table 2 Incidence of esophageal complications among high volume centers internationally [2]

Complication category	Incidence (%)
Pulmonary	27.8
Gastrointestinal	22.4
Cardiac	16.8
Infection	14.2
Neurologic/psychiatric	9.4
Urologic	8.3
Thromboembolic	5.1
Wound/Diaphragm	2.9
Other	6.8
Frequent individual complications	**Incidence (%)**
Pneumonia	14.6
Atrial dysrhythmias	14.5
Anastomotic leak	11.4
Chyle leak	4.7
Recurrent laryngeal nerve injury	4.2
Conduit necrosis	1.3

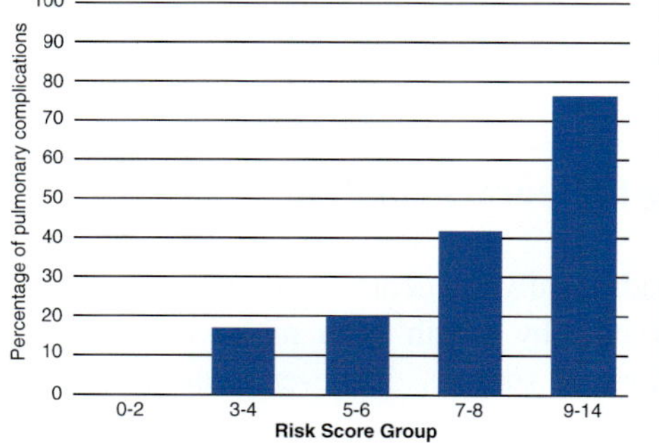

Assigned score value	0	1	2	3	4
Age	<50	51-60	61-70	71-80	>80
Performance Status (Zubrod/ECOG)	0	1	2	3	4
FEV1%		≥100	90-99.9	80-89.9	70-79.9	<70
DLCO%		≥100	90-99.9	80-89.9	70-79.9	<70

Fig. 1 Incidence postoperative pulmonary complications categorized by assigned risk score based on age, performance status zubrod/eastern cooperative oncology group (ECOG), forced expiratory volume in the first second (FEV_1), and diffusing capacity of the lung for carbon monoxide (DLCO). From Reinersman et al. with permission [42]

complications, a risk scoring system has been developed to assess relative risk of postoperative pulmonary complications based on weighted scores for FEV_1, diffusing capacity of the lung for carbon monoxide (DLCO), age, and performance status (Fig. 1) [42].

Postoperative pulmonary complications are more common in patients with reduced FEV_1, lower DLCO, and in those receiving higher doses of induction radiation [39, 43, 44]. Changes in pulmonary function following induction chemoradiation have been shown to have predictive value for patients undergoing esophagectomy. Reduced post-treatment DLCO, in particular, is associated with prolonged intubation and pulmonary complications [43]. In addition, patients with low or very high body mass index (BMI) have an increased incidence of pulmonary complications compared to patients with normal BMI [41, 45, 46]

Because of the morbidity and mortality associated with pulmonary complications, it is vital to employ measures to reduce their incidence. These measures include preoperative respiratory rehabilitation (smoking cessation, inspiratory muscle training), enhanced oral hygiene including frequent preoperative teeth brushing, postoperative pulmonary toilet maneuvers, and adequate postoperative pain management [47–49].

Cardiovascular

Atrial dysrhythmias

Atrial dysrhythmias such as atrial fibrillation (AF) occur in up to 15% of esophagectomy patients [2, 50, 51]. When AF occurs, there should be a high index of suspicion for other complications such as anastomotic leak and pneumonia. As an isolated event, AF is associated with an increase in hospital length of stay, a possible need for medical intervention, and patient distress. Prevention of postoperative AF begins with preoperative optimization of modifiable risk factors such as cardiac disease, smoking, and alcohol abuse [52]. All patients taking a preoperative beta-blocker should continue it perioperatively. Esophagectomy is classified as a high-risk procedure, and guidelines indicate that anyone who has preserved left ventricular function and is not taking a beta-blocker should be managed with perioperative prophylactic diltiazem or amiodarone [52].

Major adverse cardiac events

Assessment of activity level, along with a brief cardiac and medical history, is sufficient to determine which patients need preoperative cardiac evaluation. Level of activity is classified in terms of metabolic equivalents (METs). The risk of a major adverse cardiac event (MACE) can be calculated using the *Revised Cardiac Risk Index for Pre-Operative Risk* (Fig. 2), which incorporates the type of surgery and a history of congestive heart failure, ischemic heart disease, cerebrovascular disease, or creatinine >2 mg/

dl [53]. Patients who are low risk (< 1% risk of MACE) require no additional workup. Among patients at increased risk of MACE, no additional testing is indicated if they can climb a flight of stairs or walk on level ground at 3 to 4 mph (equivalent to ≥4 METs). For patients who are at increased risk and have an exercise ability <4 METs or that cannot be determined, further workup is suggested [53].

Venous thromboembolism (VTE)

The risk of venous thromboembolism following esophagectomy is reported to range from 3 to 8%, with the greatest risk during the initial post-operative hospitalization [54–56]. Large, population-based studies have also identified pre-operative VTE in up to 3% of patients [54]. Risk factors for in-hospital VTE are male sex, white race, prolonged ventilation, and other major complications of surgery. Risk factors for post-discharge VTE are advanced age and major postoperative complications. VTE prophylaxis includes pharmacologic and mechanical measures, should be routine, and should be started prior to induction of anesthesia. Currently, there is no consensus on the duration of postoperative prophylaxis, though elderly patients and those with major postoperative complications are most likely to benefit from extended-duration (4 to 6 weeks) chemoprophylaxis [55].

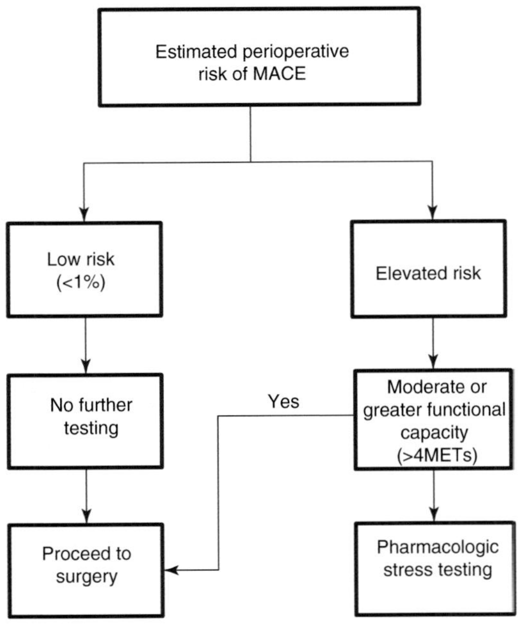

Fig. 2 Use of the revised cardiac risk index for determining which patients require preoperative cardiac evaluation. MACE: major adverse cardiac events; METs: metabolic equivalents. Modified from Fleisher et al. with permission [53]

Intraoperative Management

Fluid Administration

Perioperative fluid management to maintain euvolemia reduces morbidity and improves recovery of postoperative gastric emptying and bowel function [57–59]. This is achieved by strict intraoperative and postoperative monitoring of fluid balance, avoidance of unnecessary intravenous fluid administration including transfusions, and 'permissive oliguria' in appropriately selected patients [60].

Maintenance of Body Temperature

Maintenance of normothermia is associated with a reduction in wound infections, cardiac complications, bleeding, and transfusion requirements [61–64]. For this reason, accurate, noninvasive, and continuous intraoperative temperature monitoring is essential. Forced air heating covers should be used for all patients undergoing esophagectomy. In the event of intraoperative hypothermia, warmed intravenous fluids should be used. For rapid rewarming, infusion of warm intraperitoneally or intrapleural saline is an effective strategy.

Anesthetic Considerations

Perioperative pain management should be preemptive and multimodal. Initiation of neuroaxial blockade before surgery and its maintenance throughout surgery decreases the need for anesthetic agents, opioids and muscle relaxants in the perioperative period [65]. Non-steroidal anti-inflammatory agents in conjunction with acetaminophen and gabapentinoids reduce the need for postoperative analgesia [65]. The use of low dose propofol (<20 mcg/kg/min) with avoidance of inhalation anesthetics reduces PONV and should be considered for all patients [33].

Postoperative Management

Pain Management

The goals of pain control after esophagectomy are to permit deep breathing, prevent atelectasis, and allow unhindered ambulation, while reducing the use of opioids. This can be accomplished with the use of intraoperative local and regional anesthesia, and a multimodal perioperative regimen including acetaminophen, non-steroidal anti-inflammatories and gabapentinoids, with a limited amount of narcotic available for breakthrough pain. Patient controlled analgesia (PCA)

can be added if pain scores remain elevated following initial use of the narcotics. In patients undergoing a thoracotomy, neural blockade can be employed, and there is no clear evidence demonstrating superiority of a paravertebral block or an epidural block. Some studies suggest a reduction in minor procedure-related complications with the use of paravertebral blocks and reduced use of additional analgesic modalities with the use of epidurals [66]. Patients should be assessed early and regularly in order to make appropriate adjustments to pain medications and reinforce the importance of deep breathing and ambulation.

Early Mobilization

Early ambulation in surgical patients reduces pain scores, decreases postoperative pulmonary complications, and improves patient satisfaction [67]. Early ambulation within hours of surgery has been shown to be feasible and safe [68]. Patients can be placed in a chair upon arrival in their room and should be encouraged to ambulate with assistance as soon as possible on the day of surgery.

Diet and Nutrition

Weight loss is common both pre- and postoperatively in patients with esophageal cancer [69]. The majority of patients with esophageal malignancies present with some degree of dysphagia, which contributes substantially to pre-treatment nutritional deficiencies. Induction therapy is highly effective in decreasing tumor size, with most patients experiencing dysphagia relief during the first cycle of chemotherapy, obviating the need for surgically placed feeding tubes [70]. Nevertheless, surgeons should carefully consider nutritional status prior to undertaking esophageal resection. Gastrostomy tubes are traditionally avoided in patients who may undergo resection, preserving the stomach for conduit creation.

Early postoperative alimentation decreases time to neutral protein balance, reduces wound and pulmonary infections, and is associated with shorter length of hospital stay [71]. Postoperative management of nasogastric tubes is highly surgeon specific, however multiple groups have shown they can be removed safely on the first postoperative day if the output is minimal and there is no radiographic evidence of conduit dilation [72]. Timing of diet initiation is also highly center- and surgeon-specific, however recent publications, including a randomized controlled trial, have shown early feeding to be a safe practice. A clear liquid diet as early as post-operative day 1 is well tolerated with no difference in time to recovery or in rate of complications, including anastomotic leak and pneumonia [73, 74].

Routine Postoperative Anastomotic Evaluation

It is common practice in many centers to perform a postoperative swallow evaluation or endoscopy prior to initiating a diet, however, routine postoperative anastomotic evaluation is ineffective in diagnosing subclinical leaks and thus does not substantially change outcomes. The positive predictive value of routine postoperative endoscopy and contrast swallow are 8% and 3%, respectively [75]. In the absence of a clear indication for evaluation, anastomotic evaluation is unnecessary, costly, bears an inherent risk of aspiration, and may delay oral alimentation and discharge.

Management of Postoperative Complications

Postoperative complications after esophagectomy can result in patient distress, prolonged hospital stay, non-home discharge, delayed or incomplete recovery, delay in initiation of adjuvant treatment, and death [76]. Vigilance, early identification, and appropriate intervention in the event of postoperative complications are important to minimize the impact on the patient's recovery.

Pulmonary

Despite preventive measures, postoperative atelectasis, aspiration and pneumonia remain the most common postoperative complications in esophagectomy patients. Atelectasis may be asymptomatic or present as an increased work of breathing with hypoxemia. Treatment is guided by the presence or absence of secretions. If the patient has no secretions, first line therapy includes deep breathing exercises and incentive spirometry. If this is unsuccessful, continuous positive airway pressure reduces the incidence of reintubation and pneumonia [77]. In patients with excessive secretions, first line treatment is mucus clearance through frequent suctioning and chest physiotherapy. The use of bronchoscopy has been frequently reported but no clear benefit has been demonstrated [78].

The diagnosis of postoperative pneumonia can be challenging. The use of standard diagnostic criteria for hospital acquired pneumonia results in over diagnosis [79]. Postoperative pneumonia should be suspected in a patient with clinical signs of infection (fever, purulent sputum, leukocytosis or leukopenia and worsening oxygenation) and a new radiographic infiltrate. Treatment of hospital acquired pneumonia in high-risk patients is guided by institutional microbiological sensitivity data and infectious disease guidelines.

Atrial Fibrillation

Atrial fibrillation is one of the most common post-operative complications following esophageal resection. After ensuring patient stability, the tenants of management of AF include: (1) reducing or stopping catecholaminergic inotropic agents; (2) optimizing fluid balance; and (3) evaluating for the presence of and treating all possible correctable triggering factors. These include bleeding, pulmonary embolism, pneumothorax, pericardial irritation, myocardial infarction, and mediastinal infection secondary to anastomotic leak. In the hemodynamically unstable patient, synchronized cardioversion is indicated. In the hemodynamically stable patient, the immediate goal is rate control (heart rate <110 bpm). Intravenous esmolol, metoprolol, diltiazem, or verapamil are each recommended for use. In the presence of heart failure, esmolol is preferred. If the patient is hypotensive, esmolol or diltiazem are the drugs of choice, whereas in the presence of chronic obstructive pulmonary disease (COPD) or asthma, diltiazem or verapamil are preferred (Fig. 3) [52].

Chylothorax

Injury to the thoracic duct is associated with mortality rates as high as 18% [80, 81]. The diagnosis should be considered in association with high chest tube output or a change in the nature of the effluent—typically a milky appearance following initiation of enteral alimentation. Chyle leak is confirmed with a pleural fluid triglyceride level >110 mg/dl or a fluid triglyceride level of 50 mm/dl and the finding of chylomicrons in the pleural fluid [82, 83]. Once a diagnosis is established, the tenets of management are: (1) drainage of the pleural space; (2) reduction of lymph flow; and (3) maintenance of hydration and nutrition.

Medium chain triglyceride (MCT) diets have been used with variable success. This widely practiced approach is predicated on the fact that MCTs are taken up preferentially by the portal system and thus bypass the thoracic duct system. This effect, however, appears to be mitigated by the fact that oral intake stimulates chyle production. For this reason, many authors advocate complete bowel rest and parenteral nutrition. Octreotide, a somatostatin analog, acts on somatostatin receptors to reduce the flow of thoracic duct lymph by reducing gastric, biliary and pancreatic secretions, and to inhibit absorption from the intestine. It is an effective adjunct to operative or non-operative management [84].

A short course of nonoperative management of a chylothorax with a pleural drainage tube in place is appropriate. However, if the leak persists at >10 ml/kg for more than two to three days, it is unlikely to resolve without further intervention [85]. When non-operative management has failed, postsurgical chylothorax can be effectively managed with thoracic duct ligation. This can be performed by a thoracoscopic or open approach. This decision is based on the clinical scenario and local expertise [86, 87]. In order to identify the leak intraoperatively, dairy cream or olive oil mixed with lipophilic dye may be administered via a nasogastric or jejunal feeding tube 20 min prior to anesthetic induction.

Access to the thoracic duct injury is usually via the side with the chylothorax. However, the approach to esophageal resection, the type of reconstruction, and the unique anatomy of the patient's duct may affect the approach. When the leak is identified, direct ligation of the duct is performed with non-absorbable ligatures above and below the level of injury. If the duct injury cannot be identified then mass ligation is used, which includes all tissues located between the aorta and the azygous vein. This is most easily performed via the right chest just above the diaphragmatic hiatus. In these cases, care is taken not to injure the conduit or its blood supply.

Alternatively, thoracic duct embolization is a nonsurgical method of chylothorax treatment. There are several methods for accessing the cisterna chyli, the most common of which is direct trans-abdominal percutaneous needle cannulation [88–90]. Contrast is used to identify the source of the leak and the affected segment is embolized with coils or glue. Experience with thoracic duct embolization is limited and no randomized trials exist. Given the low morbidity rates and promising case series, this approach may be attempted prior to surgical intervention in centers with appropriate experience.

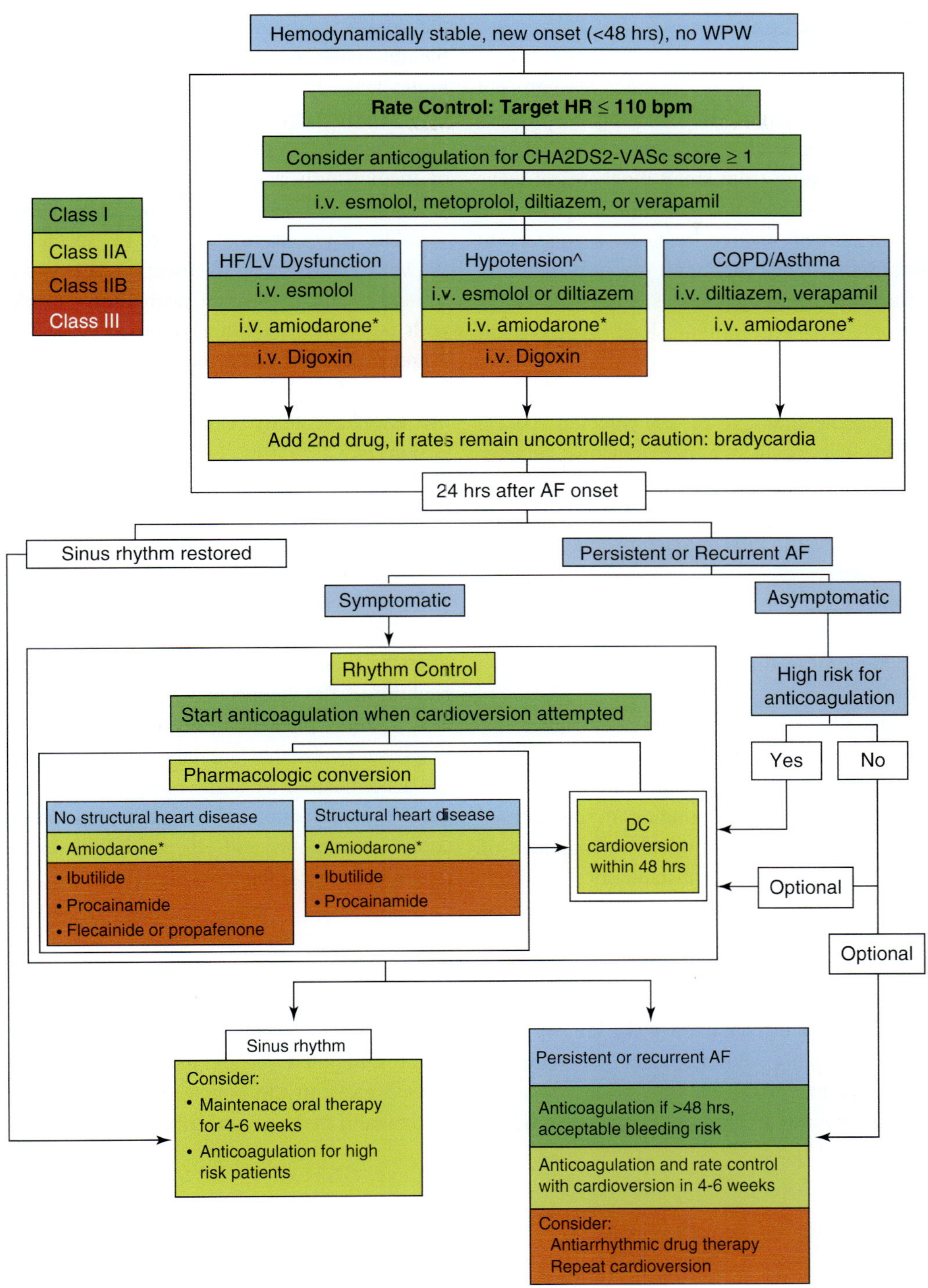

Fig. 3 Management of postoperative atrial fibrillation less than 48 h in duration in a hemodynamically stable patient. Reproduced with permission from Frendl et al. [52]. WPW: Wolff Parkinson White; HR: hear rate; i.v.: intravenous; HR: heart rate; LV: left ventricular; COPD: chronic obstructive pulmonary disease; AF: atrial fibrillation; DC: direct current; TEE: trans esophageal echocardiography

Anastomotic Leak

Anastomotic leak is a dreaded, though not uncommon complication following esophagectomy. Leaks are classified on a spectrum of severity, spanning from small biochemical leaks detected via elevations in drain amylase and minimal clinical change, to leaks secondary to anastomotic dehiscence and conduit necrosis causing life threatening sepsis. The basic tenets of esophageal anastomotic leak management include [91]:

(1) Adequate drainage of any infected spaces. This can occur via percutaneous catheter insertion, surgical exposure, pleural catheter insertion and/or intraluminal drainage such as nasogastric tube or vacuum sponge.
(2) Initiation of broad-spectrum antibiotics often including antifungal agents
(3) Optimizing nutritional status via enteral or parenteral feeding.

For clinically significant leaks, early endoscopy is often indicated to differentiate between anastomotic leaks limited to defects in the anastomosis with healthy surrounding tissues versus conduit necrosis, as the clinical management of these two entities differs substantially.

Contained anastomotic leaks are defined as leaks in which contrast material extravasates outside the alimentary lumen to a limited extent and gathers in a well-defined and small collection. Patients with contained leaks are, by definition, minimally symptomatic. Uncontained leaks are characterized by free extravasation of intraluminal contents into the space surrounding the anastomosis, often with extension into the pleural space or mediastinum. Cervical anastomotic leaks have a low morbidity and mortality rate compared to intrathoracic leaks. This is due primarily to the relatively decreased rates of mediastinitis and empyema. In contrast, the severity of thoracic anastomotic leaks is highly variable, from asymptomatic to severe sepsis with multi-organ dysfunction. Leak severity and extent of conduit necrosis is correlated with outcomes, including survival [92]. Tables 3 and 4 demonstrate a method of classification of esophageal leaks and conduit necrosis by the Esophagectomy Complications Consensus Group (ECCG) [50].

Cervical anastomotic leaks

Small contained cervical leaks are managed with observation and maintenance of a clear liquid diet. Larger contained cervical leaks can often be managed successfully by opening and packing of the wound and less commonly with closed drain placement, if one is not already in place. Leaks that are large, uncontained, or are accompanied by signs of sepsis more often require examination under general anesthesia, copious irrigation and, if possible, attempted repair and muscle flap coverage [93].

Thoracic anastomotic leaks

In the stable patient, initial work-up should include imaging and endoscopic evaluation. Chest computed tomography should be performed early in the course of the treatment to determine if there are undrained fluid collections.

Table 3 Classification of esophageal leaks [50]

Classification	Description
Type I	Local defect requiring no change in therapy or treated medically or with dietary modification
Type II	Localized defect requiring interventional but not surgical therapy; for example, interventional radiology drain, stent or bedside opening, and packing of incision
Type III	Localized defect requiring surgical therapy

Table 4 Classification of esophageal conduit necrosis [50]

Classification	Description
Type I	Conduit necrosis focal Identified endoscopically Treatment is additional monitoring or non-surgical therapy
Type II	Conduit necrosis focal Identified endoscopically and not associated with free anastomotic or conduit leak Treatment is surgical therapy not involving esophageal diversion
Type III	Conduit necrosis extensive Treated with conduit resection with diversion

Endoscopy provides an assessment of the severity of disruption and necrosis as well as enabling interventions such as covered stent placement. Conduit necrosis, if present, is classified using the ECCG grading system (Table 4) [50].

Stents have shown promise in permitting early oral feeding and reduction of leakage of intraluminal contents, while endoluminal sponge vacuum systems have shown excellent control of leaks and enhanced rates of closure [94]. Conversely, there is concern that the radial force of the expandable stent could cause worsening local ischemia [95, 96]. Stent migration occurs in up to 75% of patients, although the problem is less frequent with increased experience and with the use of endoscopic fixation techniques [97]. Stent erosion and ingrowth limit the time that they can be left in place [94, 98].

Decisions on operative management are based on clinical status, the level of extraluminal contamination, and the presence or absence of conduit necrosis. Small, contained leaks can often be managed without intervention and simple NPO status with nutritional supplementation. Conversely, the presence hemodynamic instability, extensive intrathoracic/mediastinal contamination, or Type II or III conduit necrosis requires intervention. This may include thoracostomy tube placement, stenting or other endoluminal therapies, and/or an operation. When an operation is deemed necessary and the leak is not accompanied by extensive conduit necrosis, all devitalized tissue should be debrided from the site. Primary repair of the leak should be considered, even if the diagnosis is delayed. Coverage with a vascularized pedicled flap may aid in healing. The most commonly used flaps include intercostal muscle, latissimus dorsi, serratus anterior, pericardium, pleura, and omentum. The area surrounding the repair should be widely drained. In the rare case of a type III (severe) conduit necrosis, conduit resection and proximal salivary diversion should be performed.

In all cases, if initial management is ineffective, secondary, or tertiary management strategies should be explored. Many surgeons advocate for a "step-up approach" to leak management, beginning with less invasive techniques before proceeding to operative intervention [99]. Regardless of the path chosen, new management strategies should be adopted when faced with failure of initial therapy [92].

Endoluminal vacuum assisted closure (EVAC) devices for anastomotic defects have gained popularity in recent years, offering an alternative to other non-surgical endoluminal therapies, such as stents. The EVAC is a form of negative pressure wound therapy applied to an area of the GI tract via a porous sponge connected to a negative pressure device—typically a nasogastric tube. With a mechanism of action similar to traditional negative pressure therapy, EVACs remove luminal fluid while physically shrinking the defect and driving changes in the wound environment such as angiogenesis and neurogenesis that promote healing [100, 101]. Multiple published case series have demonstrated EVAC assisted closure of anastomotic defects at rates greater than stent-based approaches and with lower morbidity [102–106]. A recent meta-analysis included 18 studies investigating EVAC therapy for esophageal defects and reported a clinical success rate of 89% with an adverse event rate of 13%; 15% of patients needed adjuvant treatment for ongoing leak or complication [107].

Delayed Gastric Emptying

Delayed gastric emptying is common after esophagectomy, occurring in approximately 20% of patients. The etiology is most often multifactorial and thought to be secondary to relative ischemia of the neoesophagus with loss of parasympathetic innervation of the pylorus and transposition of the stomach into the negatively pressured chest. It is important to rule out gastric outlet obstruction by swallow evaluation or endoscopy. When present, delayed gastric emptying can be treated with a step-up approach, utilizing medications, pyloric balloon dilation, and botulinum toxin injection. For patients who do not respond, either pyloromyotomy or peroral endoscopic myotomy is occasionally performed, with good results [108, 109].

Erythromycin is a motilin receptor agonist which induces migrating motor complexes by stimulating the motilin receptors in the gastric antrum and duodenum, resulting in improved gastric emptying. The major limitation of erythromycin is tachyphylaxis (diminishing effectiveness over time) due to down-regulation of motilin receptors. The medication can be held for 2 weeks and then resumed. Metoclopramide is a dopaminergic agonist which is a good second line therapy, although there is a 1% risk of tardive dyskinesia. Patients must be instructed to stop the medication if they develop involuntary body movements. Domperidone is another second line medication that can be prescribed with new investigational drug clearance from the Food and Drug Administration. It has been shown to be as effective as metoclopramide, with less central nervous system side effects. It can prolong the QT interval, and a baseline EKG should be performed [110].

Intermediate-term measures are most appropriate in the immediate postoperative period. Resolution of delayed gastric emptying usually occurs over time, and has been attributed to increased involvement of the myenteric plexus in pyloric function and gastric motility [111]. In instances in which delayed gastric emptying is unremitting despite pharmacologic and endoscopic intervention, pyloromyotomy or pyloroplasty can be considered.

Conclusions

Despite improvements in operative technique and the adoption of minimally invasive approaches, successful esophageal resection demands precise and high-quality perioperative care. Appropriate preoperative risk-stratification can assist in properly identifying suitable candidates for resection and recognizing potentially modifiable risk factors. The application of perioperative ERAS protocols has been shown to reduce adverse outcomes and minimize the impact of surgery on the patient, thus reducing postoperative complications, minimizing length of hospital stay, and lowering costs. Preoperative elements such as high-quality patient education, PONV screening, and minimization of the effects of preoperative fasting prepare patients for surgery. The use of multimodal analgesia, prophylactic antiemetics, judicious fluid administration, and permissive oliguria are important in the operative phase. Post-operative elements include early ambulation, multimodal pain control, and early alimentation. When postoperative complications occur, prompt identification and appropriate management can reduce their negative sequelae.

References

1. Wright CD, Kucharczuk JC, O'Brien SM, Grab JD, Allen MS. Predictors of major morbidity and mortality after esophagectomy for esophageal cancer: a society of thoracic surgeons general thoracic surgery database risk adjustment model. J Thorac Cardiovasc Surg. 2009;137(3):587–96.
2. Low DE, Kuppusamy MK, Alderson D, Cecconello I, Chang AC, Darling G, et al. Benchmarking complications associated with esophagectomy. Ann Surg. 2019;269(2):291–8.

3. Finks JF, Osborne NH, Birkmeyer JD. Trends in hospital volume and operative mortality for high-risk surgery. N Engl J Med. 2011;364(22):2128–37.

4. Greco M, Capretti G, Beretta L, Gemma M, Pecorelli N, Braga M. Enhanced recovery program in colorectal surgery: a meta-analysis of randomized controlled trials. World J Surg. 2014;38:1531–41.

5. Nicholson A, Lowe M, Parker J, Lewis S, Alderson P, Smith A. Systematic review and meta-analysis of enhanced recovery programmes in surgical patients. Br J Surg. 2014;101(3):172–88.

6. Lemanu D, Singh P, Stowers M, Hill A. A systematic review to assess cost effectiveness of enhanced recovery after surgery programmes in colorectal surgery. Colorectal Dis. 2014;16(5):338–46.

7. Joliat G-R, Labgaa I, Petermann D, Hübner M, Griesser A-C, Demartines N, et al. Cost–benefit analysis of an enhanced recovery protocol for pancreaticoduodenectomy. Br J Surg. 2015;102(13):1676–83.

8. Shewale JB, Correa AM, Baker CM, Villafane-Ferriol N, Hofstetter WL, Jordan VS, et al. Impact of a fast-track esophagectomy protocol on esophageal cancer patient outcomes and hospital charges. Ann Surg. 2015;261(6):1114–23.

9. Underwood TJ, Noble F, Madhusudan N, Sharland D, Fraser R, Owsley J, et al. The development, application and analysis of an enhanced recovery programme for major oesophagogastric resection. J Gastrointest Surg. 2017;21:614–21.

10. Munitiz V, Martinez-de-Haro LF, Ortiz A, Ruiz-de-Angulo D, Pastor P, Parrilla P. Effectiveness of a written clinical pathway for enhanced recovery after transthoracic (Ivor Lewis) oesophagectomy. Br J Surg. 2010;97(5):714–8.

11. Cao S, Zhao G, Cui J, Dong Q, Qi S, Xin Y, et al. Fast-track rehabilitation program and conventional care after esophagectomy: a retrospective controlled cohort study. Support Care Cancer. 2013;21(3):707–14.

12. Cerfolio RJ, Bryant AS, Bass CS, Alexander JR, Bartolucci AA. Fast tracking after Ivor Lewis esophagogastrectomy. Chest. 2004;126(4):1187–94.

13. Parise P, Ferrari C, Cossu A, Puccetti F, Elmore U, De Pascale S, et al. Enhanced recovery after surgery (ERAS) pathway in esophagectomy: is a reasonable prediction of hospital stay possible? Ann Surg. 2019;270(1):77–83.

14. Nishigori T, Okabe H, Tanaka E, Tsunoda S, Hisamori S, Sakai Y. Sarcopenia as a predictor of pulmonary complications after esophagectomy for thoracic esophageal cancer. J Surg Oncol. 2016;113(6):678–84.

15. Elliott JA, Doyle SL, Murphy CF, King S, Guinan EM, Beddy P, et al. Sarcopenia: prevalence, and impact on operative and oncologic outcomes in the multimodal management of locally advanced esophageal cancer. Ann Surg. 2017;266(5):822–30.

16. Boshier PR, Heneghan R, Markar SR, Baracos VE, Low DE. Assessment of body composition and sarcopenia in patients with esophageal cancer: a systematic review and meta-analysis. Dis Esophagus. 2018;31(8).

17. Halliday LJ, Boshier PR, Doganay E, Wynter-Blyth V, Buckley JP, Moorthy K. The effects of prehabilitation on body composition in patients undergoing multimodal therapy for esophageal cancer. Dis Esophagus. 2022;36(2).

18. Knops AM, Legemate DA, Goossens A, Bossuyt PM, Ubbink DT. Decision aids for patients facing a surgical treatment decision: a systematic review and meta-analysis. Ann Surg. 2013;257(5):860–6.

19. Oshima Lee E, Emanuel EJ. Shared decision making to improve care and reduce costs. N Engl J Med. 2013;368(1):6–8.

20. de Mik SML, Stubenrouch FE, Balm R, Ubbink DT. Systematic review of shared decision-making in surgery. Br J Surg. 2018;105(13):1721–30.

21. Mastracci TM, Carli F, Finley RJ, Muccio S, Warner DO, Group E-BRiS. Effect of preoperative smoking cessation interventions on postoperative complications. J Am College Surg. 2011;212(6):1094–6.

22. Mills E, Eyawo O, Lockhart I, Kelly S, Wu P, Ebbert JO. Smoking cessation reduces postoperative complications: a systematic review and meta-analysis. Am J Med. 2011;124(2):144–54.e8.

23. Wong J, Abrishami A, Matthew T, Chan V, Chung F. Short-term preoperative smoking cessation and postoperative complications: a systematic review and meta-analysis. Can J Anaesth. 2012;59(3):268–79.

24. Levett DZ, Grocott MP. Cardiopulmonary exercise testing, prehabilitation, and enhanced recovery after surgery (ERAS). Can J Anaesth. 2015;62(2):131–42.

25. Chen K-N. Managing complications I: leaks, strictures, emptying, reflux, chylothorax. J Thorac Dis. 2014;6(Suppl 3):S355–63.

26. Weissman C. The metabolic response to stress: an overview and update. Anesthesiology. 1990;73(2):308–27.

27. Ljungqvist O. Modulating postoperative insulin resistance by preoperative carbohydrate loading. Best Pract Res Clin Anaesthesiol. 2009;23(4):401–9.

28. Svanfeldt M, Thorell A, Hausel J, Soop M, Rooyackers O, Nygren J, et al. Randomized clinical trial of the effect of preoperative oral carbohydrate treatment on postoperative whole-body protein and glucose kinetics. Br J Surg. 2007;94(11):1342–50.

29. McClave SA, Heyland DK. The physiologic response and associated clinical benefits from provision of early enteral nutrition. Nutr Clin Pract. 2009;24(3):305–15.

30. Practice guidelines for preoperative fasting and the use of pharmacologic agents to reduce the risk

of pulmonary aspiration: application to healthy patients undergoing elective procedures: an updated report by the American Society of Anesthesiologists Task Force on Preoperative Fasting and the Use of Pharmacologic Agents to Reduce the Risk of Pulmonary Aspiration. Anesthesiology. 2017;126(3):376–93.

31. Bilku D, Dennison A, Hall T, Metcalfe M, Garcea G. Role of preoperative carbohydrate loading: a systematic review. Ann R Coll Surg Engl. 2014;96(1):15–22.

32. Apfel CC, Läärä E, Koivuranta M, Greim C-A, Roewer N. A simplified risk score for predicting postoperative nausea and vomiting: conclusions from cross-validations between two centers. J Am Soc Anesthesiologists. 1999;91(3):693.

33. Schaefer M, Apfel C, Sachs H-J, Stuttmann R, Bein B, Tonner P, et al. Predictors for postoperative nausea and vomiting after xenon-based anaesthesia. Br J Anaesth. 2015;115(1):61–7.

34. D'Journo XB, Boulate D, Fourdrain A, Loundou A, van Berge Henegouwen MI, Gisbertz SS, et al. Risk prediction model of 90-day mortality after esophagectomy for cancer. JAMA Surg. 2021;156(9):836–45.

35. Inoue J, Ono R, Makiura D, Kashiwa-Motoyama M, Miura Y, Usami M, et al. Prevention of postoperative pulmonary complications through intensive preoperative respiratory rehabilitation in patients with esophageal cancer. Dis Esophagus. 2013;26(1):68–74.

36. Schieman C, Wigle D, Deschamps C, Nichols Iii F, Cassivi S, Shen K, et al. Patterns of operative mortality following esophagectomy. Dis Esophagus. 2012;25(7):645–51.

37. Swanson SJ, Batirel HF, Bueno R, Jaklitsch MT, Lukanich JM, Allred E, et al. Transthoracic esophagectomy with radical mediastinal and abdominal lymph node dissection and cervical esophagogastrostomy for esophageal carcinoma. Ann Thorac Surg. 2001;72(6):1918–25.

38. Abou-Jawde RM, Mekhail T, Adelstein DJ, Rybicki LA, Mazzone PJ, Caroll MA, et al. Impact of induction concurrent chemoradiotherapy on pulmonary function and postoperative acute respiratory complications in esophageal cancer. Chest. 2005;128(1):250–5.

39. Ferguson MK, Celauro AD, Prachand V. Prediction of major pulmonary complications after esophagectomy. Ann Thorac Surg. 2011;91(5):1494–501.

40. Browner WS, Li J, Mangano DT, Hollenberg M, Tubau JF, Leung JM, et al. In-hospital and long-term mortality in male veterans following noncardiac surgery. JAMA. 1992;268(2):228–32.

41. Wightman S, Posner M, Patti M, Ganai S, Watson S, Prachand V, et al. Extremes of body mass index and postoperative complications after esophagectomy. Dis Esophagus. 2017;30(5).

42. Reinersman JM, Allen MS, Deschamps C, Ferguson MK, Nichols FC, Shen KR, et al. External validation of the Ferguson pulmonary risk score for predicting major pulmonary complications after oesophagectomy. Eur J Cardiothorac Surg. 2016;49(1):333–8.

43. Elliott JA, O'Byrne L, Foley G, Murphy CF, Doyle SL, King S, et al. Effect of neoadjuvant chemoradiation on preoperative pulmonary physiology, postoperative respiratory complications and quality of life in patients with oesophageal cancer. Br J Surg. 2019;106(10):1341–51.

44. Goense L, Meziani J, Bülbül M, Braithwaite SA, van Hillegersberg R, Ruurda JP. Pulmonary diffusion capacity predicts major complications after esophagectomy for patients with esophageal cancer. Dis Esophagus. 2018;32(3).

45. Hasegawa T, Kubo N, Ohira M, Sakurai K, Toyokawa T, Yamashita Y, et al. Impact of body mass index on surgical outcomes after esophagectomy for patients with esophageal squamous cell carcinoma. J Gastrointest Surg. 2015;19:226–33.

46. Mitzman B, Schipper PH, Edwards MA, Kim S, Ferguson MK. Complications after esophagectomy are associated with extremes of body mass index. Ann Thorac Surg. 2018;106(4):973–80.

47. Kulkarni S, Fletcher E, McConnell A, Poskitt K, Whyman M. Pre-operative inspiratory muscle training preserves postoperative inspiratory muscle strength following major abdominal surgery—a randomised pilot study. Ann R Coll Surg Engl. 2010;92(8):700–5.

48. Dettling DS, van der Schaaf M, Blom RL, Nollet F, Busch OR, van Berge Henegouwen MI. Feasibility and effectiveness of pre-operative inspiratory muscle training in patients undergoing oesophagectomy: a pilot study. Physiother Res Int. 2013;18(1):16–26.

49. Soutome S, Yanamoto S, Funahara M, Hasegawa T, Komori T, Yamada S-I, et al. Effect of perioperative oral care on prevention of postoperative pneumonia associated with esophageal cancer surgery: a multicenter case–control study with propensity score matching analysis. Medicine. 2017;96(33).

50. Low DE, Alderson D, Cecconello I, Chang AC, Darling GE, D'Journo XB, et al. International consensus on standardization of data collection for complications associated with esophagectomy. Ann Surg. 2015;262(2):286–94.

51. Murthy SC, Law S, Whooley BP, Alexandrou A, Chu K-M, Wong J. Atrial fibrillation after esophagectomy is a marker for postoperative morbidity and mortality. J Thorac Cardiovasc Surg. 2003;126(4):1162–7.

52. Frendl G, Sodickson AC, Chung MK, Waldo AL, Gersh BJ, Tisdale JE, et al. 2014 AATS guidelines for the prevention and management of perioperative atrial fibrillation and flutter for thoracic

surgical procedures. J Thorac Cardiovasc Surg. 2014;148(3):e153–93.

53. Fleisher LA, Fleischmann KE, Auerbach AD, Barnason SA, Beckman JA, Bozkurt B, et al. 2014 ACC/AHA guideline on perioperative cardiovascular evaluation and management of patients undergoing noncardiac surgery: a report of the American College of Cardiology/American Heart Association Task Force on practice guidelines. J Am Coll Cardiol. 2014;64(22):e77–137.

54. Hanna NM, Williams E, Kong W, Fundytus A, Booth CM, Patel SV, et al. Incidence, timing, and outcomes of venous thromboembolism in patients undergoing surgery for esophagogastric cancer: a population-based cohort study. Ann Surg Oncol. 2022;29(7):4393–404.

55. Martin JT, Mahan AL, Ferraris VA, Saha SP, Mullett TW, Zwischenberger JB, et al. Identifying esophagectomy patients at risk for predischarge versus postdischarge venous thromboembolism. Ann Thorac Surg. 2015;100(3):932–8.

56. De Martino RR, Goodney PP, Spangler EL, Wallaert JB, Corriere MA, Rzucidlo EM, et al. Variation in thromboembolic complications among patients undergoing commonly performed cancer operations. J Vasc Surg. 2012;55(4):1035-40.e4.

57. Gustafsson U, Scott M, Schwenk W, Demartines N, Roulin D, Francis N, et al. Guidelines for perioperative care in elective colonic surgery: enhanced recovery after surgery (ERAS®) society recommendations. World J Surg. 2013;37:259–84.

58. Fearon K, Ljungqvist O, Von Meyenfeldt M, Revhaug A, Dejong C, Lassen K, et al. Enhanced recovery after surgery: a consensus review of clinical care for patients undergoing colonic resection. Clin Nutr. 2005;24(3):466–77.

59. Lobo DN, Bostock KA, Neal KR, Perkins AC, Rowlands BJ, Allison SP. Effect of salt and water balance on recovery of gastrointestinal function after elective colonic resection: a randomised controlled trial. Lancet. 2002;359(9320):1812–8.

60. Miller TE, Roche AM, Mythen MG. Fluid management and goal-directed therapy as an adjunct to enhanced recovery after surgery (ERAS). Can J Anesth. 2016;62(2):158–68.

61. Kurz A, Sessler DI, Lenhardt R. Perioperative normothermia to reduce the incidence of surgical-wound infection and shorten hospitalization. N Engl J Med. 1996;334(19):1209–16.

62. Frank SM, Fleisher LA, Breslow MJ, Higgins MS, Olson KF, Kelly S, et al. Perioperative maintenance of normothermia reduces the incidence of morbid cardiac events. A randomized clinical trial. JAMA. 1997;277(14):1127–34.

63. Nesher N, Zisman E, Wolf T, Sharony R, Bolotin G, David M, et al. Strict thermoregulation attenuates myocardial injury during coronary artery bypass graft surgery as reflected by reduced levels of cardiac-specific troponin I. Anesth Analg. 2003;96(2):328–35.

64. Schmied H, Reiter A, Kurz A, Sessler D, Kozek S. Mild hypothermia increases blood loss and transfusion requirements during total hip arthroplasty. Lancet. 1996;347(8997):289–92.

65. Gottschalk A, Durieux ME, Nemergut EC. Intraoperative methadone improves postoperative pain control in patients undergoing complex spine surgery. Anesth Analg. 2011;112(1):218–23.

66. Yeung JH, Gates S, Naidu BV, Wilson MJ, Smith FG. Paravertebral block versus thoracic epidural for patients undergoing thoracotomy. Cochrane Database Syst Rev. 2016;2(2):CD009121.

67. Wren SM, Martin M, Yoon JK, Bech F. Postoperative pneumonia-prevention program for the inpatient surgical ward. J Am Coll Surg. 2010;210(4):491–5.

68. Giacopuzzi S, Weindelmayer J, Treppiedi E, Bencivenga M, Ceola M, Priolo S, et al. Enhanced recovery after surgery protocol in patients undergoing esophagectomy for cancer: a single center experience. Dis Esophagus. 2017;30(4):1–6.

69. D'Journo X, Ouattara M, Loundou A, Trousse D, Dahan L, Nathalie T, et al. Prognostic impact of weight loss in 1-year survivors after transthoracic esophagectomy for cancer. Dis Esophagus. 2012;25(6):527–34.

70. Cools-Lartigue J, Jones D, Spicer J, Zourikian T, Rousseau M, Eckert E, et al. Management of dysphagia in esophageal adenocarcinoma patients undergoing neoadjuvant chemotherapy: can invasive tube feeding be avoided? Ann Surg Oncol. 2015;22(6):1858–65.

71. Barlow AD, Thomas DC. Autophagy in diabetes: β-cell dysfunction, insulin resistance, and complications. DNA Cell Biol. 2015;34(4):252–60.

72. Weijs TJ, Kumagai K, Berkelmans GHK, Nieuwenhuijzen GAP, Nilsson M, Luyer MDP. Nasogastric decompression following esophagectomy: a systematic literature review and meta-analysis. Dis Esophagus. 2017;30(3):1–8.

73. Berkelmans GHK, Fransen LFC, Dolmans-Zwartjes ACP, Kouwenhoven EA, van Det MJ, Nilsson M, et al. Direct oral feeding following minimally invasive esophagectomy (NUTRIENT II trial): an international, multicenter, open-label randomized controlled trial. Ann Surg. 2020;271(1):41–7.

74. Sun H-B, Li Y, Liu X-B, Zhang R-X, Wang Z-F, Lerut T, et al. Early oral feeding following mckeown minimally invasive esophagectomy: an open-label, randomized, controlled, noninferiority trial. Ann Surg. 2018;267(3):435–42.

75. Nederlof N, de Jonge J, de Vringer T, Tran T, Spaander M, Tilanus H, et al. Does routine endoscopy or contrast swallow study after esophagectomy and gastric tube reconstruction change patient management? J Gastrointest Surg. 2017;21:251–8.

76. Biere S, Maas K, Cuesta M, Van Der Peet D. Cervical or thoracic anastomosis after esophagectomy for cancer: a systematic review and meta-analysis. Dig Surg. 2011;28(1):29–35.

77. Squadrone V, Coha M, Cerutti E, Schellino MM, Biolino P, Occella P, et al. Continuous positive airway pressure for treatment of postoperative hypoxemia: a randomized controlled trial. JAMA. 2005;293(5):589–95.

78. Milledge J. Therapeutic fibreoptic bronchoscopy in intensive care. BMJ. 1976;2(6049):1427–9.

79. Radu DM, Jauréguy F, Seguin A, Foulon C, Destable MD, Azorin J, et al. Postoperative pneumonia after major pulmonary resections: an unsolved problem in thoracic surgery. Ann Thorac Surg. 2007;84(5):1669–73.

80. Shah RD, Luketich JD, Schuchert MJ, Christie NA, Pennathur A, Landreneau RJ, et al. Postesophagectomy chylothorax: incidence, risk factors, and outcomes. Ann Thorac Surg. 2012;93(3):897–904.

81. Bolger C, Walsh T, Tanner W, Keeling P, Hennessy T. Chylothorax after oesophagectomy. Br J Surg. 1991;78(5):587–8.

82. Maldonado F, Hawkins FJ, Daniels CE, Doerr CH, Decker PA, Ryu JH. Pleural fluid characteristics of chylothorax. Mayo Clin Proc. 2009;84(2):129–33.

83. Kim D, Cho J, Kim K, Shim YM. Chyle leakage patterns and management after oncologic esophagectomy: a retrospective cohort study. Thorac Cancer. 2014;5(5):391–7.

84. Ismail NA, Gordon J, Dunning J. The use of octreotide in the treatment of chylothorax following cardiothoracic surgery. Interact Cardiovasc Thorac Surg. 2015;20(6):848–54.

85. Dugue L, Sauvanet A, Farges O, Goharin A, Le Mee J, Belghiti J. Output of chyle as an indicator of treatment for chylothorax complicating oesophagectomy. Br J Surg. 1998;85(8):1147–9.

86. Fahimi H, Casselman FP, Mariani MA, van Boven WJ, Knaepen PJ, van Swieten HA. Current management of postoperative chylothorax. Ann Thorac Surg. 2001;71(2):448–50.

87. Zabeck H, Muley T, Dienemann H, Hoffmann H. Management of chylothorax in adults: when is surgery indicated? Thorac Cardiovasc Surg. 2011;59(04):243–6.

88. Cerfolio RJ, Allen MS, Deschamps C, Trastek VF, Pairolero PC. Postoperative chylothorax. J Thorac Cardiovasc Surg. 1996;112(5):1361–6.

89. Nadolski GJ, Itkin M. Thoracic duct embolization for nontraumatic chylous effusion: experience in 34 patients. Chest. 2013;143(1):158–63.

90. Guevara CJ, Rialon KL, Ramaswamy RS, Kim SK, Darcy MD. US–guided, direct puncture retrograde thoracic duct access, lymphangiography, and embolization: feasibility and efficacy. J Vasc Interv Radiol. 2016;27(12):1890–6.

91. Martin LW, Hofstetter W, Swisher SG, Roth JA. Management of intrathoracic leaks following esophagectomy. Adv Surg. 2006;40:173–90.

92. Collaborative O-GASGobotWMR. Rates of anastomotic complications and their management following esophagectomy: results of the Oesophago-Gastric Anastomosis Audit (OGAA). Ann Surg. 2022;275(2):e382–e91.

93. Ferguson M. Reconstructive surgery of the esophagus. Wiley-Blackwell; 2002.

94. Freeman RK, Van Woerkom JM, Vyverberg A, Ascioti AJ. Esophageal stent placement for the treatment of spontaneous esophageal perforations. Ann Thorac Surg. 2009;88(1):194–8.

95. D'Cunha J, Rueth NM, Groth SS, Maddaus MA, Andrade RS. Esophageal stents for anastomotic leaks and perforations. J Thorac Cardiovasc Surg. 2011;142(1):39–46.e1.

96. Langer FB, Wenzl E, Prager G, Salat A, Miholic J, Mang T, et al. Management of postoperative esophageal leaks with the Polyflex self-expanding covered plastic stent. Ann Thorac Surg. 2005;79(2):398–403.

97. Sharma P, Kozarek R, Gastroenterology PPCotACo. Role of esophageal stents in benign and malignant diseases. Am J Gastroenterol. 2010;105(2):258–73.

98. Schweigert M, Solymosi N, Dubecz A, GonzáLez MP, Stein HJ, Ofner D. One decade of experience with endoscopic stenting for intrathoracic anastomotic leakage after esophagectomy: brilliant breakthrough or flash in the pan? Am Surg. 2014;80(8):736–45.

99. Ubels S, Matthée E, Verstegen M, Klarenbeek B, Bouwense S, van Berge Henegouwen MI, et al. Practice variation in anastomotic leak after esophagectomy: unravelling differences in failure to rescue. Eur J Surg Oncol. 2023;S0748–7983(23)00032-X.

100. Moore CB, Almoghrabi O, Hofstetter W, Veeramachaneni N. Endoluminal wound vac: an evolving role in treatment of esophageal perforation. J Visualized Surg. 2020;6. https://doi.org/10.21037/jovs.2020.01.04

101. Argenta LC, Morykwas MJ. Vacuum-assisted closure: a new method for wound control and treatment: clinical experience. Ann Plast Surg. 1997;38(6):563–77.

102. Berlth F, Bludau M, Plum PS, Herbold T, Christ H, Alakus H, et al. Self-expanding metal stents versus endoscopic vacuum therapy in anastomotic leak treatment after oncologic gastroesophageal surgery. J Gastrointest Surg. 2019;23:67–75.

103. Brangewitz M, Voigtländer T, Helfritz F, Lankisch T, Winkler M, Klempnauer J, et al. Endoscopic closure of esophageal intrathoracic leaks: stent versus endoscopic vacuum-assisted closure, a retrospective analysis. Endoscopy. 2013;45(06):433–8.

104. Mennigen R, Harting C, Lindner K, Vowinkel T, Rijcken E, Palmes D, et al. Comparison of

endoscopic vacuum therapy versus stent for anastomotic leak after esophagectomy. J Gastrointest Surg. 2015;19:1229–35.

105. Hwang JJ, Jeong YS, Park YS, Yoon H, Shin CM, Kim N, et al. Comparison of endoscopic vacuum therapy and endoscopic stent implantation with self-expandable metal stent in treating postsurgical gastroesophageal leakage. Medicine. 2016;95(16).

106. Kuckelman J, Bryan D, Wiener D. Endoluminal vacuum therapy for definitive management of an esophagobronchial fistula. Ann Thorac Surg. 2022;113(2):669–73.

107. Aziz M, Haghbin H, Sharma S, Weissman S, Saleem S, Lee-Smith W, et al. Safety and effectiveness of endoluminal vacuum-assisted closure for esophageal defects: systematic review and meta-analysis. Endoscopy Int Open. 2021;9(9):e1371–80.

108. Lanuti M, DeDelva P, Morse CR, Wright CD, Wain JC, Gaissert HA, et al. Management of delayed gastric emptying after esophagectomy with endoscopic balloon dilatation of the pylorus. Ann Thorac Surg. 2011;91(4):1019–24.

109. Zhang R, Zhang L. Management of delayed gastric conduit emptying after esophagectomy. J Thorac Dis. 2019;11(1):302–7.

110. Camilleri M, Parkman HP, Shafi MA, Abell TL, Gerson L. Clinical guideline: management of gastroparesis. Am J Gastroenterol. 2013;108(1):18–37.

111. Smith DS, Williams CS, Ferris CD. Diagnosis and treatment of chronic gastroparesis and chronic intestinal pseudo-obstruction. Gastroenterol Clin. 2003;32(2):619–58.

Quality of Life After Esophagectomy

Francisco Schlottmann, Fernando A. M. Herbella and Marco G. Patti

Abstract

Esophagectomy for esophageal cancer is a complex operation which involves working in the abdomen, chest and often in the neck. The stomach is the preferred esophageal substitute. Transhiatal esophagectomy, Ivor Lewis esophagectomy, and McKeown esophagectomy are the techniques most frequently used (open or minimally invasive). When lymph node involvement is suspected during the pre-operative staging, neoadjuvant therapy is used. While in the past the focus was mostly on survival, today importance has also been given to the quality of life as often the operation is associated to longer survival. This is particularly true when the esophagectomy is performed for early-stage tumors discovered during follow-up for Barrett's esophagus or in patients who had a complete response to neo-adjuvant therapy. This chapter will focus on the factors that may influence the quality of life after the operation.

Keywords

Esophageal cancer · Survival · Disease free survival · Complications · Quality of life · Open esophagectomy · Minimally invasive esophagectomy

Introduction

The incidence of esophageal cancer, particularly esophageal adenocarcinoma, is expected to rise dramatically in many Western countries. Surgical resection, often after neo-adjuvant therapy, is the cornerstone of curative treatment. Although there has been a significant improvement in operative techniques and postoperative care, esophagectomy remains one of the most demanding surgical procedures, with significant associated morbidity and mortality.

While in the past the focus was mostly on survival, today importance has also been given to the quality of life as often the operation is associated to a longer survival. This is particularly true when the esophagectomy is performed for early-stage tumors discovered during follow-up for Barrett's esophagus or in patients

F. Schlottmann (✉)
Department of Surgery, Hospital Alemán of Buenos Aires, Buenos Aires, Argentina
e-mail: fschlottmann@hotmail.com

F. Schlottmann
Department of Surgery, University of Illinois at Chicago, Chicago, IL, USA

F. A. M. Herbella
Escola Paulista de Medicina, Sao Paulo, Brazil

M. G. Patti
Department of Surgery, University of Virginia, Charlottesville, VA, USA

"

who had a complete response to neo-adjuvant therapy.

While overall survival and disease-free survival are easy concepts to understand and measure, health related quality of life (HRQL) is a more complex concept. HRQL is, in fact, a multidimensional concept that includes physical, emotional, mental, and social elements.

This chapter will focus on the factors that may influence the quality of life after esophagectomy.

Preoperative Comorbid Conditions

It has been shown that preoperative comorbid conditions affect the HRQL after esophagectomy. Djarv and colleagues in Sweden conducted a prospective, population based, nationwide study of patients who underwent esophagectomy for cancer between April 2001 and December 2005 [1]. Survival data were assessed through the Swedish Register of the Total Population; 56% of patients had preoperative comorbidities. Regarding the effect of any comorbidity on HRQL, the selected aspects were global quality of life, physical function, emotional function, social function, fatigue, and dyspnea. The most common comorbidities were cardiac (28%) followed by diabetes (25%) and pulmonary (22%). The study showed that patients with comorbidities had a clinically and statistically poorer global quality of life compared with those without comorbidities. Specifically, the presence of preoperative cardiac comorbidities was associated with worse postoperative dyspnea and fatigue [1]. In a similar study, Backemar and colleagues found that among 136 patients after esophagectomy, those with 3 or more comorbidities at the time of surgery had poorer global quality of life and physical function and more fatigue compared with those without comorbidities [2]. Patients with ASA III–IV reported more problems with the above aspects of the HRQL and worse social function and pain compared with those with

ASA I–II. Cardiac comorbidities were associated with worse quality of life and dyspnea, while pulmonary comorbidities were associated with coughing [2]. Both studies stress the importance of discussing with patients before surgery the potential detrimental effect of these comorbidities on the postoperative quality of life. Comorbidities, particularly previous myocardial infarction and congestive heart failure, are also associated with increase mortality after esophagectomy for cancer [3].

Preserving functional capacity is a key element in the care continuum for patients with esophagogastric cancer. In a prospective and randomized trial from McGill University, Minnella and colleagues showed that pre-habilitation (a preoperative conditioning by exercise and proper nutrition) improved the functional capacity both before surgery and after surgery, avoiding a physical and nutritional status decline [4].

Neoadjuvant Therapy

The CROSS trial clearly showed that neoadjuvant therapy (chemotherapy and radiation therapy) followed by surgery determines an increased in survival in patients with locally advanced esophageal cancer as compared to surgery alone [5]. Initially there was some concern about the effect of this regimen on postoperative HRQL, as a decline was seen in the global quality of life, physical function, fatigue, nutrition, and emotional problems one week after completion of therapy. However, an analysis of the results of the initial trial showed that there was no effect of the neoadjuvant treatment on the HRQL in the postoperative period as compared with patients who had surgery alone [6]. These findings were confirmed by other studies which showed that chemoradiation does not have an adverse effect on the postoperative quality of life after esophagectomy [7, 8], and therefore should be considered standard of care for patients with locally advanced esophageal cancer.

Postoperative Complications

Many patients experience complications after esophagectomy. A national cohort study from the Netherlands showed that complications occurred in 1046 of 1617 esophagectomy patients (65%). Of these patients, 468 (29%) had a major complication. Most common complications were pneumonia (19%), esophageal anastomotic leak, staple line, or localized conduit necrosis (19%), and atrial dysrhythmia (15%). The 30-day mortality was 1.7% [9].

There is no consensus on how postoperative complications affect long-term quality of life. Derogar and colleagues used the Swedish Esophageal and Cardia cancer register to assess the influence of major postoperative complications (respiratory failure, pneumonia, anastomotic leak, myocardial infarction, stroke) on HRQL among patients that had survived 5 years after the operation. Among 141 patients, 33% had sustained a major complication. Dyspnea, fatigue, and eating restrictions deteriorated more during the follow-up period in patients with major postoperative complications compared with patients without major complications. They concluded that the occurrence of postoperative complications exerts a long-lasting detrimental effect on HRQL in patients who survive 5 years after esophagectomy for cancer [10].

A more recent study from Sweden has assessed the effect of medical (pneumonia, respiratory failure, myocardial infarction, renal and liver insufficiency) and surgical complications (anastomotic leak, major bleeding, splenectomy, severe lymph leakage, empyema) on HRQL after esophagectomy for cancer. At long-term follow-up (up to 10 years), the HRQL was worse in patients with medical complications, while in patients with surgical complications the HRQL was worse up to 5 years after surgery but eventually the effect decreased after 5 years [11].

Other studies, however, have reached different conclusions showing that postoperative complications after esophagectomy for cancer were not associated with short- or long-term decreased HRQL [12, 13].

Operative Approach and HRQL

An Ivor Lewis esophagectomy, performed through a laparotomy and a right thoracotomy has been considered standard of care for many decades. The operation, however, was associated to some long-term problems such as development of abdominal ventral hernia or post-thoracotomy pain. During the last decade, minimally invasive techniques using laparoscopy and thoracoscopy have being slowly replacing the open approach as it has been shown that a minimally invasive esophagectomy (MIE) is associated with reduced perioperative morbidity while having the same oncologic outcomes of an open esophagectomy [14].

The effect of a MIE on quality of life is more controversial. Kauppila and colleagues recently performed a meta-analysis of HRQL after MIE versus open esophagectomy for esophageal cancer. They included in their qualitative analysis 9 studies involving 1157 patients who had MIE and 907 patients who underwent open surgery. MIE resulted in better scores for global quality of life, physical function, and pain compared with open surgery at 3 months follow-up. However, at long-term follow-up of 6 and 12 months no significant differences remained [15].

Klevebro and colleagues compared the HRQL following totally-MIE (laparoscopy and thoracoscopy), hybrid minimally invasive esophagectomy (thoracoscopic/open abdomen or laparoscopic/open chest) and open esophagectomy (open abdomen and open chest). Of the 246 patients recruited, 153 underwent a minimally invasive esophagectomy, 75 hybrid and 78 totally MIE. After adjusting for age, sex, Charlson comorbidity index, pathologic stage and neo-adjuvant therapy, at 2-year follow-up there were not clinically and statistically significant differences in overall or disease-specific HRQL among the 3 techniques [16].

Esophageal Cancer Surgery: Importance of Center and Surgeon Volume

The relationship between hospital operative volume and postoperative mortality rates after complex surgical procedures has been clearly established [17–19]. Specifically, it has been shown that operative volume is an important determinant of quality of care for esophagectomy, suggesting that centralization of esophageal cancer surgery may improve the quality of care. Schlottmann and colleagues recently determined that a spontaneous centralization of esophageal cancer surgery has occurred in the last 2 decades in the United States, determining a reduction in mortality without causing health disparities [20]. The authors found that the percentage of esophagectomies performed at high volume centers increased from 29.2 to 68.5%, while the percentage at low- and intermediate volume hospitals decreased from 24.9 to 9.6% and from 45.9 to 21.9% respectively. During the same period, the operative mortality rate decreased from 10% in 2000 to 3.5% in 2011. The lower mortality in high volume centers is probably due to the presence of experienced multidisciplinary groups and an increased ability to rescue. The high-volume hospitals were also associated with less postoperative morbidity and shorter length of hospital stay.

In addition to the hospital volume, many studies have demonstrated the importance of the surgeon's volume for both postoperative complications and survival [21–24]. Dolan and colleagues from the Brigham and Women's hospital examined the short and long-term outcomes among high volume ($\geq$7 cases/year) and low volume esophagectomy surgeons (<7/year) [24]. In total, 1029 cases were evaluated; 120 performed by low volume surgeons and 909 by high volume surgeons. Low volume surgeons did more open cases, and had more

complications than high volume surgeons, specifically, grade II and III complications were more frequent. A possible explanation for the higher complication rate is that low volume surgeons performed fewer MIE (30% vs 70%). In addition, the conversion rate to open surgery was higher among the low volume group.

Conclusions

Esophageal resection for cancer is a challenging procedure associated with significant morbidity and mortality. The best results are obtained in centers that perform a large number procedures every year, where patients are evaluated and treated by a multidisciplinary group and operated by experienced surgeons.

References

1. Djarv T, Derogar M, Lagergren P. Influence of co-morbidity on long-term quality of life after oesophagectomy for cancer. Br J Surg. 2014;101:495–501.
2. Backemar L, Johar A, Wikman A, et al. The influence of comorbidity on health-related quality of life after esophageal cancer surgery. Ann Surg Oncol. 2020;27:2637–45.
3. Backemar L, Lagergren P, Johar A, Lagergren J. Impact of comorbidity on mortality after oesophageal cancer surgery. Br J Surg. 2015;102:1097–105.
4. Minnella EM, Awasthi R, Loiselle SE, et al. Effect of exercise and nutrition prehabilitation on functional capacity in esophagogastric cancer surgery. A randomized clinical trial. JAMA Surg. 2018;153:1081–9.
5. Shapiro J, van Lanschot JB, Hulshof MCC, et al. Neoadjuvant chemoradiation plus surgery versus surgery alone for oesophageal or junctional cancer (CROSS): long-term results of a randomized controlled trial. Lancet Oncol Noor. 2015;16:1090–8.
6. Noordman BJ, Verdam MGE, Lagarde SM, et al. Effect of neoadjuvant chemoradiotherapy on health-related quality of life in esophageal or junctional cancer: results from the randomized CROSS trial. J Clin Oncol. 2018;36:268–75.
7. Blazeby JM, Sanford E, Falk SJ, Alderson D, Donovan JL. Health-related quality of life during neo-adjuvant treatment and surgery for localized esophageal carcinoma. Cancer. 2005;103:1791–9.
8. Van Meerten E, van der Gaast A, Looman CWN, et al. Quality of life during neoadjuvant treatment

and after surgery for resectable esophageal carcinoma. Int J Radiat Oncol Biol Phys. 2008;71:160–6.

9. Van der Werf LR, Busweiler LAD, van Sandick JW, et al. Reporting national outcomes after esophagectomy and gastrectomy according to the esophageal complications consensus group (ECCG). Ann Surg. 2020;271:1095–101.

10. Derogar M, Orsini N, Sadr-Azadi O, Lagergren P. Influence if major postoperative complications on health-related quality of life among long-term survivors of esophageal cancer surgery. J Clin Oncol. 2012;30:1615–9.

11. Kauppila JH, Johar A, Lagergren P. Medical and surgical complications and health-related quality of life after esophageal cancer surgery. Ann Surg. 2020;271:502–8.

12. Jezerskyte E, van Berge Henegouwen MI, van Laarhoven HWM, et al. Postoperative complications and long-term quality of life after multimodal treatment for esophageal cancer: an analysis of the prospective observational cohort study of esophageal-gastric cancer patients (POCOP). Ann Surg Oncol. 2021;28:7259–76.

13. Schuring N, Jezerskyte E, van Berge Henegouwen MI, et al. Influence of postoperative complications following esophagectomy for cancer on quality of life: a European multicenter study. Eur J Surg Oncol. 2023;49:97–105.

14. Bograd AJ, Molena D. Minimally invasive esophagectomy. Curr Probl Surg. 2021;58:1–12.

15. Kauppila JH, Xie S, Johar A, Markar SR, Lagergren P. Meta-analysis of health-related quality of life after minimally invasive versus open esophagectomy for oesophageal cancer. Br J Surg. 2017;104:1131–40.

16. Klevebro F, Kauppila JH, Johar A, Markar S, Lagergren P. Health-related quality of life following minimally invasive, hybrid minimally invasive or open esophagectomy: a population-based cohort study. Br J Surg. 2020;109:283–90.

17. Birkmeyer JD, Siewers AE, Finlayson EVA, et al. Hospital volume and surgical mortality in the United States. N Engl J Med. 2002;346:1128–37.

18. Patti MG, Corvera CU, Glasgow RE, Way LW. A hospital's annual rate of esophagectomy influences the operative mortality rate. J Gastrointest Surg. 1998;2:186–92.

19. Gasper WJ, Glidden DV, Jin C, Way LW, Patti MG. Has recognition of the relationship between mortality rates and volume for major cancer surgery in California made a difference? A follow-up analysis of another decade. Ann Surg. 2009;250:472–83.

20. Schlottmann F, Strassle PD, Charles A, Patti MG. Esophageal cancer surgery: spontaneous centralization in the US contributed to reduce mortality without causing health disparities. Ann Surg Oncol. 2018;25:1580–7.

21. Birkmeyer JD, Stukel TA, Siewers AE, et al. Surgeon volume and operative mortality in the United States. N Engl J Med. 2003;349:21172127.

22. Brusselaers N, Mattson F, Lagergren J. Hospital and surgeon volume in relation to long-term survival after oesophagetomy: systematic review and meta-analysis. Gut. 2014;63:1393–400.

23. Markar SR, Lagergren J. Surgical and surgeon-related factors related to long-term survival in esophageal cancer: a review. Ann Surg Oncol. 2020;27:718–23.

24. Dolan D, White A, Lee DN, et al. Short and long-term outcomes among high-volume versus low-volume esophagectomy surgeons at a high-volume center. Semin Thoracic Surg. 2021;34:1340–50.

Palliative Treatment of Esophageal Cancer

Simon Y. W. Che and Michael B. Ujiki

Abstract

Esophageal cancer has a rising incidence with many presenting in late stages of disease. Overall prognosis is poor and when unresectable, management focuses on palliation of symptoms and improving quality of life. Patients with locally advanced esophageal cancer most commonly presents with dysphagia, weight loss and pain. There are various modalities used for alleviation of symptoms including chemoradiation, endoluminal stenting, brachytherapy and other ablative techniques. Each option has associated risks and benefits. Patient performance status should be taken into account and choice of approach should be individualized with the aid of a multidisciplinary care team.

Keywords

Unresectable esophageal cancer · Dysphagia · Endoscopic stenting · Brachytherapy · Palliative chemoradiation

S. Y. W. Che · M. B. Ujiki (✉)
NorthShore University HealthSystem,
Evanston, USA
e-mail: mujiki@northshore.org

S. Y. W. Che
e-mail: sche@northshore.org

Introduction

Worldwide, esophageal cancer is the sixth leading cause of cancer-related deaths [1]. In the Western world, the incidence of esophageal adenocarcinoma has increased almost sevenfold from 1973 to 2006 [2]. Despite advances in medical technology, the 5-year survival rate is still less than 20%.

Most patients present with advanced disease due to delayed onset of symptoms, most commonly, dysphagia and pain. They either have surgically unresectable disease or are too malnourished from progressive dysphagia and are unfit to undergo surgery. As a result, more than 50% of patients presenting with esophageal cancer are not candidates for curative surgical resection [3]. Tumors are unresectable if they meet any of the following criteria: distant metastasis, invasion into adjacent organs (T4b disease), associated with multi-station bulky lymphadenopathy or esophagogastric junction/supraclavicular lymphadenopathy [1]. Even amongst those who undergo surgical resection, 70–80% have regional lymph node metastasis. On the other hand, cancer related cachexia is seen in 52.9% of patients in esophageal cancer [4]. Cachexia is associated with decreased survival, poorer outcomes and may preclude patients from undergoing chemotherapy and/or surgery. Despite optimal treatment, most patients develop disease progression or recurrence. When this occurs, care focuses primarily on mitigation of symptoms.

The sequelae of late-stage esophageal cancer include dysphagia, odynophagia and aspiration. Around 70% of patients with inoperable esophageal malignancy develop dysphagia [3]. Malnutrition and psychological difficulties from prolonged fasting also occur. Palliation is an individualized approach and aims to maximize quality of life. Active communication is necessary and identifies patient goals. Multidisciplinary care teams consider tumor pathology and patient physiology to ascribe a proper treatment plan.

There is a wide array of modalities in the treatment of unresectable esophageal cancer. Palliative chemotherapy is standard in patients with unresectable esophageal cancer. Pain and nausea are best treated with opioid analgesics, anti-emetics and anxiolytics. Malnutrition can be abated with gastrostomy tube feeds. Radiation therapy and endoscopic stenting are the most common methods for palliation of dysphagia. Often a combination of modalities is used to obtain maximum quality of life.

Palliative Treatment of Esophageal Cancer

Chemotherapy and External Beam Radiation

Systemic chemoradiotherapy is standard in most cases of unresectable or metastatic esophageal cancer. Radiation therapy can decrease tumor bulk and symptoms, but has little survival benefit as a sole modality. The addition of chemotherapy can help to ameliorate tumor growth, extend survival and improve quality of life. Initiation of radiation therapy and systemic chemotherapy should be individualized based on patient performance status.

Prior to the advent of modern chemotherapy, external beam radiation therapy was used for controlling tumor growth and local regional disease. Today, advances in radiation therapy,

including three-dimensional conformal radiation therapy and intensity-modulated radiation therapy are able to obtain similar effects on tumor growth while diminishing radiation toxicity. Historical studies show an overall 5-year survival rate of 9.0% and median survival of 8.9 months in patients with locally advanced esophageal cancer treated by radiation alone [5, 6]. Dysphagia improved in 66% of patients treated with radiation alone [7]. Best results are seen in high-dose radiation with no improvement with dose escalation past 50.4 Gray [8, 9].

The addition of chemotherapy to conventional radiation increases overall survival with a moderate increase is adverse events. Combined therapy is recommended in all patients with good performance status. The Eastern Cooperative Oncology Group Performance Status Scale (ECOG) and Karnofsky Performance Status Scale are most commonly used to assess overall fitness. A Karnofsky Score of $\geq 60\%$ or ECOG score ≤ 2 typically indicates patient tolerance of combined therapy [10].

A phase III, randomized study showed combined chemotherapy with radiation was superior to radiation alone. One hundred and twenty-three patients with primarily squamous cell carcinoma were randomized in each arm. Those undergoing combined therapy had a median survival of 14.1 months and a 5-year survival rate of 27% compared to median survival of 9.3 months and 0% 5-year survival rate in the isolated radiation therapy group. However, as expected, systemic side effects such as nausea, emesis and myelosuppression were more common in the combined group [11]. A similar randomized trial reported survival benefit of combined therapy with a 44% and 20% rate of severe and life-threatening side effects respectively [7].

Current National Comprehensive Cancer Network (NCCN) guidelines recommend a two-agent regiment in combination with a total radiation dose of 50.4 Gray [10]. Primary agents include paclitaxel and carboplatin for adenocarcinoma and 5-fluorouracil and cisplatin for squamous cell carcinoma.

Palliative systemic therapy increases overall survival compared to best supportive care with a modest increase in formation of tracheoesophageal fistulas, ulcers and strictures [12, 13]. Radiation is important in reducing tumor bulk and improving dysphagia with 50% of all patients having improvement in dysphagia score [14]. Additional study is ongoing regarding the addition of immunotherapy and targeted therapies. Trastuzumab or pembrolizumab can be added to standard regiments in adenocarcinomas that overexpress the Herceptin-2 receptor. However, response rate to systemic therapy is still only 35% and overall survival is less than one year [15]. Furthermore, patient's tolerance and performance status can limit initiation of chemoradiotherapy.

Management of dysphagia and the sequelae of late-stage esophageal cancer remains paramount. With combined chemoradiation, symptom improvement occurs at median of two weeks with maximum improvement at four weeks [16]. For those who present with severe dysphagia or who cannot tolerate or do not respond to chemotherapy or radiation therapy, other palliative modalities including endoscopic stenting or brachytherapy may improve quality of life.

Endoscopic Dilation and Stenting

Endoscopic stenting is one of the most valuable modalities in the palliation of dysphagia from esophageal cancer. It has since replaced endoscopic dilation in the management of malignant strictures and palliation of dysphagia. Compared with dilation, esophageal stenting produces more durable results with fewer procedural related complications.

Endoscopic dilation typically involves the use of a weighted bougie (Maloney or Hurst bougie) or a wire-guided balloon dilated (Savory-Gillard dilator). Placement of a bougie or dilator can be completed under fluoroscopic guidance. There is an associated perforation rate of 0.4% up to 2.6% and a 1% associated mortality [17, 18]. In general, no more than three dilations in

1 mm increments should be completed in a single session. This may require multiple attempts at dilation in order to obtain symptomatic improvement. Today, dilation is still sometimes performed in high-grade strictures as a means to safely performing stenting or when endoscopic stenting is not available.

Endoscopic stenting is indicated in inoperable tumors or patients who are unable to tolerate chemotherapy. Modern endoscopic stents have evolved from rigid plastic tubes to self-expanding metal stents (SEMS). These advances are meant to reduce tissue ingrowth, migration and obstruction. Compared to other modalities, stenting can result in immediate relief of dysphagia and initiation of oral feeds. SEMS can be either fully covered, partially covered or uncovered. Uncovered stents are rarely used due to the high rates of tissue ingrowth. Meanwhile, fully covered stents are associated with high rates of migration, but low rates of tissue ingrowth and recurrent dysphagia. Partially covered stents are uncovered at the proximal and distal phalanges to prevent migration and are the primary choice for the palliation of malignant dysphagia. Newer evolutions include stents with anti-reflux valves or stents with implanted radioiodine seeds. Radioactive SEMS have reported higher rates of survival with more durable relief of dysphagia at three and six months with similar rate of complications [19].

Esophageal stenting can be performed under moderate sedation. Upper endoscopy is completed to identify the lesion and determine the length of obstruction and degree of narrowing. SEMS are typically deployed under either endoscopic or fluoroscopic guidance two ensure at least a 2 cm overlap. Following stent placement, fibrous foods are avoided to prevent stent obstruction and patients are encouraged to eat in an upright position to prevent associated reflux when the stent is deployed across the gastroesophageal junction.

SEMS are associated with relief of dysphagia within 1–2 days after placement [12, 20]. Of those who undergo endoscopic stenting, 95% are able to tolerate a liquid diet [21]. SEMS placement has been shown to increase quality of life when compared to gastrostomy or jejunostomy tube feeds.

Placement of a SEMS is also useful in the management of malignant tracheoesophageal fistulas, a late sequalae of esophageal cancer. Around 5–15% of patients develop fistula and present with symptoms of aspiration, dyspnea and dysphagia [22]. Proper placement of a stent can occlude the fistula. Sometimes, an additional stent in the airway is also used. Endoscopic stenting has also been utilized in the palliation of dysphagia for cervical lesions as well. Despite anatomic constraints of the hypopharynx, placement of covered stents is feasible and leads improvement in dysphagia [23].

Placement of SEMS are best reserved for individuals with a short life expectancy due to associated adverse events. The most common complication of endoscopic stenting if migration with a rate of 0% to 23% with 25% to 50% of patients requiring reintervention [12, 24]. Pain is also frequent following endoscopic stenting. Esophageal perforation (2%), hemorrhage (8%), aspiration pneumonia (5%), fever (5%), fistula formation (3%), pressure necrosis (2%) are less common adverse events related to stent placement [25]. Stent associated mortality is between 0 and 2% [22]. Placement of stents may also lead to extraluminal compression of the airways, ulceration of severe gastroesophageal reflux.

When compared to radiation therapy alone, endoscopic stenting has a 51% increased risk of adverse events. Adverse events also occurred sooner, at a median of 43 days, after esophageal stenting than with radiation therapy, a median of 114 days [24]. Retrospective studies show comparable relief of pain and more durable management of dysphagia with radiation therapy [24]. Furthermore, endoscopic stenting should not be performed following radiation therapy as stent associated mortality increases from 0–6% to 0–54% [22]. Prior radiation leads to tissue destruction, fibrosis and ischemic changes resulting in higher rates of perforation and necrosis.

Placement of a SEMS can immediately improve malignant dysphagia. Current guidelines recommend esophageal stenting for palliation of malignant dysphagia over other ablative techniques [22]. However, this procedure is associated with significant adverse events and need for additional procedures. Esophageal stent placement should be reserved for those who are unable to undergo radiation therapy and have a short-expected survival. SEMS can also be combined with other adjuncts such as brachytherapy to improve efficacy and durability.

Brachytherapy

Brachytherapy can provide effective palliation of malignant dysphagia. It consists of an intraluminal application of a radioactive substance providing effect directly to the tumor site minimizing further exposure to surrounding tissues. Brachytherapy can be used alone or in conjunction with other modalities. The European Society for Gastrointestinal Endoscopy (ESGE) recommends the use of brachytherapy in conjunction with SEMS placement to improve quality of life [22].

Brachytherapy is performed at specialized centers. Unlike external beam radiation therapy, endoluminal application of a radioactive substance, typically iridium based, provides therapeutic effect over a three-to-eight-week time span. Its effects are not as immediate as endoscopic stenting, but it may provide more durable results and local control in 25 to 35% on all individuals [26].

A randomized control trial showed brachytherapy has equal long-term outcomes in the palliation of malignant dysphagia when compared to SEMS. Brachytherapy was also associated with improved quality of life and fewer adverse effects. Adverse events and acute toxicity occurred in up to 21% to 58% of individuals [27, 28]. Brachytherapy is associated with a 12% risk of esophageal fistula formation and should be reserved for palliation in individuals with short life expectancy. The main limitations of initiating brachytherapy include limited availability, technical difficulty as well as logistical challenges [22].

Endoscopic Ablative Techniques

The most common mechanisms for management of malignant dysphagia include radiation induced tumor necrosis and mechanical stenting of tumor related stenosis. Endoscopic ablation can achieve destruction of tumor cells to allow for passage of intraluminal contents. Different techniques have been developed including laser ablation, argon plasma coagulation, cryotherapy and photodynamic therapy.

Laser ablation was one of the first ablative techniques developed. It uses a high-energy laser light delivered endoscopically with a probe resulting in heating and vaporization of tumor cells. Laser therapy achieves improvement in dysphagia in 70 to 80% of individuals. Longer strictures were associated with poor outcomes due to an increase risk of disorientation and adverse events including perforation. Laser therapy has since fallen out of favor due to high rates of adverse events.

Argon plasma coagulation (APC) uses monopolar electrocautery conducted by argon gas to achieve tumor destruction. Improvement in dysphagia is seen in up to 94% of patients [29]. A median of three APC sessions were required to obtain patency with as many as two thirds requiring repeat treatments every three to four weeks [30, 31]. APC does show some promise and is found to have statistically significant improvement in median survival days for both stage III and stage IV disease as well as reduction in 30-day mortality [30].

Other ablative techniques include the used of liquid nitrogen cryotherapy resulting in cryonecrosis of tumor cells. Cryotherapy has shown the potential to obtain complete luminal response in treatment of T1 and T2 esophageal cancers. More recently, cryotherapy has been proposed as a salvage technique in the palliation of malignant dysphagia. Each cryotherapy treatment consists of multiple freeze and thaw cycles and can be repeated as needed. Retrospective studies have shown a 0.7 point improvement in dysphagia score with a median of 2.5 cryotherapy treatments. Despite only modest improvement in dysphagia, cryotherapy has a low adverse event rate of 6.7% with a majority being minor [32].

Photodynamic Therapy (PDT) represents a more targeted ablative technique. Patients initially undergo infusion with a photosensitizing agent (Photofrin) which is absorbed by malignant cells. In another session, tumor cells are exposed to a low power laser. A unique wave length (630 nm) causes a photooxidative reaction and tumor necrosis.

Surgical Palliation

Surgical management including palliative resection or bypass has fallen out of favor due to high associated morbidity and mortality. These techniques have been widely replaced with endoscopic modalities. Palliative surgery is associated with an in-hospital mortality ranging from 10 to 35%. Furthermore, a database review of 2812 patients receiving palliative surgery showed a median overall survival of 6 months, about 5.5 months less than non-palliative approaches [33].

Newer surgical techniques, though not widely adopted, have been shown to preserve oral intake up to one year. A study from Japan reports the use of a modified bypass procedure, the drainless tubeless (DRESS) surgery, in patients with unresectable cancers. This procedure creates a Y-shaped gastric tube. The esophagus remains in continuity with the lesser curvature of the stomach while the tubularized greater curvature is used to create an esophagogastric anastomosis often in combination with an esophagostomy. They reported two of three patients alive at one year and tolerating oral intake [34]. However, surgical palliation is still not recommended in the palliation of esophageal cancer.

Conflicts of Interest

The authors have no conflicts of interest.

References

1. Ajani JA, et al. Esophageal and esophagogastric junction cancers, version 2.2019, NCCN clinical practice guidelines in oncology. J Natl Compr Canc Netw. 2019;17:855–83. https://doi.org/10.6004/jnccn.2019.0033

2. Wheeler JB, Reed CE. Epidemiology of esophageal cancer. Surg Clin North Am. 2012;92:1077–87. https://doi.org/10.1016/j.suc.2012.07.008

3. Diamantis G, et al. Quality of life in patients with esophageal stenting for the palliation of malignant dysphagia. World J Gastroenterol. 2011;17:144–50. https://doi.org/10.3748/wjg.v17.i2.144

4. Sun L, Quan XQ, Yu S. An epidemiological survey of cachexia in advanced cancer patients and analysis on its diagnostic and treatment status. Nutr Cancer. 2015;67:1056–62. https://doi.org/10.1080/01635581.2015.1073753

5. Okawa T, Kita M, Tanaka M, Ikeda M. Results of radiotherapy for inoperable locally advanced esophageal cancer. Int J Radiat Oncol Biol Phys. 1989;17:49–54. https://doi.org/10.1016/0360-3016(89)90369-6

6. Newaishy GA, Read GA, Duncan W, Kerr GR. Results of radical radiotherapy of squamous cell carcinoma of the oesophagus. Clin Radiol. 1982;33:347–52. https://doi.org/10.1016/s0009-9260(82)80288-2

7. Herskovic A, et al. Combined chemotherapy and radiotherapy compared with radiotherapy alone in patients with cancer of the esophagus. N Engl J Med. 1992;326:1593–8. https://doi.org/10.1056/NEJM199206113262403

8. Minsky BD, et al. INT 0123 (Radiation Therapy Oncology Group 94-05) phase III trial of combined-modality therapy for esophageal cancer: high-dose versus standard-dose radiation therapy. J Clin Oncol. 2002;20:1167–74. https://doi.org/10.1200/JCO.2002.20.5.1167

9. Kachnic LA, et al. Longitudinal quality-of-life analysis of RTOG 94-05 (Int 0123): a phase III trial of definitive chemoradiotherapy for esophageal cancer. Gastrointest Cancer Res. 2011;4:45–52.

10. Ajani JA, et al. Esophageal and esophagogastric junction cancers, version 2.2023, NCCN clinical practice guidelines in oncology. J Natl Compr Canc Netw. 2023;21:393–422. https://doi.org/10.6004/jnccn.2023.0019

11. al-Sarraf M, et al. Progress report of combined chemoradiotherapy versus radiotherapy alone in patients with esophageal cancer: an intergroup study. J Clin Oncol. 1997;15:277–84. https://doi.org/10.1200/JCO.1997.15.1.277

12. van Rossum PSN, Mohammad NH, Vleggaar FP, van Hillegersberg R. Treatment for unresectable or metastatic oesophageal cancer: current evidence and trends. Nat Rev Gastroenterol Hepatol. 2018;15:235–49. https://doi.org/10.1038/nrgastro.2017.162

13. Janmaat VT, et al. Palliative chemotherapy and targeted therapies for esophageal and gastroesophageal junction cancer. Cochrane Database Syst Rev. 2017;11:CD004063. https://doi.org/10.1002/14651858.CD004063.pub4

14. Harvey JA, et al. Chemoradiation therapy is effective for the palliative treatment of malignant dysphagia. Dis Esophagus. 2004;17:260–5. https://doi.org/10.1111/j.1442-2050.2004.00420.x

15. Ueda H, et al. Clinical evaluation of palliative chemoradiotherapy for metastatic esophageal cancer. Oncotarget. 2017;8:80286–94. https://doi.org/10.18632/oncotarget.17925

16. Coia LR, Soffen EM, Schultheiss TE, Martin EE, Hanks GE. Swallowing function in patients with esophageal cancer treated with concurrent radiation and chemotherapy. Cancer. 1992;71:281–6. https://doi.org/10.1002/1097-0142(19930115)71:2<281::aid-cncr2820710202>3.0.co;2-0

17. Standards of Practice C, et al. Esophageal dilation. Gastrointest Endosc. 2006;63:755–60. https://doi.org/10.1016/j.gie.2006.02.031

18. Mocanu A, Barla R, Hoara P, Constantinoiu S. Endoscopic palliation of advanced esophageal cancer. J Med Life. 2015;8:193–201.

19. Chen HL, Shen WQ, Liu K. Radioactive self-expanding stents for palliative management of unresectable esophageal cancer: a systematic review and meta-analysis. Dis Esophagus. 2017;30:1–16. https://doi.org/10.1093/dote/dow010

20. Spaander MCW, et al. Esophageal stenting for benign and malignant disease: European society of gastrointestinal endoscopy (ESGE) guideline—update 2021. Endoscopy. 2021;53:751–62. https://doi.org/10.1055/a-1475-0063

21. Halpern AL, McCarter MD. Palliative management of gastric and esophageal cancer. Surg Clin North Am. 2019;99:555–69. https://doi.org/10.1016/j.suc.2019.02.007

22. Spaander MC, et al. Esophageal stenting for benign and malignant disease: European society of gastrointestinal endoscopy (ESGE) clinical guideline. Endoscopy. 2016;48:939–48. https://doi.org/10.1055/s-0042-114210

23. Battaglia G, et al. Feasibility, efficacy and safety of stent insertion as a palliative treatment for malignant strictures in the cervical segment of the esophagus and the hypopharynx. Surg Endosc. 2016;30:159–67. https://doi.org/10.1007/s00464-015-4176-z

24. Martin EJ, et al. Palliative radiotherapy versus esophageal stent placement in the management of patients with metastatic esophageal cancer. J Natl Compr Canc Netw. 2020;18:569–74. https://doi.org/10.6004/jnccn.2019.7524

25. Vermeulen BD, Siersema PD. Esophageal stenting in clinical practice: an overview. Curr Treat

Options Gastroenterol. 2018;16:260–73. https://doi.org/10.1007/s11938-018-0181-3

26. Sur RK, Donde B, Levin VC, Mannell A. Fractionated high dose rate intraluminal brachytherapy in palliation of advanced esophageal cancer. Int J Radiat Oncol Biol Phys. 1998;40:447–53. https://doi.org/10.1016/s0360-3016(97)00710-4

27. Homs MY, et al. Single-dose brachytherapy versus metal stent placement for the palliation of dysphagia from oesophageal cancer: multicentre randomised trial. Lancet. 2004;364:1497–504. https://doi.org/10.1016/S0140-6736(04)17272-3

28. Gaspar LE, et al. A phase I/II study of external beam radiation, brachytherapy and concurrent chemotherapy in localized cancer of the esophagus (RTOG 92-07): preliminary toxicity report. Int J Radiat Oncol Biol Phys. 1997;37:593–9. https://doi.org/10.1016/s0360-3016(96)00591-3

29. Eickhoff A, et al. Prospective nonrandomized comparison of two modes of argon beamer (APC) tumor desobstruction: effectiveness of the new pulsed APC versus forced APC. Endoscopy. 2007;39:637–42. https://doi.org/10.1055/s-2007-966571

30. Sigounas DE, et al. Argon plasma coagulation compared with stent placement in the palliative treatment of inoperable oesophageal cancer. United Eur Gastroenterol J. 2017;5:21–31. https://doi.org/10.1177/2050640616650786

31. Heindorff H, Wojdemann M, Bisgaard T, Svendsen LB. Endoscopic palliation of inoperable cancer of the oesophagus or cardia by argon electrocoagulation. Scand J Gastroenterol. 1998;33:21–3. https://doi.org/10.1080/00365529850166158

32. Kachaamy T, et al. Liquid nitrogen spray cryotherapy for dysphagia palliation in patients with inoperable esophageal cancer. Gastrointest Endosc. 2018;88:447–55. https://doi.org/10.1016/j.gie.2018.04.2362

33. Coffey MR, et al. Palliative surgery outcomes for patients with esophageal cancer: an national cancer database analysis. J Surg Res. 2021;267:229–34. https://doi.org/10.1016/j.jss.2021.05.013

34. Takeno S, et al. Drainage tubeless (DRESS) bypass surgery as the best palliative care for unresectable thoracic esophageal cancer with and without esophago-respiratory fistula. Ann Thorac Cardiovasc Surg. 2019;25:82–6. https://doi.org/10.5761/atcs.oa.18-00170

Index

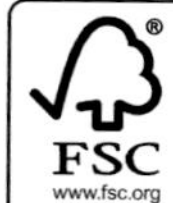

MIX
Papier aus verantwortungsvollen Quellen
Paper from responsible sources
FSC® C105338

If you have any concerns about our products,
you can contact us on
ProductSafety@springernature.com

In case Publisher is established outside the EU,
the EU authorized representative is:
Springer Nature Customer Service Center GmbH
Europaplatz 3, 69115 Heidelberg, Germany

Printed by Libri Plureos GmbH
in Hamburg, Germany